LYMPHOCYTE UPDATES - CANCER, AUTOIMMUNITY AND INFECTION

Edited by **Gheorghita Isvoranu**

Lymphocyte Updates - Cancer, Autoimmunity and Infection
http://dx.doi.org/10.5772/66613
Edited by Gheorghita Isvoranu

Contributors

Simone Bürgler, Won Fen Wong, Hamiyet Donmez-Altuntas, Ahmet Eken, Tatsuaki Tsuruyama, Teodora Karan-Djurasevic, Sonja Pavlovic, Cadiele Oliana Reichert, Joel Da Cunha, Débora Levy, , Luciana Morganti Ferreira Maselli, Sérgio Bydlowski, Celso Spada, Luciana Marti, Julieta Luna-Herrera, Jorge Ismael Castañeda-Sánchez, Ana Rosa Muñóz-Duarte, María Lilia Domínguez-López, Juan José De La Cruz-López

Published by InTech

Janeza Trdine 9, 51000 Rijeka, Croatia

Publishing Process Manager Dajana Pemac
Technical Editor SPi Global
Cover InTech Design team

First published July, 2017
Printed in Croatia
Legal deposit, Croatia: National and University Library in Zagreb

Additional hard copies can be obtained from orders@intechopen.com

Lymphocyte Updates - Cancer, Autoimmunity and Infection, Edited by Gheorghita Isvoranu
p. cm.
Print ISBN 978-953-51-3343-8
Online ISBN 978-953-51-3344-5

For EU product safety concerns :
IN TECH d . o . o . , Prolaz Marije Krucifikse Kozulić 3 , 51000 Rijeka , Croatia ,
info@intechopen . com or visit our website at intechopen . com .

Meet the editor

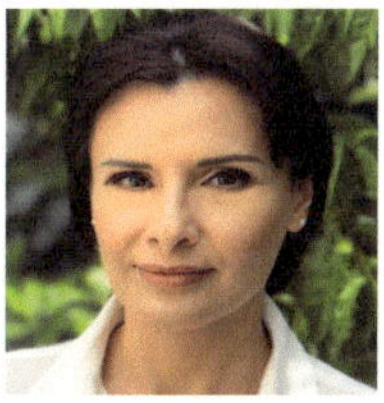

Gheorghita Isvoranu, PhD, is currently a research scientist at "Victor Babeş" National Institute of Pathology, Bucharest, Romania. In 2012, she got her PhD degree in Biology, at the University of Bucharest. She is author and/or coauthor of over 20 scientific papers and conference abstracts and also a book chapter. Her major areas of scientific interest include immunology, ancer therapy, and regenerative medicine. Gheorghita Isvoranu is also a member of the Romanian Society of Immunology and Romanian Association for Laboratory Animal Science.

Contents

Preface

This book represents a synergic effort of an international team of specialists in immunology to expand the scientific achievements in the field of lymphocytes. It offers important and specific updated information to researchers, students, teachers, and medical professionals. Moreover, considering the remarkable dynamics of immunology and immunotherapy, this book *"Lymphocyte Updates - Cancer, Autoimmunity, and Infection"* aims to represent a significant source of concise scientific data and advancement of knowledge in this field. The chapters offer new insights into the latest scientific progress on lymphocyte roles in protective immunity, as well as their involvement in pathogenesis of various disorders. Last, but not least, I would like to extend all my gratitude to InTech for the special opportunity offered to me to be the editor of this book and also for the valuable collaboration in realizing this achievement.

Gheorghita Isvoranu,
"Victor Babeş" National Institute of Pathology,
Bucharest, Romania

Chapter 1

Lymphoid Hematopoiesis and Lymphocytes Differentiation and Maturation

Luciana Cavalheiro Marti, Nydia Strachman Bacal, Laiz Camerão Bento, Rodolfo Patussi Correia and Fernanda Agostini Rocha

Additional information is available at the end of the chapter

http://dx.doi.org/10.5772/intechopen.69058

Abstract

Lymphocytes belong to the lymphoid lineage and are considered as divergent from other blood cells lineages as those from the myeloid or erythroid lineage. Lymphoid hematopoiesis is not trivial, because although lymphocytes are found in the bloodstream and their precursor originates in the bone marrow, they mainly belong to the separate lymphatic system, which interacts with the blood circulation. We will discuss B cell differentiation in the bone marrow and the later stages of maturation in secondary lymphoid tissues, besides the B cell profiles in interfollicular, perifollicular, and follicular areas. In addition, we will also discuss T-cell precursor and natural killer cells derivation in the marrow. Furthermore, we will also discuss T-cell precursor migration to thymus, differentiation, rearrangement, thymic selection, involved transcription factors, and, finally, T-cell profiles and subsets in secondary lymphoid organs. We will provide flow cytometry plots showing strategies to identify and characterize NK, T and B lymphocytes and their subsets in circulation. Furthermore, we will provide illustrations to help the reader to understand and visualize the information provide over the chapter. Furthermore, the comprehension about lymphocytes and their contribution to the immune response will favor their application in developmental hematology and immunology. These topics are very important for the continuous development of knowledge.

Keywords: hematopoiesis, B cells, T cells, differentiation

1. Introduction

Lymphocytes belong to the lymphoid lineage and are considered as divergent from other blood cells lineages as those from the myeloid or erythroid lineage. Lymphoid hematopoiesis is not trivial, because although lymphocytes are found in the bloodstream and their precursor originates in the bone marrow, they mostly belong to the separate lymphatic system, which interacts with the blood circulation. Lymphoid and myeloid lineages are separated at the progenitor level; the common lymphoid progenitors (CLPs) can differentiate into all types of lymphocytes but lack the myeloid potential under physiological conditions, although some myeloid-related genes can be detected in CLPs depending on experimental conditions [1, 2].

After transplanting a single hematopoietic stem cell (HSC) into an irradiated mouse, long-term reconstitution of both lymphoid and myeloid compartments was achieved demonstrating that the HSC is the common predecessor of all blood cells [3–5].

Hematopoiesis studies, mainly in the fetal liver indicated that the difference between the lymphoid and myeloid lineages may not be as simple as imagined. Nevertheless, a corresponding adult common myeloid progenitor (CMP) has been recognized in a fetal liver, but the presence of a lymphoid-committed progenitor (CLPs) has not yet been demonstrated [6, 7].

The bi-directional T and B cell derivation from a single cell was not found in the fetal liver progenitors at clonal levels, but T cell and granulocytes and macrophages (GM) or B cell and GM progenitor ability of differentiation were present [8]. Regarding these findings, it has been wondered whether these differences observed in fetal and adult hematopoiesis are due to different intrinsic mechanisms in fetal and adult progenitors or due to the liver and bone marrow environmental differences.

Several hematopoietic and lymphoid progenitors, such as multipotent progenitors (MPPs) and CLPs, are mobilized from bone marrow and initiate T-cell development in the thymus [9]. MPPs CCR9+ are the major bone marrow population that transit to the thymus. Once the hematopoietic progenitor cell home to the thymus, B cell development potential is immediately turned off by stimulation through Notch, while B cell differentiation will be regulated by several transcription factors in the bone marrow.

Next, we will discuss B lymphocyte differentiation in the bone marrow and later their stages of maturation in secondary lymphoid tissues and profiles in interfollicular, perifollicular and follicular areas. In addition, we will also discuss T-cell precursor and natural killer cell derivation in the marrow. Furthermore, we will also discuss T-cell precursor migration to thymus, differentiation, rearrangement, thymic selection, involved transcription factors, and, finally, T-cell profiles and subsets in secondary lymphoid organs.

1.1. B Lymphocytes

1.1.1. B Lymphocytes ontogeny

Lymphocytes are cells from the adaptive immune system and are derived from hematopoietic progenitor cells. These cells are first produced in the yolk sac, next, they are formed in the liver during the fetal phase and lastly in the bone marrow [10]. B cell development is dependent of several specific cytokines and contact with a favorable microenvironment [11, 12].

The hematopoietic progenitor cell differentiates into a CLP and depending on stimuli they will give rise to a T or a B lymphocyte [13]. B cell differentiation from a CLP is regulated by several factors such as E-box binding protein 2A (E2A), early B cell factor-1 (EBF1), purine box factor 1 (PU.1), Ikaros, paired box protein-5 (Pax5) and CXCL12. These factors are resulting from the interaction of interleukin 7 (IL-7) and their receptor CD127 (IL-7Rα) existent in the B lymphocyte. Together, these factors are crucial for the hematopoietic progenitor cell commitment to B lymphocyte differentiation and gene rearrangement to the immunoglobulin heavy chain [14–21].

The first cell committed to B-lymphoid differentiation is the pro-B cell. The presence of stromal cells and IL-7 also favors the B lymphocyte differentiation. These cells begin to express CD45^{dim}, CD22, CD34, terminal deoxynucleotidyl transferase (TdT) and CD38^{high} [19]. The Pax5 factor activates the CD19 expression, one of the most premature B lymphocyte antigens [18, 22]. In the next step of differentiation, these cells express CD10^{high}, CD38^{high}, CD34, CD79a, TdT and start being called pre-B I [19, 20]. Immunoglobulin (Ig) gene recombination in the heavy chain locus starts in this phase. The heavy chain gene is present in segments that code for the variable (V), diversity (D), joining (J), and constant (C) regions [23, 24]. Gene recombination is initiated by recombinase activating gene proteins RAG1 and RAG2; these proteins have the ability to bind and cleave DNA at specific recombination signal sequences called RSSs.

These RSSs surround each genic segment V, D and J. During recombination, D and J gene segments are drawn closer, excluding the intermediary DNA, and this DJ segment is joined to a V segment originating VDJ rearranged exon. Pre-B I cells also express TdT, which is responsible for catalyzing the random addition of junctional (N) nucleotides [24, 25]. The VDJ rearrangement is now adjacent to the constant Cμ region and creates an active gene which codes for the heavy chain, whose synthesis originates the μ intracytoplasmic chain (IgM) and from now these cells become termed pre-B II [19].

During pre-B II cells, they gain heterogeneous CD20 expression and lack the expression of CD34 and TdT [19, 20, 26]. Besides, B lymphocyte expresses a complex known as a pre-B cell receptor (pre-BCR) that is formed by the heavy chain μ (Igμ) associated to a light chain (λ5 and pre-B V) joined to a heterodimer Igα (CD79a) and Igβ (CD79b) [27]. If the pre-BCR is able to bind to the bone marrow microenvironment, the *immune-receptor tyrosine*-based *activation motif* (ITAMs) domains of Igα and Igβ are phosphorylated and their signaling rescues these cells from apoptosis. This positive selection confirms that the Igμ chain generated is functional, and the pre-B II cells detected with Igμ not functional are deleted [19]. The signals generated by the pre-BCR also stimulated the pre-B II differentiation and are responsible for their proliferation in the bone marrow, inhibiting the heavy chain recombination and stimulating the light chain recombination [28, 29]. The light chain rearrangement comprises the junction of a V with a J segment forming a VJ exon associated with an Igμ chain. This association activates the translation of kappa and lambda proteins leading to a formation of a complete IgM molecule [30, 31]. The B cell that expresses an IgM molecule on the cell membrane is denominated immature B cell [19].

Immature B lymphocytes begin to express some immunophenotypic markers of still naïve but mature B lymphocytes; among these characteristics we can quote the CD20 expression, enhanced expression of CD45, CD10^{dim} and CD38^{high}, low expression of CD21, CD5 (homogeneous), and high levels of CD81 [19, 26].

These cells undergo a positive and negative selection process before completing their maturation status. During this process, the B lymphocytes that complete, successfully, the gene rearrangement program are positively selected, there are the shut-down of RAG genes and these cells will receive survival signals to proceed in the maturation process [32]. Though, when the B lymphocyte recognizes self-antigens, their receptor is modified, the genes RAG are reactivated and another rearrangement in the light chain V-J is initiated allowing the B cell to develop a non-self-reactive BCR [32–34]. However, if this rearrangement did not succeed this cell undergo through apoptosis in a process known as negative selection. The positively selected cells leave the bone marrow and complete their maturation status in the secondary lymphoid organs.

Mature B lymphocytes lack CD10 and CD38 and express IgD and IgM on their membrane (**Figure 1**) [19]. IgD expression happens when the VDJ segment is trasncribed with Cδ exon instead of Cμ [35]. B lymphocyte differentiation in the bone marrow is heterogeneous and goes through several maturation stages that can be observed by analysis of immunophenotypic characteristics (**Figure 2**).

1.1.2. Mature B lymphocytes

Mature B cells are usually divided into three subgroups known as follicular B cells, marginal zone (MZ) B-cell and B1 cells. The follicular B lymphocytes are the majority of mature B cells and are located in the lymphoid follicle of the lymph node and spleen. These cells will stimulate the T lymphocyte response and this can occur in two different locations, extra-follicular and in the germinal center [36]. B cells in the extra-follicular can be activated by the T-helper

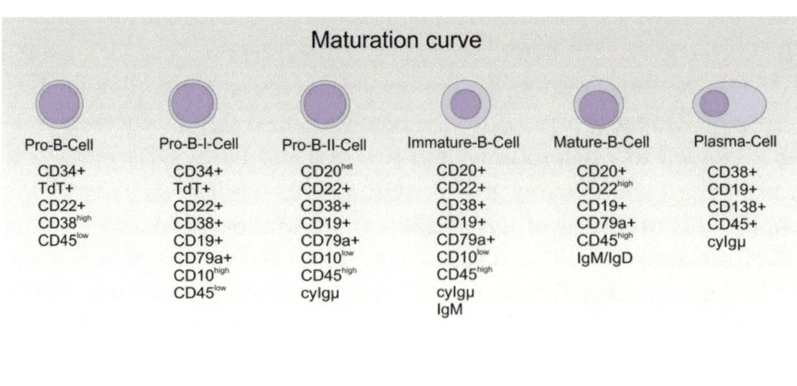

Figure 1. Schematic B cell regular development.

http://dx.doi.org/10.5772/intechopen.69058

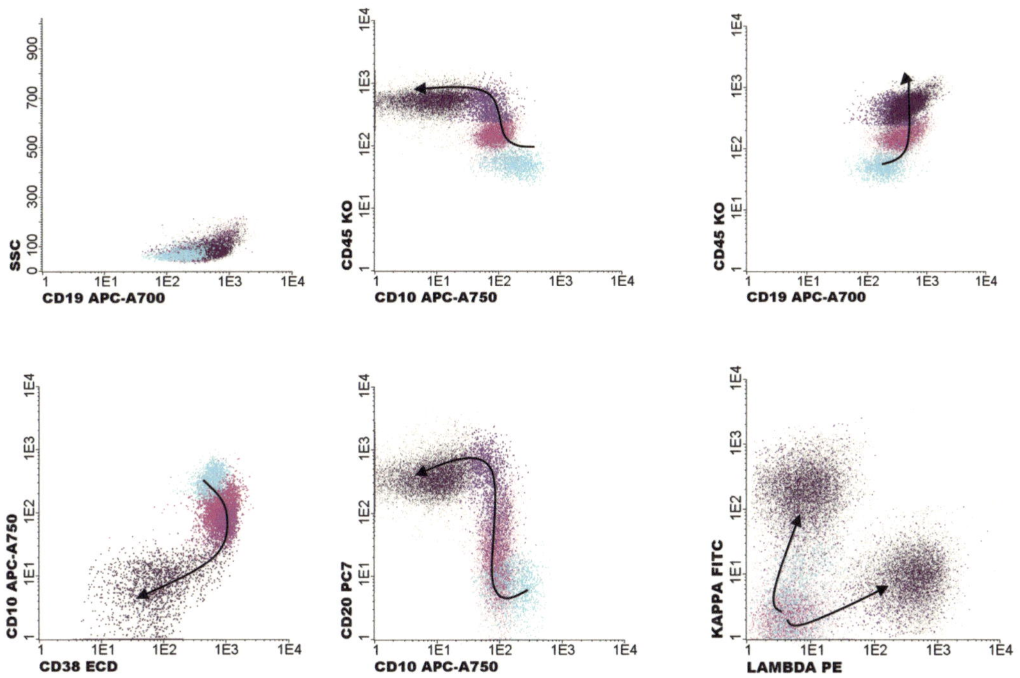

Figure 2. Bone marrow expression profile of B cells in different stages of maturation. The B cells maturation states are represented by the colors displayed in the flow cytometry plots figures: light blue represents immature B cells, purple represents intermediate stage and brown the mature B cells. Analysis performed with the Infinicyt software (Cytognos).

lymphocytes and differentiate into short-lived plasmablasts which secrete antibodies. On the other hand, some activated B cells migrate back to the follicles and under follicular helper T cell (T_{FH}) influence proliferate vigorously to form the germinal centers (GC) [37, 38]. Inside a GC, in the dark zone region, the B cells, now called centroblasts, goes through a rapid cellular division, somatic hypermutation, and isotypes class switching. Centroblasts express CD10 and Bcl-6. Next, these cells migrate to the light zone region and become centrocytes. These centrocytes in the light zone will be in contact with follicular dendritic cells (FDC) and T_{FH} through the interactions between CD23 and CD40L (**Figure 3**). B cells with high affinity for the antigens in this microenvironment will differentiate into plasmablasts (plasma cells) or memory B cells and will express CD27. Plasma cells return to the bone marrow and display well-defined characteristics expressing CD19, CD27, CD38, CD45, CD138 and intracytoplasmic Ig [10, 19, 37–39].

MZ B cells are located in the spleen MZ and are responsible by the T independent-responses (polysaccharides, glycolipids, and nucleic acid). These cells express pan-B markers, lack CD10 and show weak IgD expression [39]. B-1 cells represent another B cell lineage located mainly in the peritonea and mucosa [40]. These cells are also responsive to T cell-independent antigens and can be recognized by the expression of CD27 and CD43, even though this phenotype remains controversial [40, 41].

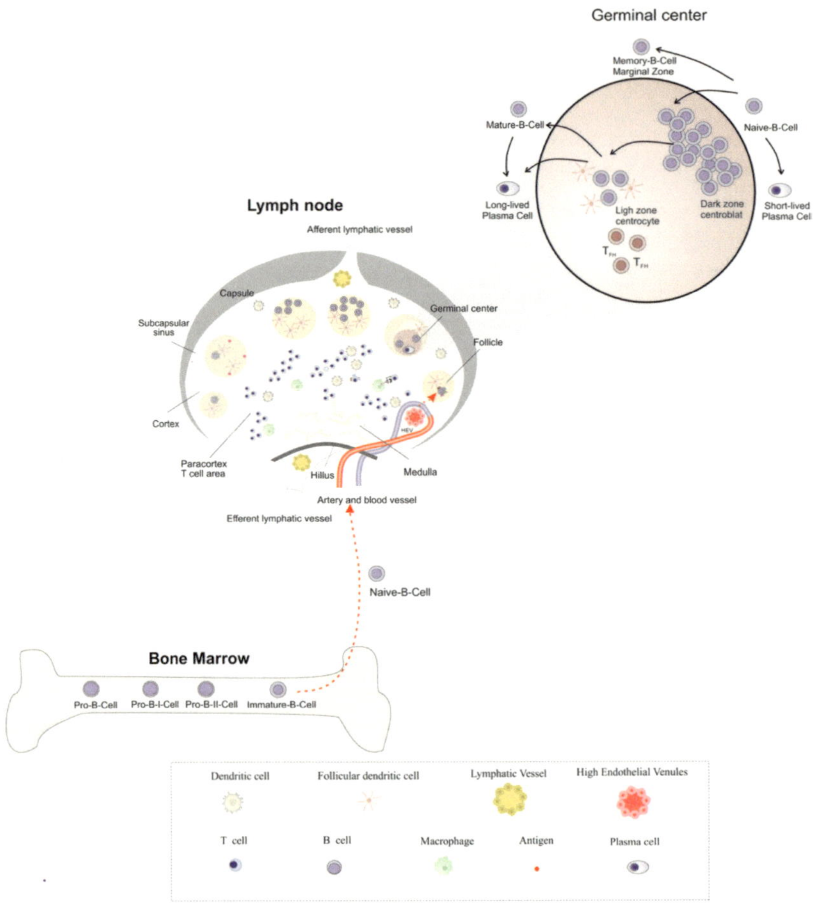

Figure 3. Schematic representation of B cell maturation in bone marrow and their differentiation in the lymph node [19, 35].

1.2. T Lymphocytes

1.2.1. T Lymphocytes ontogeny

Currently, we will discuss the origin and differentiation of T and natural killer (NK) cells, as well the migration of T cell precursors from the bone marrow to the thymus. In addition, we will discuss stages of T cells maturation and immunological development such as differentiation and proliferation, T cell receptor (TCR) genic rearrangement, thymic positive and negative selection and T cells with different phenotypes. These steps summarize the requisites for T cells to become immunologically competent and populate the peripheral lymphoid tissues.

It is well known and scientifically accepted that all blood cells are derived from a hematopoietic stem cell (HSC), defined as pluripotent and capable of self-renewal. HSCs express the CD34 antigen and account only for 0.1% of the all bone marrow nucleated cells. The first phase of HSC differentiation is the cell commitment to specific lineages. The lymphoid lineage commitment is dependent on several environmental factors such as stromal cells signaling, growth factors, cytokines, and kinases (Janus-JAK), tyrosine kinases (Kit-L) and surface molecules such as Notch-1. Notch-1 is very important since their collaboration with GATA-3 will contribute to the T lymphocytes lineage commitment, mainly to the αβ receptor T cells [21]. Radtke et al. have shown that the deletion of Notch-1 in murine models resulted in the T lymphocytes impaired development in the thymus [42].

The interleukins (IL) are also fundamental for HSC differentiation into lymphoid precursors and the key ILs involved in this process are IL-1, IL-2, IL-3, IL6, and IL-7. IL-7 is produced by the bone marrow stromal cells and by the thymic epithelial cells, and IL-7 plays a role in T cell development, proliferation and survival of lymphoid precursors. The IL-7 receptor is composed of two chains, IL-7Rα, and the gamma common (γc), the last is shared by several cytokines receptors such as IL-2, IL-4, IL-9, IL15 and IL-21. Alterations in the genes that codify IL-7Rα or the γc result in an immunodeficiency X-linked named severe combined immunodeficiency (SCID), which is characterized by the significant reduction or absence of T lymphocytes and NK cells, revealing the roles of IL-7 in humans [43–46].

Lymphoid progenitors can be characterized phenotypically by the expression of CD7 and CD34. Some studies define the lymphoid progenitors by the CD7 expression since this antigen has a lower expression in myeloid cells and is not expressed in other cell lineages [47].

A key event on T lymphocyte development is the gene rearrangement that is responsible for the generation of a diverse antigen receptor repertoire. The genes involved in the T cell receptor (TCR) rearrangement are present in the germ cell lineage and are located in the chromosomes 7 and 14. As seen in B lymphocytes, the heavy chain genes are present in the segments that code for the variable (V), diversity (D), joining (J) and constant (C) regions, and this recombination is known as V(D)J. In humans and mice, the γδ T cells have a limited repertoire of V and J segments that are involved in the TCR genic rearrangement [48, 49]. In humans, the δ-locus is clustered inside the α-locus, and there are only three true Vδ, they are Vδ1, Vδ2, and Vδ3. The human Vγ repertoire is situated in the γ-locus with 12 Vγ genes, of which only seven are identified as functional, since Vγ1, Vγ5P, Vγ6, Vγ7, and Vγ10 are considered pseudogenes. The difference between the low diversity in γ-δ loci and the high diversity of the α-β loci suggest that the γδ TCRs low diversity accompanies their recognition of preserved self-proteins with low variability.

The TCR V(D)J recombination is very similar to the B lymphocytes BCR recombination, involving also the enzymes Rag-1 and Rag-2, endonuclease *Artemis* and terminal deoxynucleotidyl transferase (TdT), Ku70, Ku80, DNA-dependent protein kinase (DNA-PK) and *XRCC4-DNA ligase IV.* Functional defects on these enzymes can result in immune deficiency such as SCID that can be derived of Rag-1 or Rag-2 mutations [50–52]. The higher TCR diversity generated during V(D)J recombination is a result of two combined mechanisms of diversity that involve random combination of gene segments and junctional diversity that results from the nucleotides addition or removal, complementary or not, within the junctions between V(D)J segments. These mechanisms of diversity can generate around of 10^7 different T lymphocyte clones. Each clone represents a unique TCR, the number of T cells clones is not higher as expected, but can be explained by the large number of T cells depleted during the thymic selection [51, 53].

1.2.2. Thymocytes and thymic selection

Different from B lymphocytes, the precursors of T lymphocytes migrate from the bone marrow to the thymus to complete their maturation status and undergo the positive and negative selections. The thymus colonization by immature lymphocytes, also known as thymocytes, enrolls chemokines, mainly CC-chemokine ligand 21 (CCL21) and CCL25, and their respective receptors CCR7 and CCR9 [54]. The thymic maturation is very important and only 1–3% of thymocytes that enter in the thymus survive the selection steps and gain the circulation [55–57].

Initially, the T cell precursor migrates to the corticomedullary region of the thymus, then inside the cortex and the double negative cells (DN) CD4-CD8- (**Figures 4** and **5**) [58]. The DN cells in development receive Notch-1 and IL-7 mediates signals, usually derived from the cortical thymic epithelial cells (cTECs) [59, 60]. Most thymocytes rearrange the V(D)J genes efficiently to express TCR αβ from DN3, at this stage, the TCR was not tested for their specificity and is termed pre-TCRαβ, which is associated with the protein complex CD3/ζ for the signal transduction [61]. Following maturation, thymocytes begin to express CD4 and CD8 co-receptors, initially expressing CD8, and then expressing CD4 to form the thymocyte double positives (DP) CD4+CD8+ (**Figures 4** and **5**). This DP population is present in the thymic cortex, expresses TCRαβ and consists of most lymphocytes inside the thymus of young individuals [62].

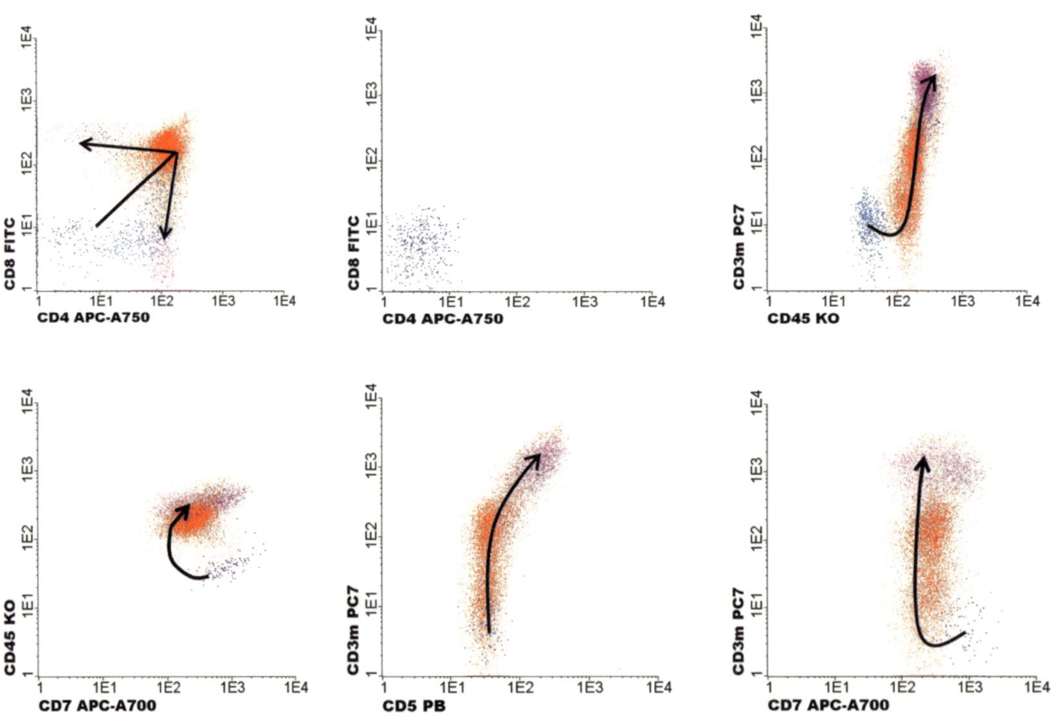

Figure 4. Thymus expression profile of T cells in different stages of maturation. The maturation states are represented by the colors displayed in the flow cytometry plots figures: dark blue represents immature double negative T cells, orange represents double positive cells in intermediate stage and purple represents the single positive mature T cells. Analysis performed with Infinicyt software (Cytognos).

http://dx.doi.org/10.5772/intechopen.69058

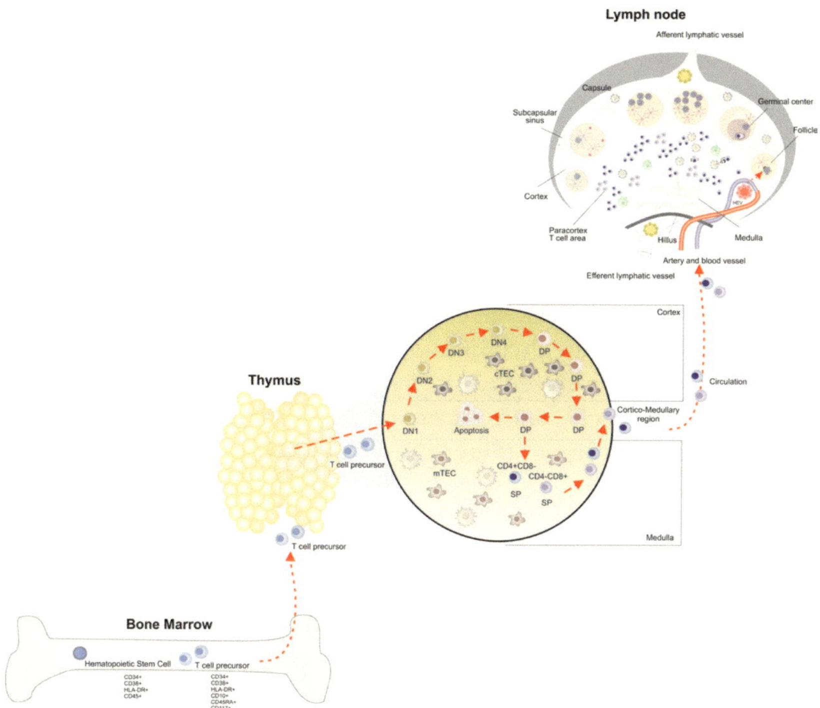

Figure 5. Schematic representation of T lymphocytes thymic selection [54, 59–63].

In the cortex, the TCRs from DP thymocytes interact with peptides via major histocompatibility complex (MHC) molecules expressed by the cTECs and dendritic cells and go through steps of positive and negative selections, thymocytes that interacting properly (low avidity interaction) are positively selected and receive survival signals (**Figure 5**). Thymocytes that fail in this interaction or interact with high avidity are selected negatively by the mechanism of apoptosis (death by neglect). This process is important so that thymocytes that continue their development are able to recognize foreign antigens but not self-antigens, thus avoiding autoimmunity. Interestingly, approximately 90% of DP thymocytes express ineffective TCRs and do not pass through cortex checkpoints and end dying due to the absence of positive selection (**Figure 5**) [54, 61, 63]. The positively selected DP thymocytes migrate to the thymus medulla, guided primarily by the expression of CCR7 and the chemoattraction of CCL19 and CCL21 produced by the medullar thymic epithelial cells (mTECs) and are induced initiate differentiation for CD4+CD8- or CD8+CD4-positive single (SP) thymocytes (**Figure 4**) per the MHC molecule involved (MHC class II for SP CD4+and MHC class I for SP CD8+) (**Figure 5**) [64].

The thymocytes that have escaped negative selection by cTECs and are self-reactive to tissue-specific antigens expressed by mTECs are also depleted [65, 66]. TThe expression of tissue-specific antigens by mTECs is controlled by the transcriptional factor autoimmune regulator (AIRE) and AIRE deficiency results in the disease, in humans, called autoimmune polyendocrinopathy – candidiasis - ectodermal dystrophy (APECED) [67, 68]. Interestingly, some thymocytes CD4+ that recognize self-antigens with high avidity into the thymus may develop in a CD4+ population of peripheral regulatory lymphocytes, which have the function of controlling and preventing autoimmune reactions.

Phenotypically, SP thymocytes express CD62 L and CD69 and also acquire the functional capacity of mature T lymphocytes, but are still naïve, not having yet experienced antigens during an adaptive immune response [69, 70]. Expression of sphingosine-1-phosphate receptor 1 (S1P1), one of the S1P receptors, is required for the outflow of the mature T lymphocytes from the thymus and in addition to S1P1, CCR7, CCL19 and CXCL12 also participate in this process [71]. This stage of differentiation and maturation in the thymus lasts approximately 12 days and is critical for the establishment of central tolerance [56]. Finally, immunologically competent lymphocytes leave the thymus and become part of the pool of mature and naive peripheral T lymphocytes, which remain in the cell cycle interphase for extended periods until they encounter with specific antigens presented by antigen-presenting cells (APCs) via MHC in secondary lymphoid organs (**Figure 5**).

1.2.3. Mature T lymphocytes

Once lymphocytes have left the thymus, they are carried in the blood to the peripheral lymphoid tissues such as lymph nodes, where the cells organize themselves to facilitate the encounter with antigenic particles and consequent lymphocytic activation. Immune cell-cell interactions are usually rolling interfaces that undergo continuous architectural change. The contact between T and B lymphocytes and the antigen-presenting cells (APCs) favors the information exchange among the cells, contributing to the assembly, type, and scope of immune responses [72].

Now, we will describe different classes of lymphocytes based on transcription factors expression and their cytokine secretion profile, associated to their differentiation status, functional profile and plasticity. It is important to highlight that each lymphocyte has a unique antigen receptor that is generated by somatic recombination and recognizes a different foreign component, and thus collectively, lymphocytes provide an almost limitless defense against a wide range of antigens. Recent evidences have demonstrated that a lymphocyte can produce daughter cells with different fates that carry out different functions. Based on these indications, it seems as if a single lymphocyte typically produces a diversity of functional daughter cells and manages to renew itself [73–76]. Successful immune responses often require more than one type of differentiated cell fate. Kelso and collaborators had already demonstrated in 1995 that biased T helper (Th) Th2 responses contained traces of Th1-type cytokines expression [77].

Activated $CD4^+$ T cells differentiate into immune suppressive regulatory T (Treg) cells or inflammatory T effector cells, such as T helper Th1, Th2, Th9, Th17, Th22 and follicular helper T (Tfh), each one with distinct characteristic metabolic programs (**Figure 5**). These different $CD4^+$ subsets play a critical role in the immune and effector response functions of T cells [78]. In response to distinct antigen challenge and extracellular cytokines signals, each $CD4^+$ T cell subset has distinct abilities in producing cytokine and chemokine receptors and expressing

http://dx.doi.org/10.5772/intechopen.69058

polarizing transcription factors, along with their association with specific forms of immune defense. New tools and techniques have revealed the capacity of polarized cells change their phenotype and repolarize towards mixed or alternative fates. The same cytokines that drive the polarization of each T helper cell subset during initial priming also drive the plasticity of established T helper cell subsets [79, 80].

1.2.3.1. CD4 Cell subsets

Since the establishment of the Th1-Th2 dogma in the 1980s [81, 82], different lineages of effector T cells have been identified that not only promote but also suppress immune responses.

Th1 cells are defined based on the production of pro-inflammatory cytokines such as interferon (IFN)-γ, and tumor necrosis factor (TNF)-α or TNF-β to stimulate innate and T cell immune responses. These cells are induced by natural killer (NK) and/or dendritic cells, through IFN-γ producing, which activate signal transducer and activator of transcription (STAT) STAT1, resulting in activation of lineage-specific transcription factor encoded by T-box transcription factor—TBX21 (T-bet) [83]. IL-27, a cytokine from IL-12 family, contributes to STAT1 phosphorylation and T-bet activation. T-bet enhances the synthesis of the IL-12 receptor, which activates STAT4 and consequent transcription and production of IFN-γ. Th1-type cytokines are responsible for the death of intracellular antigens and for the autoimmune response maintenance (**Figure 6**) [84, 85].

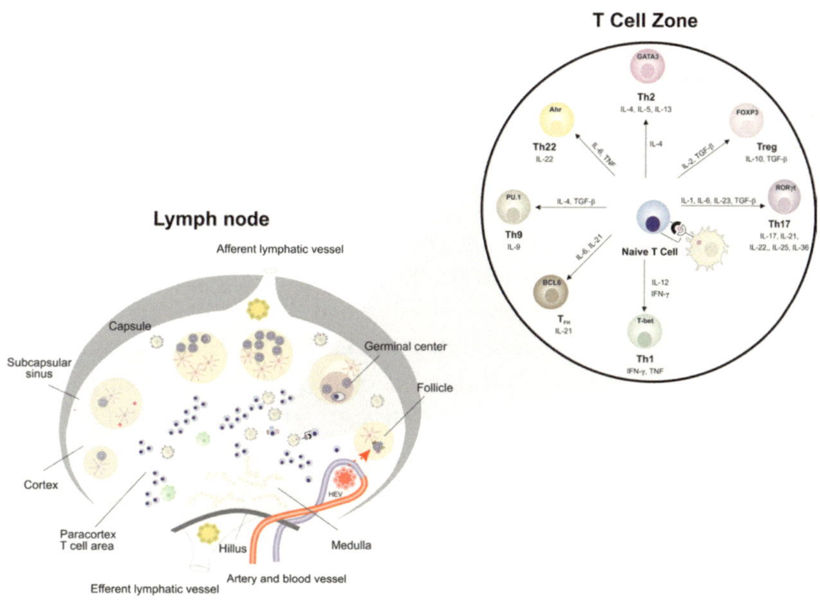

Figure 6. CD4 subsets differentiation, cytokines and transcription factors [78, 84–90, 121].

On the one hand, Th2 cells are defined as producers of IL-4, IL-5, and IL-13, which are associated with the production of IgE and eosinophilic responses in atopy. Differentiation of the Th2 subset requires IL-4 produced by Notch ligand activation of dendritic cells, inducing STAT6, which activates GATA-3. This transcription factor activates the production of the Th2 the lineage-specifying cytokines. Th2 cells control immunity to extracellular parasites and all forms of allergic inflammatory responses (**Figure 6**) [85, 86].

In recent years, it became evident that more functional subsets of T helper cells can be induced by various stimuli *in vivo* and *in vitro.* Induction of the Th17 lineage occurs when IL-6, IL-23, and TGF-β are present in the inflammatory milieu without Th1 or Th2 cytokines (**Figure 6**) [87]. Toll-like receptor signaling, leading to MyD88 signaling, is another innate immune signal fostering Th17 differentiation [88]. The cytokine IL-6 promotes STAT3, which induces retinoic orphan receptor (ROR) transcription factors, RORα and RORγT, leading to production of Th17 cytokines IL-17, IL-17F, and IL-22 [89, 90]. Functionally, Th17 cells play a role in host defense against extracellular pathogens by mediating the recruitment of neutrophils and macrophages to infected tissues. Moreover, it has become evident that abnormal regulation of Th17 cells may play a significant role in the pathogenesis of a variety of autoimmune and inflammatory diseases, because these cells can cause tissue injury when aber¬rantly regulated [85].

Another recently reported T helper population includes Th9 cells. This subset of cell undergoes a maturation program similar to Th2 cells, with IL-4 inducing STAT6 activation, and produces the Th2 cytokines IL-9 and IL-10, but unlike Th2 cells, they require TGF-β for maturation (**Figure 6**) [91, 92]. The IL-2-STAT5 signaling including interferon regulatory factor **(IRF)4** expression is critical for Th9 cell differentiation. Additionally, the lineage-specific transcription factor for Th9 development may be the activator protein 1 family transcription factor, BATF, leading to a transcriptional program, which results in increased IL-9 and IL-10 production [85, 91, 93]. There is a requirement as well for TGF-β-induced SMAD proteins and the SMAD-independent induction the transcription factor PU.1 in the generation of IL-9-secreting T cells. Although the GATA3 expression is lower in Th9 cells than Th2 cells, STAT6 is an important target gene involved in Th9 differentiation. These cells can exacerbate the immune response by enhancing antibody production and increasing immune cell infiltration and activity within the respiratory tract, contributing to asthmatic disease. In addition, IL-9 mediates anti-parasitic activity by altering epithelial cell function, increasing immune cell infiltration into infected locations, and augmenting leukocyte immune function. Besides that, the production of IL-9 by Th9 cells impairs tissue repair process during colitis, in contrast, can limit tumor growth by stimulating lymphocyte anti-tumor activity (**Figure 6**).

Th22 cells are promoted by IL-6 and TNF-α, which induces STAT3, and expression of the aryl hydrocarbon receptor [94]. Th22 cells have a specific profile of Th1 and Th17-associated genes, such as IFN-γ, IL17a, T-bet and RORγt [95]. In addition the counterpart maturation between Th17 and Th22 subsets, numerous phenotypic markers are expressed in both cell populations, including CCR6, CCR4, dipeptidyl peptidase IV, CD26, and CD90. But, differently from Th17, the Th22 cells expresses CCR10 and represents a distinct subtype of T cells that is involved in the epidermis immunity. IL-22, a cytokine from the IL-10 family, is not exclusively produced by the Th22 cells, then also by Th1 and Th17 cells (**Figure 6**) [85, 96].

A subset of human CD4⁺ T cells that specifically express IL-22 has been identified in the skin where the synthesis of active vitamin D enhances IL-22 expression, contributing to skin homeostasis, but also to the pathogenesis of skin disease, observed in psoriasis patients [97, 98].

Follicular helper CD4+T (Tfh) cells were first found in human tonsils, but now it is clear that are localized in the B-cell follicle and germinal center (GC) and is specialized in facilitating B-cell responses, enhancing immunoglobulin production [98, 99]. Tfh cells require a strong TCR signal for induction, which is also required for Treg responses [85, 100]. Tfh specification requires activation of the inducible co-stimulator (ICOS), a CD28-related co-stimulatory signal provided by activated dendritic cells or B cells, which initiates transcription of MAF, one transcription factor that induces IL-21 activation. The OX-40/CD134 co-stimulatory signal ligation is necessary to down-regulates CTLA-4, a dominant suppressor molecule of T cell activation (**Figure 6**) [101]. IL-6 and STAT3 are required for Tfh development like Th17 cells, yet Tfh cells can be generated in the absence of Th17 cytokines, IL-17, IL-17F, or TGF-β [102].

In order to understand how Tfh cells are identified, first is necessary to comprehend T and B cells migration for their interaction sites, which usually takes place in secondary lymphoid organs such as lymph nodes (LNs). Naive T cells migrate to the T cell zone in LNs responding to CCL19 and CCL21 gradients. After dendritic cells antigen stimulation, Tfh cells up-regulate CXCR5, down-regulate CCR7 and migrate to the interfollicular regions within LNs, where they interact with activated B cells. These interactions result in antibody production by the short-lived plasmablasts, which take place in extrafollicular regions or in the germinal center. In both regions, Tfh cells support B-cell maturation, class switch and affinity selection, via cytokines secretion or by expressing surface molecules. The germinal center responses drive memory B cell and plasma cell development. Then, Tfh cells are characterized according to patterns of receptor expression that enables their movements, as well as the expression of other surface proteins associated with migratory processes [103–107].

Regulatory T-cells (Treg) represent a heterogeneous population of CD4+T-cells characterized by suppressive capacity, which can be generated in the thymus, termed natural Tregs (nTregs) or adaptive regulatory T cells, induced in the periphery, involved in maintaining oral tolerance (Th3 cells), and T regulatory type 1 cells (Tr1 cells), stimulated by IFN-α secreted by neighboring plasmacytoid dendritic cells (pDCs). According to the literature, the nTregs need a strong TCR signal for their development. They are formed by low co-stimulation, so the T cell antigen recognition without a robust second signal provide by the CD28 family members leads to tolerance [85, 108]. Differentiation of induced Tregs, Th3 cells, and Tr1 cells happens in the periphery and needs high TGF-β concentrations and absence of pro-inflammatory cytokines [109]. Cell-cell interaction and IL-10 secretion are essential for the Treg suppressor function, mediated by the transcription factor Foxp3 through STAT5 activation (**Figure 6**), and simultaneous RORγt down regulation, which is the Th17 transcription factor [85, 110, 111].

Human T cells can be divided into functionally distinct subsets. Two primary categories are naïve T cells (TN) that have not been exposed to antigen and those that are antigen-experienced (memory). Naive T cells are usually characterized by the expression of CD45RA+, CD62L+ and CCR7+. CD45RA and CD45RO are high and low molecular weight protein derived from the CD45 gene splice variant, distinctly, with CD45RO being mainly expressed by memory cells. CD45RO+ cells are rarely found in neonates and gradually increased with age. The analysis of homing receptors revealed that T cells are heterogeneous and in particular naïve T cells express high levels of the lymph-node homing receptor CD62 L (L-selectin). Long-lived memory CD4+ lymphocytes are a hallmark feature of the adaptive immune system in response to pathogens and tumors [112]. The memory T cell compartment is heterogeneous and has been conventionally divided into two subsets on the basis of the lymph node homing molecules CD62 L and CCR7 expression [113]. Central memory T cells (TCM cells) highly express CD45RO+, CD45RA−, CD62L+ and CCR7+, whereas CD45RO+, CD45RA−, CD62L− CCR7− effector memory T cells (TEM cells) are considered to be committed progenitor cells that undergo terminal differentiation after a limited number of divisions (**Figure 7**) [114]. CCR7 and CD62 L are mostly co-expressed on the surface of CD4+ and CD8+T cells, and cells expressing these markers nearly uniformly express CD27 and CD28—but the inverse is not true. CD27 and CD28 are the main co-stimulatory molecules required to induce T cell activation, although memory T cells seem to be less dependent on CD27 and CD28 for their reactivation than naïve T cells [115, 116]. CCR7−/CD62L−, CD28+ cells are found in the peripheral blood of healthy individuals and known as a subset of transitional memory (TM) cells. TM cells seem to be more mature than TCM cells, but not as totally mature as TEM cells [117]. IL-15 administration increases a cell subset that re-expresses CD45RA (named terminal effector cells–TEMRA). The TEMRA cells express senescence markers, such as KLRG-1, CD57, and H2AX phosphorylation, have low functional and proliferative ability, indicating their terminal differentiation [118].

1.2.3.2. CD8⁺ cytotoxic T lymphocytes (CTLs) subsets

Similar to T $CD4^+$ cells, naïve $CD8^+$ T cells differentiate into effector T cells (CD62L- CD127-) upon TCR engagement with antigen and costimulation by an APC, but the antigen recognition occurs by MHC class I in peripheral lymphatic organs. Additionally, $CD8^+$ T cells also acquire different profiles according to co-stimulatory molecules and cytokines presents in the environmental, contributing to transcription factors induction and specific differentiation into Tc1, Tc2, Tc9, Tc17 or $CD8^+$ T regulatory fate, as we observe in $CD4^+$ T cells [119].

Cytotoxic T lymphocytes (CTLs) also named Tc1 are the best-characterized subset of $CD8^+$ T cells that are responsible for the direct killing of infected, damaged, and dysfunctional cells, including tumor cells. Once differentiated, these cells are IL-2 and IL-12 dependent and highly cytotoxic, rapidly expressing high levels of IFN-γ, TNF-α, perforin, and granzymes, into immunological synapse, following activation [120]. IL-12 promotes expression of T-bet and Id2, and IL-2 down-regulates BCL-6 [121]. The initial activation of $CD8^+$ T cells is related with the up-regulation of CD44 and CD69, killer cell lectin-like receptor G1 (KLRG1) and IL-2 receptor subunit-α (CD25), though the L-selectin (CD62 L), the IL-7 receptor subunit-α (CD127) and CD27 are diminished in comparison with naïve cells [119, 121].

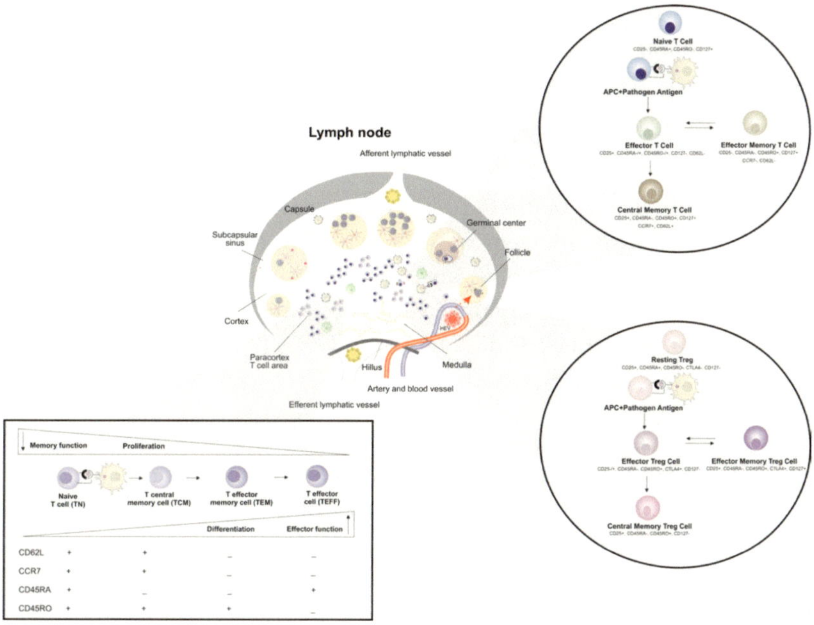

Figure 7. CD4 and CD8 subsets of memory [113, 114, 155].

While most CD8⁺ T cells die by apoptosis after antigen clearance, there are rare cells that survive as long-lived memory T cells. Memory CD8⁺ T cells were subdivided into two broad subsets [113, 122], central memory (CD62L+ CD127+ CCR7+) and effector memory (CD162L-CD127+CCR7-), distinguished by the relative expression of two homing molecules, CD62 L and CCR7. T effector memory cells have a phenotype more similar to that of effector cells, characterized by a loss of CCR7 expression and intermediate to no CD62 L expression (**Figure 7**). These cells exhibit rapid effector function, readily differentiating into T effector cells that secrete high amounts of IFN-γ and are highly cytotoxic upon re-exposure to cognate antigen. In contrast, T central memory cells are less differentiated, have increased proliferative potential and greater self-renewal capability, can produce high amounts of IL-2, and acquire effector functions less rapidly [120, 123, 124].

Tc2 cells, similarly to Th2 cells, produce IL-5, IL-13, but the limited extent of IL-4, besides granzymes and perforin, and express the lineage-specific transcription factor GATA3. This profile is associated with propagation of Th2-mediated allergy and probably contributes to rheumatoid arthritis [119, 125].

The differentiation of CD8⁺ T cells into IL-9 producers (Tc9 cells), in agreement with low expression of granzyme B, occurs mostly in the intestinal epithelium by IL-4 and TGF-β induction, favoring their greater anti-tumor activity. The transcription factors STAT6 and IRF4 are important for IL-9 production while Foxp3 for inhibition [119, 126].

The IL-17-producing CD8⁺ T (Tc17) cells are differentiated by IL-6 or IL-21 along with TGF-β while IL-23 stabilizes their phenotype. Similar to Th17 cells, they produce IL-17 and IL-21, express the receptor for IL-23 and the lineage-specific transcription factors IRF-4, RORγt and RORα [127]. Tc17 presents impaired cytotoxic activity because of a low IFN-γ, perforin, and granzyme B production. In contrast, they are able to enhance anti-tumor immunity due to their pro-inflammatory properties, which, on the other hand, may contribute to autoimmune processes [119, 128].

The suppressor $CD8^+$ Treg cells restricted by the non-classical MHC class Ib molecules Qa-1 (mouse) or HLA-E (human) represent a well-defined subpopulation. These cells present $CD44^{hi}$ $CD122^+$ $Ly49^+$ $Foxp3^+$ phenotype and IL-15 is important to their activity [129]. For suppression, these $CD8^+$ Treg cells rely on diverse mechanisms including TGF-β, IL-10, granzymes, perforin and indoleamine 2, 3-dioxygenase (IDO) [129].

1.3. Natural killer cells (NK)

Natural killer (NK) cells are an important piece of the innate immunity and provide a first-line defense against tumors and viral infections. NK cells were identified in the 1970s by the ability of kill tumor cells without previous activation [130]. The precursor cell able to differentiate towards NK cells was originally identified in the bone marrow, the main organ of hematopoiesis in adult life. However, subsequent experiments revealed that hematopoietic progenitor cell and/or NK cell committed precursors (NKPs) can traffic from bone marrow to peripheral sites, and it is now clear that the NK cell development occurs not only in the bone marrow but also in peripheral lymphoid and non-lymphoid organs [131]. In addition, Yu et al. demonstrated that precursor cells isolated from different sites of tissues can differentiate *in vitro* into mature NK cells [132]. The HSC commitment to NK cells differentiation includes transcription factors such as ID2, PU.1, Ets-1, TOX and NFIL3, and their maturation involves Eomes and Tbet [133–136].

Later studies demonstrated the cytotoxic ability of these cells against virus-infected cells and their participation into early inflammatory response secreting cytokines and chemokines [51, 137]. Particularly, upon activation, NK cells may also sense various bacterial products via toll-like receptors, an event resulting in a significant and rapid increase in their cytolytic activity and cytokine production [138]. Human NK cell function is regulated by several inhibitory and activating receptors. Among the various inhibitory NK cell receptors, an important role is played by Killer Ig-like Receptors (KIRs) that recognize allotypic determinants of HLA-A, -B, -C molecules and by the heterodimer NKG2A specific for the non-classical HLA-E molecule [139]. Regarding the activating NK cell receptors, the examples are NKp46, NKp44, and NKp30 that have been together named Natural Cytotoxicity Receptors (NCRs). The NCRs ligands are only partially known and possibly include pathogen-derived molecules and cellular ligands. In addition to NCR, other activating receptors and co-receptors are involved in NK cell function. These include NKG2D (recognizing MICA/B and ULBPs molecules), DNAM-1 (specific for CD155 and CD112), CD16 (FcRIII), NKp80 (specific for AICL), CD244 (that binds CD48), and NTBA (mediating hemophilic interaction) (**Figure 8**) [140].

Peripheral blood NK cells are not a uniform population. Consequently, two main subsets are identified regarding levels of CD56 expression, $CD56^{dim}$ and $CD56^{bright}$ NK cells [141]. $CD56^{dim}$

http://dx.doi.org/10.5772/intechopen.69058

NK cells are mainly in peripheral blood and show potent cytolytic activity and fast release of IFN-γ and other cytokines or chemokines upon cell activation through NK receptors. A large fraction of CD56^{dim} co-expresses CD16. CD56^{bright} NK cells represent a smaller population in peripheral blood while they are predominant in tissues and secondary lymphoid organs and are supposed to be responsible for the long-lasting production of chemokines and cytokines [137]. Several soluble factors participate on the NK cells development, and they are listed in **Table 1**.

1.4. Innate lymphoid cells (ILCs)

While NK cells have been known for almost four decades and have been extensively studied, other innate lymphoid cells (ILCs) have been better characterized in recent years. ILCs play a significant role in innate defenses against pathogens in different sites and in lymphoid tissue organization, primarily during fetal life. ILCs are emerging as a family of effectors and regulators of innate immunity and tissue remodeling and express neither somatically recombined

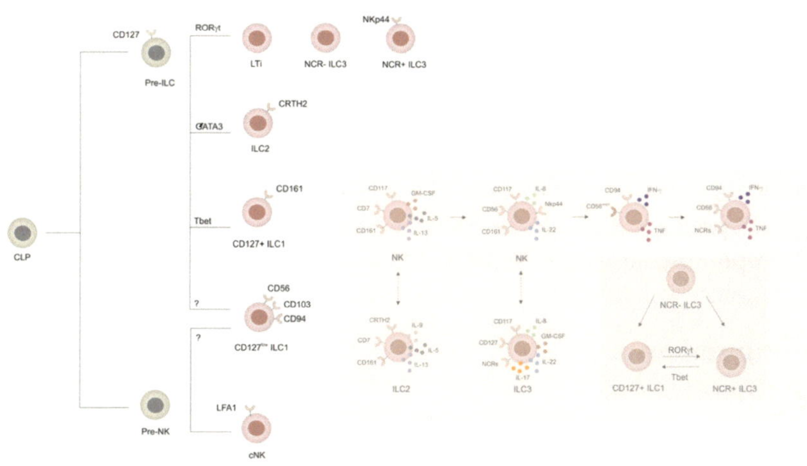

Figure 8. Developmental relationship between NK cells and other ILCs [137, 144, 156].

Cytokine	Role	Reference
IL-15	Central role in the development, maturation, survival, proliferation and differentiation	[142]
IL-7, SCF and Flt3-L	NK cells differentiation	[142]
IL-21	*killer immunoglobulin-like receptors* (KIR) expression on final stage of NK cell differentiation	[143]
IL-8 and MIP-1α	Favor the precursor to differentiate into NK cell, inhibiting the development of myeloid precursors	[144]

Table 1. Soluble factors involved in the NK cell development.

antigen receptors nor phenotypical markers of myeloid cells [145]. These subsets of cells require the transcriptional repressor Id2 and the interleukin 7 (IL-7) for their development, and they generate cytokine secretion patterns that mirror those of helper T cells of the adaptive immune system [146, 147]. ILCs have been classified in three main groups ILC1, ILC2, and ILC3 according to their cytokine profile and to the transcription factors required for their differentiation.

Similar to pro-inflammatory T helper type 1 cells, ILCs of group 1 (ILC1) release IFN-γ and require the transcription factor T-bet for their development, as do NK cells of the innate immune system. ILC1 cells were distinct from natural killer (NK) cells as they lacked perforin, granzyme B and the NK cell markers CD56, CD16 and CD94 (**Figure 8**) [148].

ILCs of group 2, which include natural helper cells and nuocytes, secrete IL-5 and IL-13 and require the transcription factor GATA-3 and thus resemble pro-inflammatory T helper type 2 cells. ILC2s mediate parasite expulsion but also contribute to airway inflammation, emphasizing the functional similarity between these cells and Th2 cells (**Figure 8**) [149–151]. Finally, ILCs of group 3 (ILC3 cells) require the transcription factors RORγt and AhR and include not only mucosal 'NK-22' cells, which secrete IL-22 and thus mimic non-inflammatory cells of the Th22 subset of helper T cells. ILC22 cells include NKp46 (+) and lymphoid tissue inducer (LTi)-like subsets that express the aryl hydrocarbon receptor (AHR). These cells were heterogeneous in their requirement for Notch and their effect on the generation of fetal and mucosal intestinal lymphoid tissues (LTi cells) (**Figure 8**) [152, 153], which produce IL-22 and IL-17 and thus resemble pro-inflammatory cells of the Th17 subset of helper T cells. Interleukin 22 (IL-22)- and IL-17-producing ILCs, which depend on the transcription factor RORγt, express CD127 (IL-7 receptor α-chain) and the natural killer cell marker CD161 [147, 154].

2. Concluding remarks

Herein, we have discussed B lymphocyte differentiation in the bone marrow and their stages of maturation in secondary lymphoid tissues and profiles in interfollicular, perifollicular, and follicular areas. In addition, we also have discussed derivation of T-cell precursors, natural killer cells, and other innate lymphoid cells. Moreover, T-cell precursor migration to thymus, differentiation, rearrangement, thymic selection, transcription factors, their profile and subsets in secondary lymphoid organs are also included. These topics are very important for the comprehension of the complex processes involved in forming a functional, consistently efficient immune response.

Acknowledgements

This work was funded by FAPESP, process number - 2014/15504-7 and by National Council of Technological and Scientific Development (CNPq) process number - 441665/2014-4. We are grateful to the contribution of Dr. Gilmar Santos, also to Dra. Anna Carla Goldberg for proofreading and to Sociedade Beneficente Israelita Brasileira Hospital Albert Einstein and the Clinical Pathology Laboratory for all their support.

Author details

Luciana Cavalheiro Marti[1]*, Nydia Strachman Bacal[2], Laiz Camerão Bento[2], Rodolfo Patussi Correia[2] and Fernanda Agostini Rocha[2]

*Address all correspondence to: luciana.marti@einstein.br

1 Experimental Research—Hospital Israelita Albert Einstein, São Paulo, Brazil

2 Hospital Israelita Albert Einstein, São Paulo, Brazil

References

[1] Kondo M, Scherer DC, Miyamoto T, King AG, Akashi K, Sugamura K, Weissman IL. Cell-fate conversion of lymphoid-committed progenitors by instructive actions of cytokines. Nature. 2000;**407**(6802):383-386. DOI: 10.1038/35030112

[2] Delogu A, Schebesta A, Sun Q, Aschenbrenner K, Perlot T, Busslinger M. Gene repression by Pax5 in B cells is essential for blood cell homeostasis and is reversed in plasma cells. Immunity. 2006;**24**(3):269-281. DOI: 10.1016/j.immuni.2006.01.012

[3] Smith LG, Weissman IL, Heimfeld S. Clonal analysis of hematopoietic stem-cell differentiation in vivo. Proceedings of the National Academy of Sciences of the United States of America. 1991;**88**(7):2788-92.

[4] Osawa M, Hanada K, Hamada H, Nakauchi H. Long-term lymphohematopoietic reconstitution by a single CD34-low/negative hematopoietic stem cell. Science. 1996; **273**(5272):242-245. DOI: 10.1126/science.273.5272.242

[5] Lai AY, Kondo MT, B. Lymphocyte differentiation from hematopoietic stem cell. Semin Immunol. 2008;**20**(4):207-212. DOI: 10.1016/j.smim.2008.05.002

[6] Traver D, Miyamoto T, Christensen J, Iwasaki-Arai J, Akashi K, Weissman IL. Fetal liver myelopoiesis occurs through distinct, prospectively isolatable progenitor subsets. Blood. 2001;**98**(3):627-635. DOI: doi.org/10.1182/blood. V98.3.627

[7] Mebius RE, Miyamoto T, Christensen J, Domen J, Cupedo T, Weissman IL, Akashi K. The fetal liver counterpart of adult common lymphoid progenitors gives rise to all lymphoid lineages, CD45+CD4+CD3- cells, as well as macrophages. Journal of Immunology. 2001;**166**(11):6593-6601. DOI: https://doi.org/10.4049/jimmunol.166.11.6593

[8] Kawamoto H, Ohmura K, Katsura Y. Presence of progenitors restricted to T, B, or myeloid lineage, but absence of multipotent stem cells, in the murine fetal thymus. Journal of Immunology. 1998; **161**(8):3799-3780

[9] Petrie HT, Kincade PW. Many roads, one destination for T cell progenitors. The Journal of Experimental Medicine. 2005;**202**(1):11-13. DOI: 10.1084/jem.20050990

[10] Melchers F. Checkpoints that control B cell development. The Journal of Clinical Investigation. 2015;**125**(6):2203-2210. DOI: 10.1172/JCI78083

[11] Dorshkind K. Regulation of hemopoiesis by bone marrow stromal cells and their products. Annual Review of Immunology. 1990;**8**:111-137. DOI: 10.1146/annurev.iy.08.040190.000551

[12] Hentges F. B lymphocyte ontogeny and immunoglobulin production. Clinical and Experimental Immunology. 1994;**97** Suppl 1:3-9. DOI: 10.1111/j.1365-2249. 1994.tb06252.x

[13] Ramirez J, Lukin K, Hagman J. From hematopoietic progenitors to B cells: mechanisms of lineage restriction and commitment. Current Opinion in Immunology. 2010;**22**(2):177-184. DOI: 10.1016/j.coi.2010.02.003

[14] Nutt SL, Heavey B, Rolink AG, Busslinger M. Commitment to the B-lymphoid lineage depends on the transcription factor Pax5. Nature. 1999;**401**(6753):556-562. DOI: 10.1038/44076

[15] Busslinger M. Transcriptional control of early B cell development. Annual review of immunology. 2004; **22**:55-79. DOI: 10.1146/annurev.immunol.22.012703.104807

[16] Ikawa T, Kawamoto H, Wright LY, Murre C. Long-term cultured E2A-deficient hematopoietic progenitor cells are pluripotent. Immunity. 2004;**20**(3):349-360. DOI: http://dx.doi.org/10.1016/S1074-7613(04)00049-4

[17] Yoshida T, Ng SY, Zuniga-Pflucker JC, Georgopoulos K. Early hematopoietic lineage restrictions directed by Ikaros. Nature Immunology. 2006;**7**(4):382-391. DOI: 10.1038/ni1314

[18] Hardy RR, Kincade PW, Dorshkind K. The protean nature of cells in the B lymphocyte lineage. Immunity. 2007;**26**(6):703-714. DOI: 10.1016/j.immuni.2007.05.013

[19] Perez-Andres M, Paiva B, Nieto WG, Caraux A, Schmitz A, Almeida J, et al. Human peripheral blood B-cell compartments: a crossroad in B-cell traffic. Cytometry Part B, Clinical Cytometry. 2010;**78** Suppl 1:S47-S60. DOI: 10.1002/cyto.b.20547

[20] Nagasawa T. Microenvironmental niches in the bone marrow required for B-cell development. Nature Reviews Immunology. 2006;**6**(2):107-116. DOI: 10.1038/nri1780

[21] Blom B, Spits H. Development of human lymphoid cells. Annual Review of Immunology. 2006;**24**:287-320. DOI: 10.1146/annurev.immunol.24.021605.090612

[22] Roessler S, Gyory I, Imhof S, Spivakov M, Williams RR, Busslinger M, Fisher AG, Grosschedl R. Distinct promoters mediate the regulation of Ebf1 gene expression by interleukin-7 and Pax5. Molecular and Cellular Biology. 2007;**27**(2):579-594. DOI: 10.1128/MCB.01192-06

[23] Stewart AK, Schwartz RS. Immunoglobulin V regions and the B cell. Blood. 1994;**83**(7): 1717-1730

[24] Schatz DG, Ji Y. Recombination centres and the orchestration of V(D)J recombination. Nature Reviews Immunology. 2011;**11**(4):251-263. DOI: 10.1038/nri2941

[25] Motea EA, Berdis AJ. Terminal deoxynucleotidyl transferase: the story of a misguided DNA polymerase. Biochimica et Biophysica acta. 2010;**1804**(5):1151-1166. DOI: 10.1016/j.bbapap.2009.06.030

[26] van Lochem EG, van der Velden VH, Wind HK, Marvelde JG, Westerdaal NA, van Dongen JJ. Immunophenotypic differentiation patterns of normal hematopoiesis in human bone marrow: reference patterns for age-related changes and disease-induced shifts. Cytometry Part B, Clinical Cytometry. 2004;**60**(1):1-13. DOI: 10.1002/cyto.b.20008

[27] Wang LD, Clark MR. B-cell antigen-receptor signalling in lymphocyte development. Immunology. 2003;**110**(4):411-420. DOI: 10.1111/j.1365-2567.2003. 01756.x

[28] Kitamura D, Rajewsky K. Targeted disruption of mu chain membrane exon causes loss of heavy-chain allelic exclusion. Nature. 1992;**356**(6365):154-156. DOI: 10.1038/356154a0

[29] Miosge LA, Goodnow CC. Genes, pathways and checkpoints in lymphocyte development and homeostasis. Immunology and Cell Biology. 2005;**83**(4):318-335. DOI: 10.1111/j.1440-1711.2005. 01353.x

[30] Brauninger A, Goossens T, Rajewsky K, Kuppers R. Regulation of immunoglobulin light chain gene rearrangements during early B cell development in the human. European Journal of Immunology. 2001;**31**(12):3631-3637. DOI: 10.1002/1521-4141(200112)31:12<3631::AID-IMMU3631>3.0.CO;2-L

[31] Pieper K, Grimbacher B, Eibel H. B-cell biology and development. The Journal of Allergy and Clinical Immunology. 2013;**131**(4):959-971. DOI: 10.1016/j.jaci.2013.01.046

[32] Sandel PC, Monroe JG. Negative selection of immature B cells by receptor editing or deletion is determined by site of antigen encounter. Immunity. 1999;**10**(3):289-299. http://dx.doi.org/10.1016/S1074-7613(00)80029-1

[33] Burrows PD, Cooper MD. B cell development and differentiation. Current Opinion in Immunology. 1997;**9**(2):239-244. DOI: 10.1016/S0952-7915(97)80142-2

[34] Ghia P, ten Boekel E, Rolink AG, Melchers F. B-cell development: a comparison between mouse and man. Immunology Today. 1998;**19**(10):480-485. DOI: http://dx.doi.org/10.1016/S0167-5699(98)01330-9

[35] Geisberger R, Lamers M, Achatz G. The riddle of the dual expression of IgM and IgD. Immunology. 2006;**118**(4):429-437. DOI: 10.1111/j.1365-2567.2006. 02386.x

[36] Allman D, Pillai S. Peripheral B cell subsets. Current Opinion Immunology. 2008;**20**(2):149-157. DOI: 10.1016/j.coi.2008.03.014

[37] Nutt SL, Hodgkin PD, Tarlinton DM, Corcoran LM. The generation of antibody-secreting plasma cells. Nature Reviews Immunology. 2015;**15**(3):160-171. DOI: 10.1038/nri3795

[38] Pillai S, Cariappa A. The folicular versus marginal zone B lymphocyte cell fate decision. Nature. 2009;**9**:767-777. DOI: 10.1038/nri2656

[39] Cerutti A, Cols M, Puga I. Marginal zone B cells: virtues of innatelike antibody-producing lymphocytes. Nature Reviews Immunology. 2013;**13**(2):118-132. DOI: 10.1038/nri3383

[40] Bemark M. Translating transitions - how to decipher peripheral human B cell development. Journal of Biomedical Research. 2015;**29**(4):264-284. DOI: 10.7555/JBR.29.20150035

[41] Perez-Andres M, Grosserichter-Wagener C, Teodosio C, van Dongen JJ, Orfao A, van Zelm MC. The nature of circulating CD27+CD43+ B cells. The Journal of Experimental Medicine. 2011;**208**(13):2565-2566. DOI: 10.1084/jem.20112203

[42] Radtke F, Wilson A, Stark G, Bauer M, van Meerwijk J, MacDonald HR, Aguet M. Deficient T cell fate specification in mice with an induced inactivation of Notch1. Immunity. 1999;**10**(5):547-558. DOI: http://dx.doi.org/10.1016/S1074-7613(00)80054-0

[43] Noguchi M, Yi H, Rosenblatt HM, Filipovich AH, Adelstein S, Modi WS, McBride OW, Leonard WJ. Interleukin-2 receptor gamma chain mutation results in X-linked severe combined immunodeficiency in humans. Cell. 1993;**73**(1):147-157. DOI: http://dx.doi.org/10.1016/0092-8674(93)90167-O

[44] Russell SM, Keegan AD, Harada N, Nakamura Y, Noguchi M, Leland P. et al. Interleukin-2 receptor gamma chain: a functional component of the interleukin-4 receptor. Science. 1993;**262**(5141):1880-1883. DOI: 10.1126/science.8266078

[45] Puel A, Ziegler SF, Buckley RH, Leonard WJ. Defective IL7R expression in T (-) B (+) NK(+) severe combined immunodeficiency. Nature Genetics. 1998;**20**(4):394-397. DOI: 10.1038/3877

[46] Giliani S, Mori L, de Saint Basile G, Le Deist F, Rodriguez-Perez C, Forino C, Mazzolari E, Dupuis S, Elhasid R, Kessel A, Galambrun C, Gil J, Fischer A, Etzioni A, Notarangelo LD. Interleukin-7 receptor alpha (IL-7Ralpha) deficiency: cellular and molecular bases. Analysis of clinical, immunological, and molecular features in 16 novel patients. Immunological Reviews. 2005;**203**:110-126. DOI: 10.1111/j.0105-2896.2005. 00234.x

[47] Barcena A, Muench MO, Galy AH, Cupp J, Roncarolo MG, Phillips JH, Spits H. Phenotypic and functional analysis of T-cell precursors in the human fetal liver and thymus: CD7 expression in the early stages of T- and myeloid-cell development. Blood. 1993;**82**(11):3401-3414

[48] Schwarz K, Gauss GH, Ludwig L, Pannicke U, Li Z, Lindner D, Friedrich W, Seger RA, Hansen-Hagge TE, Desiderio S, Lieber MR, Bartram CR. RAG mutations in human B cell-negative SCID. Science. 1996;**274**(5284):97-99. DOI: 10.1126/science.274.5284.97

[49] Santagata S, Gomez CA, Sobacchi C, Bozzi F, Abinun M, Pasic S, Cortes P, Vezzoni P, Villa A. N-terminal RAG1 frameshift mutations in Omenn's syndrome: internal methionine usage leads to partial V(D)J recombination activity and reveals a fundamental role

in vivo for the N-terminal domains. Proceedings of the National Academy of Sciences of the United States of America. 2000;**97**(26):14572-14577. DOI: 10.1073/pnas.97.26.14572

[50] Villa A, Sobacchi C, Notarangelo LD, Bozzi F, Abinun M, Abrahamsen TG, et al. V(D)J recombination defects in lymphocytes due to RAG mutations: severe immunodeficiency with a spectrum of clinical presentations. Blood. 2001;**97**(1):81-88. DOI: https://doi.org/10.1182/blood.V97.1.81

[51] Abbas AK, Lichtman AH, Pillai S. Cellular and Molecular Immunology. 7th ed; 2011

[52] Kazen AR, Adams EJ. Evolution of the V, D, and J gene segments used in the primate gammadelta T-cell receptor reveals a dichotomy of conservation and diversity. Proceedings of the National Academy of Sciences. U S A. 2011;**108**(29):E332-40. DOI: 10.1073/pnas.1105105108

[53] Schlissel MS. Regulating antigen-receptor gene assembly. Nature Reviews Immunology. 2003;**3**(11):890-899. Review. DOI: 10.1038/nri1225

[54] Takahama Y. Journey through the thymus: stromal guides for T-cell development and selection. Nature reviews Immunology. 2006;**6**(2):127-135. DOI: 10.1038/nri1781

[55] Scollay RG, Butcher EC, Weissman IL. Thymus cell migration. Quantitative aspects of cellular traffic from the thymus to the periphery in mice. European Journal of Immunology. 1980;**10**(3):210-218. DOI: 10.1002/eji.1830100310

[56] Egerton M, Scollay R, Shortman K. Kinetics of mature T-cell development in the thymus. Proceedings of the National Academy of Sciences of the United States of America. 1990;**87**(7):2579-2582

[57] Goldrath AW, Bevan MJ. Selecting and maintaining a diverse T-cell repertoire. Nature. 1999;**402**(6759):255-262. DOI: 10.1038/46218

[58] Godfrey DI, Kennedy J, Suda T, Zlotnik A. A developmental pathway involving four phenotypically and functionally distinct subsets of CD3-CD4-CD8- triple-negative adult mouse thymocytes defined by CD44 and CD25 expression. Journal of Immunology. 1993;**150**(10):4244-4252

[59] von Freeden-Jeffry U, Vieira P, Lucian LA, McNeil T, Burdach SE, Murray R. Lymphopenia in interleukin (IL)-7 gene-deleted mice identifies IL-7 as a nonredundant cytokine. The Journal of Experimental Medicine. 1995;**181**(4):1519-1526. DOI: 10.1084/jem.181.4.1519

[60] Peschon JJ, Morrissey PJ, Grabstein KH, Ramsdell FJ, Maraskovsky E, Gliniak BC, Park LS, Ziegler SF, Williams DE, Ware CB, Meyer JD, Davison BL. Early lymphocyte expansion is severely impaired in interleukin 7 receptor-deficient mice. The Journal of Experimental Medicine. 1994;**180**(5):1955-1960. DOI: 10.1084/jem.180.5.1955

[61] Germain RN. T-cell development and the CD4-CD8 lineage decision. Nature reviews Immunology. 2002;**2**(5):309-322. DOI: 10.1038/nri798

[62] Allman D, Sambandam A, Kim S, Miller JP, Pagan A, Well D, Meraz A, Bhandoola A. Thymopoiesis independent of common lymphoid progenitors. Nature Immunology. 2003;**4**(2):168-174. DOI: 10.1038/ni878

[63] Zuniga-Pflucker JC. T-cell development made simple. Nature Reviews Immunology. 2004;**4**(1):67-72. DOI: 10.1038/nri1257

[64] Ueno T, Saito F, Gray DH, Kuse S, Hieshima K, Nakano H, Kakiuchi T, Lipp M, Boyd RL, Takahama Y. CCR7 signals are essential for cortex-medulla migration of developing thymocytes. The Journal of Experimental Medicine. 2004;**200**(4):493-505. DOI: 10.1084/jem.20040643

[65] Zuklys S, Balciunaite G, Agarwal A, Fasler-Kan E, Palmer E, Hollander GA. Normal thymic architecture and negative selection are associated with aire expression, the gene defective in the autoimmune-polyendocrinopathy-candidiasis-ectodermal dystrophy (APECED). Journal of Immunology. 2000;**165**(4):1976-1983. DOI: https://doi.org/10.4049/jimmunol.165.4.1976

[66] Derbinski J, Pinto S, Rosch S, Hexel K, Kyewski B. Promiscuous gene expression patterns in single medullary thymic epithelial cells argue for a stochastic mechanism. Proceedings of the National Academy of Sciences of the United States of America. 2008;**105**(2):657-662. DOI: 10.1073/pnas.0707486105

[67] Nagamine K, Peterson P, Scott HS, Kudoh J, Minoshima S, Heino M, Krohn KJ, Lalioti MD, Mullis PE, Antonarakis SE, Kawasaki K, Asakawa S, Ito F, Shimizu N. Positional cloning of the APECED gene. Nature Genetics. 1997;**17**(4):393-398. DOI: 10.1038/ng1297-393

[68] Finnish-German AC. An autoimmune disease, APECED, caused by mutations in a novel gene featuring two PHD-type zinc-finger domains. Nature Genetics. 1997;**17**(4):399-403. DOI: 10.1038/ng1297-399

[69] Reichert RA, Weissman IL, Butcher EC. Phenotypic analysis of thymocytes that express homing receptors for peripheral lymph nodes. Journal of Immunology. 1986; **136**(10):3521-3528

[70] Ramsdell F, Jenkins M, Dinh Q, Fowlkes BJ. The majority of CD4+8- thymocytes are functionally immature. Journal of Immunology. 1991;**147**(6):1779-1785

[71] Matloubian M, Lo CG, Cinamon G, Lesneski MJ, Xu Y, Brinkmann V, Allende ML, Proia RL, Cyster JG. Lymphocyte egress from thymus and peripheral lymphoid organs is dependent on S1P receptor 1. Nature. 2004;**427**(6972):355-360. DOI: 10.1038/nature02284

[72] Basu R and Huse M. Mechanical Communication at the Immunological Synapse. Trends in Cell Biology. 2016. DOI: 10.1016/j.tcb.2016.10.005. [Epub ahead of print]

[73] Tubo NJ, Pagán AJ, Taylor JJ, Nelson RW, Linehan JL, Ertelt JM, Huseby ES, Way SS, Jenkins MK.. Single naive CD4+ T cells from a diverse repertoire produce different effector cell types during infection. Cell. 2013;**153**:785-796. DOI: 10.1016/j.cell.2013.04.007

[74] Gerlach, C. Rohr JC, Perié L, van Rooij N, van Heijst JW, Velds A, Urbanus J, Naik SH, Jacobs H, Beltman JB, de Boer RJ, Schumacher TN. Heterogeneous differentiation patterns of individual CD8+ T cells. Science. 2013;**40**:635-639. DOI: 10.1126/science.1235487

[75] Gerlach, C. van Heijst JW, Swart E, Sie D, Armstrong N, Kerkhoven RM, Zehn D, Bevan MJ, Schepers K, Schumacher TN. One naive T cell, multiple fates in CD8+ T cell differentiation. The Journal of Experimental Medicine. 2010;**207**:1235-1246. DOI: 10.1084/jem.20091175

[76] Reiner, SL, Adams, WC. Lymphocyte fate specification as a deterministic but highly plastic process. Nature Reviews Immunology. 2014;**14**(10):699-704. DOI: 10.1038/nri3734

[77] Kelso A, Groves P, Troutt AB, Francis K. Evidence for the stochastic acquisition of cytokine profile by CD4+ T cells activated in a T helper type 2-like response in vivo. European Journal of Immunology. 1995;**25**:1168-1175. DOI: 10.1002/eji.1830250506

[78] Raphael I, Nalawade S, Eagar TN, Forsthuber TG. T cell subsets and their signature cytokines in autoimmune and inflammatory diseases. Cytokine. 2015;**74**: 5-17. DOI: 10.1016/j.cyto.2014.09.011

[79] DuPage M, Bluestone JA. Harnessing the plasticity of CD4+ T cells to treat immune-mediated disease. Nature Reviews Immunology. 2016;**16**(3):149-163. DOI: 10.1038/nri.2015.18

[80] Slack M, Wang T, Wang R. T cell metabolic reprogramming and plasticity. Molecular Immunology. 2015;68:507-512. DOI: 10.1016/j.molimm.2015.07.036

[81] Coffman RL, Carty J. A T cell activity that enhances polyclonal IgE production and its inhibition by interferon-γ. The Journal of Immunology. 1986;**136**:949-954

[82] Mosmann T.R, Cherwinski H, Bond MW, Giedlin MA, Coffman RL. Two types of murine helper T cell clone. I. Definition according to profiles of lymphokine activities and secreted proteins. The Journal of Immunology. 1986;**136**:2348-2357

[83] Szabo SJ, Kim ST, Costa GL, Zhang X, Fathman CG, Glimcher LH. A novel transcription factor, T-bet, directs Th1 lineage commitment. Cell. 2000;**100** (6):655-669. DOI: http://dx.doi.org/10.1016/S0092-8674(00)80702-3

[84] Amsen D, Antov A, Flavell RA. The different faces of Notch in T-helper-cell differentiation. Nature Reviews Immunology. 2009;**9**(2):116-124. DOI: 10.1038/nri2488

[85] Caza T, Landas S. Functional and Phenotypic Plasticity of CD4(+) T Cell Subsets. Biomed Res Int. 2015; 2015:521957. doi: 10.1155/2015/521957. Epub 2015 Oct 25.

[86] Amsen D, Spilianakis CG, Flavell RA. How are TH1 and TH2 effector cells made? Current Opinion in Immunology. 2009;**21**(2):153-160. DOI: 10.1016/j.coi.2009.03.010

[87] Brucklacher-Waldert V, Steinbach K, Lioznov M, Kolster M, Hölscher C, and Tolosa E. Phenotypical characterization of human Th17 cells unambiguously identified by surface IL-17A expression. Journal of Immunology. 2009;**183**(9):5494-8501. DOI: 10.4049/jimmunol.0901000

[88] Davila E, Kolls J. A 'toll' for Th17 cell expansion. Journal of Leukocyte Biology. 2010; **88**(1):5-7. DOI: 10.1189/jlb.0110057

[89] Romano M, Sironi M, Toniatti C Polentarutti N, Fruscella P, Ghezzi P, Faggioni R, Luini W, van Hinsbergh V, Sozzani S, Bussolino F, Poli V, Ciliberto G, Mantovani A. Role of IL-6 and its soluble receptor in induction of chemokines and leukocyte recruitment. Immunity. 1997;**6**(3):315-325. DOI: http://dx.doi.org/10.1016/S1074-7613(00)80334-9

[90] Yang XO, Pappu BP, Nurieva R, Akimzhanov A, Kang HS, Chung Y, Ma L, Shah B, Panopoulos AD, Schluns KS, Watowich SS, Tian Q, Jetten AM, Dong C. T helper 17 lineage differentiation is programmed by orphan nuclear receptors RORα and RORγ. Immunity. 2008;**28**(1):29-39. DOI: 10.1016/j.immuni.2007.11.016

[91] Veldhoen M, Uyttenhove C, van Snick J, Helmby H, Westendorf A, Buer J, Martin B, Wilhelm C, Stockinger B. Transforming growth factor-β "reprograms" the differentiation of T helper 2 cells and promotes an interleukin 9-producing subset. Nature Immunology. 2008;**9**(12):1341-1346. DOI: 10.1038/ni.1659

[92] Dardalhon V, Awasthi A, Kwon H, Galileos G, Gao W, Sobel RA, Mitsdoerffer M, Strom TB, Elyaman W, Ho IC, Khoury S, Oukka M, Kuchroo VK. IL-4 inhibits TGF-β-induced Foxp3+ T cells and, together with TGF-β, generates IL-9+ IL-10+ Foxp3− effector T cells. Nature Immunology. 2008;**9**(12):1347-1355. DOI: 10.1038/ni.1677

[93] Jabeen R, Goswami R, Awe O, Kulkarni A, Nguyen ET, Attenasio A, Walsh D, Olson MR, Kim MH, Tepper RS, Sun J, Kim CH, Taparowsky EJ, Zhou B, Kaplan MH. Th9 cell development requires a BATF-regulated transcriptional network. Journal of Clinical Investigation. 2013;**123**(11):4641-4653. DOI: 10.1172/JCI69489

[94] Pickert G, Neufert C, Leppkes M Zheng Y, Wittkopf N, Warntjen M, Lehr HA, Hirth S, Weigmann B, Wirtz S, Ouyang W, Neurath MF, Becker C. STAT3 links IL-22 signaling in intestinal epithelial cells to mucosal wound healing. The Journal of Experimental Medicine. 2009;**206**(7):1465-1472. DOI: 10.1084/jem.20082683

[95] Duhen T, Geiger R, Jarrossay D, Lanzavecchia A, Sallusto F. Production of interleukin 22 but not interleukin 17 by a subset of human skin-homing memory T cells. Nature Immunology. **10**:857-863, 2009. DOI: 10.1038/ni.1767

[96] Trifari S, Kaplan CD, Tran EH, Crellin NK, Spits H. Identification of a human helper T cell population that has abundant production of interleukin 22 and is distinct from TH17, TH1 and TH2 cells. Nature Immunology. 2009;**10**(8):864-871. DOI: 10.1038/ni.1770

[97] Kagami S, Rizzo HL, Lee JJ, Koguchi Y, Blauvelt A. Circulating Th17, Th22, and Th1 cells are increased in psoriasis. Journal of Investigative Dermatology. 2010;**130**:1373-1383. DOI: 10.1038/jid.2009.399

[98] Sun B, Zhang Y. Overview of orchestration of CD4+ T cell subsets in immune responses. Advances in Experimental Medicine and Biology. 2014;**841**:1-235. DOI: 10.1007/978-94-017-9487-9_1

[99] Breitfeld D, Ohl L, Kremmer E, Ellwart J, Sallusto F, Lipp M, Förster R. Follicular B helper T cells express CXC chemokine receptor 5, localize to B cell follicles, and support immunoglobulin production. The Journal of Experimental Medicine. 2000;**192**:1545-1552. DOI: 10.1084/jem.192.11.1545

[100] Hogquist KA. Signal strength in thymic selection and lineage commitment. Current Opinion in Immunology. 2001;**13**(2):225-31. DOI: http://dx.doi.org/10.1016/S0952-7915(00)00208-9

[101] King C. New insights into the differentiation and function of T follicular helper cells. Nature Reviews Immunology. 2009;**9**(11):757-766. DOI: 10.1038/nri2644

[102] Nurieva RI, Chung Y, Hwang D, Yang XO, Kang HS, Ma L, Wang YH, Watowich SS, Jetten AM, Tian Q, Dong C. Generation of T follicular helper cells is mediated by interleukin-21 but independent of T helper 1, 2, or 17 cell lineages. Immunity. 2008;**29**(1):138-149. DOI: 10.1016/j.immuni.2008.05.009

[103] Willimann K, Legler DF, Loetscher M, Roos RS, Delgado MB, Clark-Lewis I, Baggiolini M, Moser B. The chemokine SLC is expressed in T cell areas of lymph nodes and mucosal lymphoid tissues and attracts activated T cells via CCR7. European Journal of Immunology. 1998;**28**:2025-2034. DOI: 10.1002/(SICI)1521-4141(199806)28:06<2025::AID-IMMU2025>3.0.CO;2-C

[104] Nagira M, Imai T, Yoshida R, Takagi S, Iwasaki M, Baba M, Tabira Y, Akagi J, Nomiyama H, Yoshie O. A lymphocyte-specific CC chemokine, secondary lymphoid tissue chemokine (SLC), is a highly efficient chemoattractant for B cells and activated T cells. European Journal of Immunology. 1998;**28**:1516-1523. DOI: 10.1002/(SICI)1521-4141(199805)28:05<1516::AID-IMMU1516>3.0.CO;2-J

[105] Luther SA, Bidgol A, Hargreaves DC, Schmidt A, Xu Y, Paniyadi J, Matloubian M, Cyster JG. Differing activities of homeostatic chemokines CCL19, CCL21, and CXCL12 in lymphocyte and dendritic cell recruitment and lymphoid neogenesis. The Journal of Immunology. 2002;**169**:424-433. DOI: https://doi.org/10.4049/jimmunol.169.1.424

[106] Haynes NM, Allen CD, Lesley R, Ansel KM, Killeen N, Cyster JG. Role of CXCR5 and CCR7 in follicular TH cell positioning and appearance of a programmed cell death gene-1High germinal center-associated subpopulation. The Journal of Immunology. 2007;**179**:5099-5108. DOI: https://doi.org/10.4049/jimmunol.179.8.5099.

[107] Craft JE. Follicular helper T cells in immunity and systemic autoimmunity Nature Reviews Rheumatology. 2012;**8**:337-347. DOI: 10.1038/nrrheum.2012.58

[108] Zhou X, Jeker LT, Fife BT, Zhu S, Anderson MS, McManus MT, Bluestone JA. Selective miRNAdisruption in T reg cells leads to uncontrolled autoimmunity. Journal of Experimental Medicine. 2008;**205**(9):1983-1991. DOI: 10.1084/jem.20080707

[109] Weaver CT, Harrington LE, Mangan PR, Gavrieli M, Murphy KM.Th17: an effector CD4 T cell lineage with regulatory T cell ties. Immunity. 2006;**24**(6):677-688. DOI: 10.1016/j.immuni.2006.06.002

[110] Zhou X, Bailey-Bucktrout S, Jeker LT, Bluestone JA. Plasticity of CD4+ FoxP3+ T cells. Current Opinion in Immunology. 2009;**21**(3):281285. DOI: 10.1016/j.coi.2009.05.007

[111] Lee YK, Mukasa R, Hatton RD, Weaver CT. Developmental plasticity of Th17 and Treg cells. Current Opinion in Immunology. 2009;**21**(3):274-280. DOI: 10.1016/j.coi.2009.05.021

[112] Wakim LM, Bevan MJ. From the thymus to longevity in the periphery. Current Opinion in Immunology. 2010;**22**(3):274-278. DOI: 10.1016/j.coi.2010.03.003

[113] Sallusto F, Lenig D, Förster R, Lipp M, Lanzavecchia A. Two subsets of memory T lymphocytes with distinct homing potentials and effector functions. Nature. 1999;**401**(6754):708-712. DOI:10.1038/44385

[114] Fearon DT, Manders P, Wagner SD. Arrested differentiation, the self-renewing memory lymphocyte, and vaccination. Science. 13 Jul 2001;**293**(5528):248-250. DOI: 10.1126/science.1062589

[115] Tortorella C, Schulze-Koops H, Thomas R, Splawski JB, Davis LS, Picker LJ, Lipsky PE. Expression of CD45RB and CD27 identifies subsets of CD4+ memory T cells with different capacities to induce B cell differentiation. The Journal of Immunology. 1995;**155**(1):149-162

[116] Bryl E, Vallejo AN, Weyand CM, Goronzy JJ. Down-regulation of CD28 expression by TNF-alpha. Journal of Immunology. 2001;**167**(6):3231-3238. DOI: https://doi.org/10.4049/jimmunol.167.6.3231

[117] Picker LJ, Reed-Inderbitzin EF, Hagen SI, Edgar JB, Hansen SG, Legasse A, Planer S, Piatak M Jr, Lifson JD, Maino VC, Axthelm MK, Villinger F. IL-15 induces CD4 effector memory T cell production and tissue emigration in nonhuman primates. Journal of Clinical Investigation. 2006;**116**(6):1514-1524. DOI: 10.1172/JCI27564

[118] Geginat J, Lanzavecchia A, Sallusto F. Proliferation and differentiation potential of human CD8+ memory T-cell subsets in response to antigen or homeostatic cytokines. Blood. 2003;**101**(11):4260-4266. DOI: 10.1182/blood-2002-11-3577

[119] Mittrücker HW, Visekruna A, Huber M. Heterogeneity in the Differentiation and Function of CD8+ T Cells. Archivum Immunologiae et Therapia Experimentalis. 2014;**62**:449-458. DOI: 10.1007/s00005-014-0293-y

[120] Reiser J, Banerjee A. Effector, Memory, and Dysfunctional CD8(+) T Cell Fates in the Antitumor Immune Response. J Immunol Res. 2016;2016:8941260. doi:10.1155/2016/8941260. Epub 2016 May 22.

[121] Yang CY, Best JA, Knell J, Yang E, Sheridan AD, Jesionek AK, Li HS, Rivera RR, Lind KC, D'Cruz LM, Watowich SS, Murre C, Goldrath AW. The transcriptional regulators Id2 and Id3 control the formation of distinct memory CD8? T cell subsets. Nature Immunology. 2001;**12**:1221-1229. DOI: 10.1038/ni.2158

[122] Förster R, Schubel A, Breitfeld D, Kremmer E, Renner-Müller I, Wolf E, Lipp M. CCR7 coordinates the primary immune response by establishing functional microenvironments in secondary lymphoid organs. Cell. 1999;**99**(1):23-33

[123] Arbonés ML, Ord DC, Ley K, Ratech H, Maynard-Curry C, Otten G, Capon DJ, Tedder TF. Lymphocyte homing and leukocyte rolling and migration are impaired in L-selectin deficient mice. Immunity. 1994;**1**(4):247-260. DOI: 10.1016/1074-7613(94)90076-0

[124] Bachmann MF, Wolint P, Schwarz K, Jäger P, Oxenius A. Functional properties and lineage relationship of CD8+ T cell subsets identified by expression of IL-7 receptor α and CD62L. The Journal of Immunology. 2005;**175**(7):4686-4696. DOI: https://doi.org/10.4049/jimmunol.175.7.4686

[125] Tang Y, Guan SP, Chua BY, Zhou Q, Ho AW, Wong KH, Wong KL, Wong WS, Kemeny DM. Antigen-specific effector CD8 T cells regulate allergic responses via IFN-gamma and dendritic cell function. Journal of Allergy and Clinical Immunology. 2012;**129**(1611-1620):e4. DOI: 10.1016/j.jaci.2011.12.976

[126] Visekruna A, Ritter J, Scholz T, Campos L, Guralnik A, Poncette L, Raifer H, Hagner S, Garn H, Staudt V, Bopp T, Reuter S, Taube C, Loser K, Huber M. Tc9 cells, a new subset of CD8(+) T cells, support Th2-mediated airway inflammation. European Journal of Immunology. 2013;**43**:606-618. DOI: 10.1002/eji.201242825

[127] Huber M, Heink S, Pagenstecher A, Reinhard K, Ritter J, Visekruna A, Guralnik A, Bollig N, Jeltsch K, Heinemann C, Wittmann E, Buch T, Prazeres da Costa O, Brüstle A, Brenner D, Mak TW, Mittrücker HW, Tackenberg B, Kamradt T, Lohoff M. IL-17A secretion by CD8+ T cells supports Th17-mediated autoimmune encephalomyelitis. Journal of Clinical Investigation. 2013;**123**:247-260. DOI: 10.1172/JCI63681

[128] Hamada H, Garcia-Hernandez Mde L, Reome JB, Misra SK, Strutt TM, McKinstry KK, Cooper AM, Swain SL, Dutton RW. Tc17, a unique subset of CD8 T cells that can protect against lethal influenza challenge. The Journal of Immunology. 2009;**182**:3469-3481. DOI: 10.4049/jimmunol.0801814

[129] Kim HJ, Cantor H. Regulation of self-tolerancebyQa-1-restricted CD8+ regulatory T cells. Seminars in Immunology. 2011;**23**:446-452. DOI: 10.1016/j.smim.2011.06.001

[130] Herberman RB, Nunn ME, Holden HT, Lavrin DH. Natural cytotoxic reactivity of mouse lymphoid cells against syngeneic and allogeneic tumors. II. Characterization of effector cells. International Journal of Cancer. 1975;**16**(2):230-239

[131] Di Santo JP. Natural killer cell developmental pathways: A question of balance. Annual Review of Immunology. 2006;**24**:257-286. DOI: 10.1146/annurev.immunol.24.021605.090700

[132] Yu J, Freud AG, Caligiuri MA. Location and cellular stages of natural killer cell development. Trends in Immunology. 2013;**34**(12):573-582. DOI: 10.1016/j.it.2013.07.005

[133] Yokota Y, Mansouri A, Mori S, Sugawara S, Adachi S, Nishikawa S, Gruss P. Development of peripheral lymphoid organs and natural killer cells depends on the helix-loop-helix inhibitor Id2. Nature. 1999;**397**(6721):702-706. DOI: 10.1038/17812

[134] Colucci F, Samson SI, DeKoter RP, Lantz O, Singh H, Di Santo JP. Differential requirement for the transcription factor PU.1 in the generation of natural killer cells versus B and T cells. Blood. 2001; **97**(9):2625-2632. DOI: https://doi.org/10.1182/blood.V97.9.2625

[135] Yun S, Lee SH, Yoon SR, Kim MS, Piao ZH, Myung PK, Kim TD, Jung H, Choi I. TOX regulates the differentiation of human natural killer cells from hematopoietic stem cells in vitro. Immunology letters. 2011;**136**(1):29-36. DOI: 10.1016/j.imlet.2010.11.008

[136] Gordon SM, Chaix J, Rupp LJ, Wu J, Madera S, Sun JC, Lindsten T, Reiner SL. The transcription factors T-bet and Eomes control key checkpoints of natural killer cell maturation. Immunity. 2012;**36**(1):55-67. DOI: 10.1016/j.immuni.2011.11.016

[137] Montaldo E, Vacca P, Moretta L, Mingari MC. Development of human natural killer cells and other innate lymphoid cells. Seminars in immunology. 2014;**26**(2):107-113. DOI: 10.1016/j.smim.2014.01.006

[138] Marcenaro E, Ferranti B, Falco M, Moretta L, Moretta A. Human NK cells directly recognize Mycobacterium bovis via TLR2 and acquire the ability to kill monocyte-derived DC. International Immunology. 2008;**20**(9):1155-1167. DOI: 10.1093/intimm/dxn073

[139] Moretta A, Bottino C, Vitale M, Pende D, Biassoni R, Mingari MC, Moretta L. Receptors for HLA class-I molecules in human natural killer cells. Annual Review of Immunology. 1996;**14**:619-648. DOI: 10.1146/annurev.immunol.14.1.619

[140] Bottino C, Castriconi R, Pende D, Rivera P, Nanni M, Carnemolla B, Cantoni C, Grassi J, Marcenaro S, Reymond N, Vitale M, Moretta L, Lopez M, Moretta A. Identification of PVR (CD155) and Nectin-2 (CD112) as cell surface ligands for the human DNAM-1 (CD226) activating molecule. The Journal of Experimental Medicine. 2003;**198**(4):557-567. DOI: 10.1084/jem.20030788

[141] Caligiuri MA. Human natural killer cells. Blood. 2008;**112**(3):461-469. DOI: 10.1182/blood-2007-09-077438

[142] Freud AG, Caligiuri MA. Human natural killer cell development. Immunological reviews. 2006;**214**:56-72. DOI: 10.1111/j.1600-065X.2006. 00451.x

[143] Sivori S, Cantoni C, Parolini S, Marcenaro E, Conte R, Moretta L, Moretta A. IL-21 induces both rapid maturation of human CD34+ cell precursors towards NK cells and acquisition of surface killer Ig-like receptors. European journal of immunology. 2003;**33**(12):3439-3447. DOI: 10.1002/eji.200324533

[144] Montaldo E, Vitale C, Cottalasso F, Conte R, Glatzer T, Ambrosini P, Moretta L, Mingari MC. Human NK cells at early stages of differentiation produce CXCL8 and express CD161 molecule that functions as an activating receptor. Blood. 2012;**119**(17):3987-3996. DOI: 10.1182/blood-2011-09-379693

[145] Walker JA, Barlow JL, McKenzie AN. Innate lymphoid cells–how did we miss them? Nature Reviews Immunology. 2013;**13**:75-87. DOI: 10.1038/nri3349

[146] Satoh-Takayama N, Lesjean-Pottier S, Vieira P, Sawa S, Eberl G, Vosshenrich CA, Di Santo JP. IL-7 and IL-15 independently program the differentiation of intestinal CD3– NKp46+ cell subsets from Id2-dependent precursors. The Journal of Experimental Medicine. 2010;**207**:273-280. DOI: 10.1084/jem.20092029

[147] Magri G, Miyajima M, Bascones S, Mortha A, Puga I, Cassis L, Barra CM et al. Innate lymphoid cells integrate stromal and immunological signals to enhance antibody production by splenic marginal zone B cells. Nature Immunology. 2014;**15**(4):354-364. DOI:10.1038/ni.2830

[148] Bernink JH, Peters CP, Munneke M, te Velde AA, Meijer SL, Weijer K, Hreggvidsdottir HS, Heinsbroek SE, Legrand N, Buskens CJ, Bemelman WA, Mjösberg JM, Spits H. Human type 1 innate lymphoid cells accumulate in inflamed mucosal tissues. Nature Immunology. 2013;**14**:221-229. DOI: 10.1038/ni.2534

[149] Neill DR, Wong SH, Bellosi A, Flynn RJ, Daly M, Langford TK, Bucks C, Kane CM, Fallon PG, Pannell R, Jolin HE, McKenzie AN. Nuocytes represent a new innate effector leukocyte that mediates type-2 immunity. Nature. 2010; **464**:1367-1370. DOI: 10.1038/nature08900

[150] Mjösberg J, Bernink J, Golebski K, Karrich JJ, Peters CP, Blom B, te Velde AA, Fokkens WJ, van Drunen CM, Spits H. The transcription factor GATA3 is essential for the function of human type 2 innate lymphoid cells. Immunity. 2012;**37**:649-659. DOI: 10.1016/j.immuni.2012.08.015

[151] Mjösberg JM, Trifari S, Crellin NK, Peters CP, van Drunen CM, Piet B, Fokkens WJ, Cupedo T, Spits H. Human IL-25- and IL-33-responsive type 2 innate lymphoid cells are defined by expression of CRTH2 and CD161. Nature Immunology. 2011;**12**:1055-1062. DOI: 10.1038/ni.2104

[152] Cella M, Otero K, Colonna M. Expansion of human NK-22 cells with IL-7, IL-2, and IL-1β reveals intrinsic functional plasticity. Proceedings of the National Academy of Sciences. USA 2010;**107**:10961-10966. DOI: 10.1073/pnas.1005641107

[153] Lee JS, Cella M, McDonald KG, Garlanda C, Kennedy GD, Nukaya M, Mantovani A, Kopan R, Bradfield CA, Newberry RD, Colonna M. AHR drives the development of gut ILC22 cells and postnatal lymphoid tissues via pathways dependent on and independent of Notch. Nature Immunology. 2012;**13**:144-151. DOI: 10.1038/ni.2187

[154] Takatori H, Kanno Y, Watford WT, Tato CM, Weiss G, Ivanov II, Littman DR, O'Shea JJ. Lymphoid tissue inducer-like cells are an innate source of IL-17 and IL-22. The Journal of Experimental Medicine. 2009;**206**:35-41. DOI: 10.1038/nri1781

[155] Golubovskaya V, Wu L. Different subsets of T cells, memory, effector functions, and CAR-T immunotherapy. Cancers (Basel). 2016;**8**(3). pii: E36. DOI: 10.3390/cancers8030036

[156] Hazenberg MD, Spits H. Human innate lymphoid cells. Blood. 2014;**124**(5):700-709. DOI: 10.1182/blood-2013-11-427781

Chapter 2

Signal Pathway in Precursor B-Cell Lymphoblastic Leukemia/Lymphoma

Tatsuaki Tsuruyama and Takuya Hiratsuka

Additional information is available at the end of the chapter

http://dx.doi.org/10.5772/intechopen.68892

Abstract

Stat5, c-myc, Hipk2, Fiz1, and ZFP521 to lymphomagenesis precursor B-cell lymphoblastic lymphoma/leukemia have been previously identified as a putative gene involved in the induction of B-cell lymphomagenesis. In this review, we summarize the role of ZFP521 in B-cell lymphomagenesis. Zinc finger protein 521 (Zfp521) is a novel identified gene that is responsible for pre–B-lymphoblastic lymphomagenesis through activation of pre–B-cell receptor (pre-BCR)-signaling by upregulation of adaptor genes and related kinases in the signaling downstream. The pre-BCR-signaling molecules, FLT3, CD43, and IL-7 receptor (IL-7R) were positively regulated by these genes. Stimulation of pre-BCR and/or IL-7R signaling caused aberrant upregulation of other oncogene sets such as cyclin genes, thereby inducing the growth of pre–B cells. IL-7R/Janus kinase (JAK)/STAT signaling cascade is one of the key signaling pathways that are activated in precursor B-cell lymphoblastic lymphoma/leukemia. FLT3, CD43, and pre-BCR cascades crosstalk with JAK/STAT cascade. FLT3 and CD43 cascades have the potential to enhance JAK/STAT cascade effect on pre-B cell growth. On the other hand, pre-BCR and interleukin (IL)-7 receptor exerted competitive effects on pre–B-cell growth; thus, precursor B-cell lymphoblastic lymphomagenesis is a consequence through interaction with these cascades.

Keywords: pre–B-cell receptor, Stat/Jak pathway, Zfp521

1. Introduction

1.1. Summary

B-cell lymphoblastic leukemia/lymphoma (B-LBL) is a neoplasm that exhibits immature phenotype of the B-cell lineage with on-going immunoglobulin rearrangement. Understanding the activation of signal pathways in tumor cells provides significant knowledge on tumorigenesis.

Surface markers interleukin-7 receptor (IL-7R), FLT3, CD43, and phenotypic marker pre–B-cell receptor are aberrantly activated in tumor cells. IL-7R is one of the developmental stage markers and is closely associated with immunoglobulin gene rearrangement in mice. In addition, these IL-7R, FLT3, and CD43 signal pathways interact with each other. The signaling molecules, JAK3, Stat5a, Fiz1, and Hipk2, play pivotal roles in these signaling pathways. In this review, we summarize the activation networks of these pathways from the perspective of the activation of adaptor molecules and immunoglobulin rearrangement.

1.2. Introduction

B-LBL is a neoplasm of B-lymphoid precursors and it is essentially identical to acute lymphocytic leukemia as it involves the bone marrow and peripheral blood [1, 2]. These lymphomas and leukemias are composed of medium-sized blast cells with scant cytoplasm, an oval nucleus, transparent nucleus, condensed chromatin, and often multiple nucleoli. The lymphoma tissues exhibit mitotic figures and are phagocytosed by macrophages after apoptosis—this histology is called "Starry sky" and is well known in Burkitt lymphoma. Distinguishing B-precursor types from T-precursor types is impossible because they share similar cytological features. Immunophenotypes of pre–B LBL resemble the normal immature B-cell lineages, primarily including pre–B cells, because pre–B LBL consists of ongoing immunoglobulin gene (*Ig*) rearrangements of heavy chains (*Igh*) or light chains (*Igl*). This rearrangement depends on the activity of recombination-activating gene 1 (*RAG1*) and *RAG2* under the high expression of the interleukin 7 receptor (IL-7R) [3]. In addition, pre–B receptors consist of lambda5 and Vpreb component, which are surrogate light-chain components at the time of completion of *Igh* rearrangement (**Figure 1**) [4, 5].

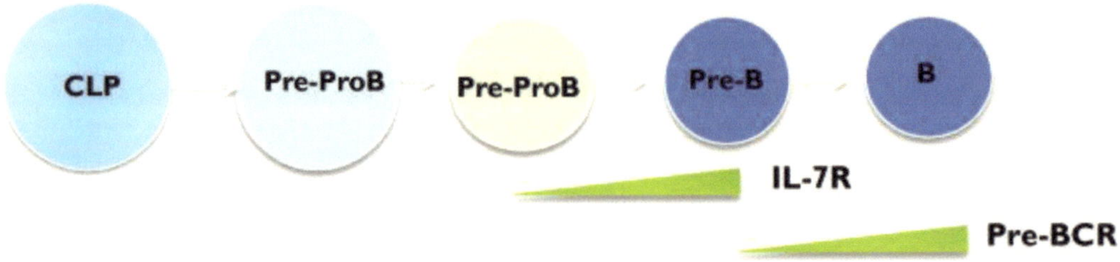

Figure 1. Scheme of B-cell development stage and IL-7R/pre–B-cell receptor (BCR) expression. CLP, common lymphocyte precursor.

2. The characterization of spontaneous pre–B-cell lymphoma in SL/Kh mice

2.1. Experimental mouse model of spontaneous lymphoma

We established an inbred strain of mouse called the spontaneous lymphoma mouse strain (SL/Kh) as a model of murine leukemia virus (MLV) integration-induced B-LBL lymphomagenesis. In the experimental model, transgenic mice carrying chimera genes, such as Emu-myc mice, MT-BCR-ABL mice, [6, 7], and TEL/AML1 mice rapidly develop pre-B LBL [8–10]. Unlike these models, the SL/Kh mouse develops spontaneously in the absence of artificially introduced gene mutation; however, Zfp521 is the gene that is spontaneously and constitutively mutated by MLV insertion after the birth [11, 12].

These mice share MLV with AKR-strain mice that are susceptible to T lymphoma [13, 14]. SL/Kh mice were found to have multiple copies of the pathogenic endogenous proviral genome that are genetically transmitted through the germ line on chr 7 [12, 15]. A type of MLV expressed from this provirus infects the hematopoietic cells and MLV genome is somatically re-integrated into the host cell genome. Subsequently, B-LBL spontaneously develops with a high frequency of 95% after 6 months of birth. These lymphoma cells are positive for lambda5 and Vpreb, which are a part of the pre-BCR. Myeloid leukemia, mature B-cell lymphoma, and T-cell lymphoma are known to occur in the inbred strain of mouse [16]. Such high occurrence of identical B-lymphoblastic lymphoma/leukemia phenotypes has not been reported in other mice. The initial growth of pre–B cells in SL/Kh was proven to be independent of the provirus integration, but dependent on the bone marrow pre-B1 (*Bomb1)* locus that includes BANK1 and the *enpep* gene that involves a glutamyl aminopeptidase (*BP-1*) (Mm.1193, UniGeneID) [17]. Clinically, the mice present with hepatosplenomegaly in which pre–B LBL invades via the portal tract and replace the splenocytes. In addition, the spinal bone becomes deformed, because of bone structure remodeling. As described later, the identified signal cascade promoting the MLV proviral element gives the clue for understanding of the development of lymphomagenesis through upregulation of signaling pathways and can serve as a model of clinical intervention by administration of anti-tumor drugs because of stable susceptibility for lymphomagenesis.

2.2. Flow cytometry analysis of B-LBL experimental lymphomas

Flow cytometric analysis is the one of the most important methods for analyzing pre–B cells. BP1, B220, IL-7R, CD24, and CD43 are the classical phenotypic markers of pre–B cells as well as λ5 and Vpreb. These markers were available for Hardy's classification for murine B cell lineage (**Figures 2** and **3**) [18, 19]. These markers are a little different from those that are used for the classification of human B-cell lineages, because B220 , BP-1, CD43, and CD24 are included.

2.3. Genetic background of pre–B lymphomagenesis

Bomb1, a quantitative trait locus (QTL), on *Mus musculus* (MMU) chromosome 3 is responsible for pre–B-cell expansion [20, 21] (**Figure 4**). In analysis of the congenic mice carrying SL/Kh alleles of *Bomb1*, polyclonal expansion of pre–B cells is observed. BANK1, an adaptor molecule of pre-BCR, is located near the *Bomb1* locus. We generated a congenic strain, NFS. SL/Kh-Bomb1 mice, with the replacement of this locus with SL/Kh *Bomb1*, without pre–B-induced provirus. The congenic mice showed pre–B-cell expansion, but pre–B lymphomagenesis were not observed. Therefore, the pre–B-cell lymphomagenesis is probably induced by multiple genes, including MLV integration into the proto-oncogenes. Notably, this locus is

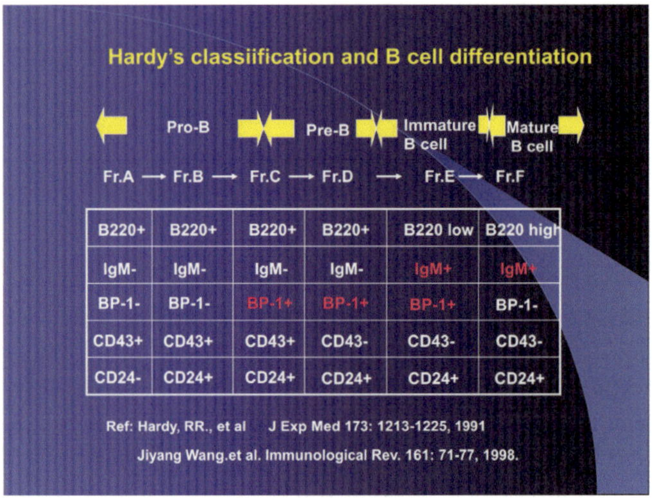

Figure 2. Surface phenotypic markers and Hardy's classification. BP-1 and IgM are notable markers. Fr., fraction.

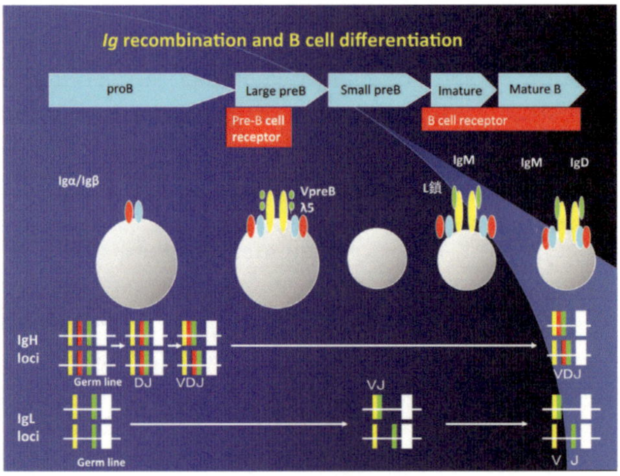

Figure 3. *Ig* recombination and B-cell development stage. VpreB and λ5 are components of surrogate light change in the pre-BCR. Igα and β are adaptor molecules that are identical to CD79a and CD79b. Pre-BCR is tentatively formed in the stage of large pre-B.

also susceptible to high-frequency microsatellite instability (MSI) in the pre–B LBL in mouse chromosome 3 including the *Bomb1* [17] (**Figure 5**). MSI is confirmed at ≥2 markers in DNA derived from tumor tissues in 93.7% of SL/Kh mice. To date, there have been only few systematic analyses of MSI and our data are significant in the hematopoietic tumors. Irregular deletion and insertion are observed within *Bomb1* in the course of lymphoma tissue with a high frequency.

http://dx.doi.org/10.5772/intechopen.68892

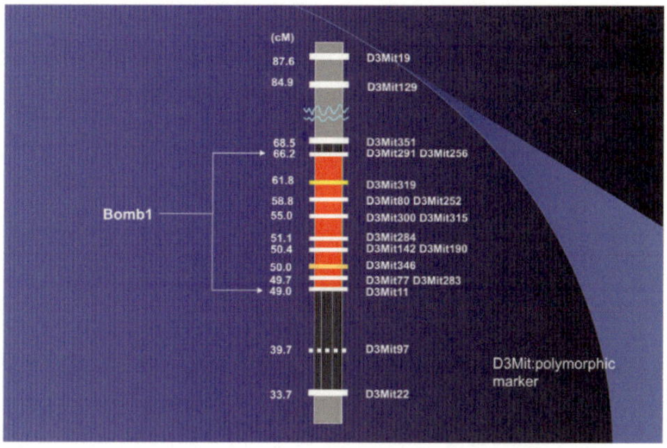

Figure 4. *Bomb1* locus and microsatellite markers on chromosome 3.

D3Mit129 Sequence Results

Lane	Sample
1	Ladder 100bp
2	NFS (control)
3	Congenic (control)
4	30 (spleen)
5	42 (spleen)
6	72 (spleen)
7	74 (spleen)
8	76 (spleen)
9	79 (spleen)
10	217 (lymphoma)
11	218 (lymphoma)
12	219 (lymphoma)
13	221 (lymphoma)

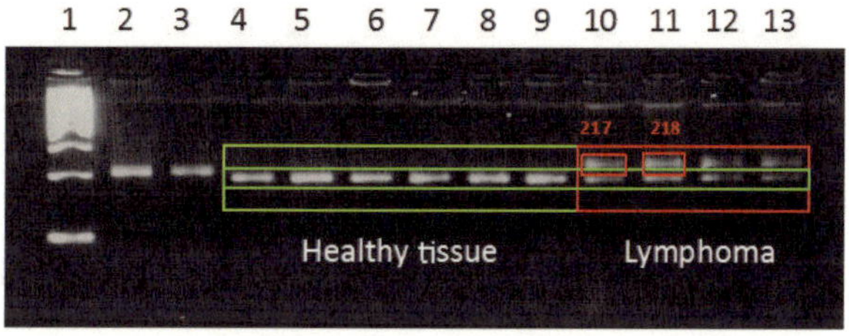

217

```
                 10         20         30         40         50
Control     CAGGGGCTTG ATACAGCAGT AGGATAAGTC ATCTCTGTCT CTCTCTCTCT
Sample 217  CAGGGGCTTG ATACAGCAGT AGGATAAGTC ATCTCTGTCT CTCTCTCTCT

            ....|....| ....|....| ....|....| ....|....| ....|....|
                 60         70         80   10 bp 90        100
Control     CTGTCTGTCT CTGTCTGTCT CTGTCTGT-- --------CT CTGTCTCTCT
Sample 217  CTGTCTGTCT CTGTCTGTCT CTGTCTGTTT CTCTCTCTCT CTGTCTCTCT
```

218

```
                 10         20         30         40         50
Control     CAGGGGCTTG ATACAGCAGT AGGATAAGTC ATCTCTGTCT CTCTCTCTCT
Sample 218  CAGGGGCTTG ATACAGCAGT AGGATAAGTC ATCTCTGTCT CTCTCTCTCT
            ....|....| ....|....| ....|....| ....|....| ....|....|
                 60         70         80   12 bp 90        100
Control     CTGTCTGTCT CTGTCTGTCT CTGTCTGT-- ---------- CTCTGTCTCT
Sample 218  CTGTCTGTCT CTGTCTGTCT CTGTCTGTTT CTCTCTCTCT CTCTGTCTCT
```

Figure 5. Microsatellite instability in the genome of lymphoma cells in the lane of healthy lymph node tissue [17]. Dinucleotide CT is deleted in the lymphoma genomes.

3. Upregulation of proto-oncogenes in pre–B lymphomas

Retroviral tagging, such as MLV insertion, is considered as a useful method for the identification of proto-oncogenes. RTCGD (Retrovirus and Transposon-tagged Cancer Gene Database, http://variation.osu.edu/rtcgd/) is one of the established registration systems of MLV integration, and many genes were identified as the common integration site (CIS) [16].

There many identified genes that are involved in the development of hematopoietic tumors. We summarize the signaling pathways that are associated with the target genes as described in the subsequent text.

3.1. IL-7R-signaling pathway and Stat5a

In both humans and mice, the IL-7R (also known as CD127) is expressed by early B-cell progenitors, and signaling via IL-7Rα activates signal transducer and activator of transcription 5 (STAT5) and drives pro-B-cell proliferation, while inhibiting Igκ recombination [22, 23].

Stat5a gene is one of the target genes of MLV integration in B-cell tumors (**Table 1**). The encoded STAT5 protein is a member of the signal inducer and activator of transcription (STAT) family and includes STAT5A and STAT5B subtypes. They are encoded by separate genes—the proteins are 90% identical at the amino acid level. These encoding genes are both targets of MLV. STAT5 proteins are activated by Janus kinases (JAKs) associated with transmembrane receptors such as interleukin receptor. Because, deletion of *Stat5a* and *Stat5b* arrests B-cell development at the pre–pro-B cell stage [24].

Binding of the cytokine ligands to these receptors on the outside of the cell activates the JAK3 [25]. Subsequently, the activated kinases add a phosphate group to tyrosine residues (Y449) on the IL-7Rα chain of the receptor. STAT5 then binds to these phosphorylated tyrosines. STAT5 is subsequently phosphorylated by the JAK3. The phosphorylated STAT5 forms either homodimer. Phosphorylated STAT proteins have the potential to form a dimer that can translocate into the nucleus and upregulate transcriptional activity by binding to the gamma interferon activation site palindromic (GAS) element in the promoters of the target genes. The targets encode *c-Myc, Pim-1* [26], *Bcl-xL,* and *Cyclin D1* [27], which promote proliferation and apoptosis in hematopoietic cells [28]. STAT5A, in particular, contributes to IL-7–induced B-cell precursor expansion. IL-7R is highly expressed in pre–B cells during *Igh* recombination, and therefore Stat5a has been one of the responsible molecules for *Igh* recombination [29]. Attenuation of IL-7R signaling in both human and mouse pre–B cells is associated with the expression of *RAG1* and *RAG2*.

Gene	Mean interval (bp)	Number of integration sites
Stat5a	26.2	92
c-myc	55.5	16
N-myc	6	8
Fiz1	89.1	8
Hipk2	101.1	7
Stat5b	121.7	3
MHC class heavy chain	100	2

Table 1. Common integration site.

A comparison of the phenotype of SL/Kh lymphomas showed that when the *Stat5a* was highly expressed, clones completed *Igh* $D_H J_H$ recombination but not *Igh* variable segment—D_H recombination; on the other hand, when the *Stat5a* was relatively less expressed in clones, both $D_H J_H$ and *Igh* variable segment, D_H recombination, are completed. On the other hand, *Stat5a*-high clones highly express λ5 but low for *Vpreb*; by contrast, *Stat5a*-low clones were constitutively high for both λ5 and *Vpreb*. In summary, the *Stat5a*-high lymphoma clones are more immature than other lymphomas. Stat5a may contribute to the lymphomagenesis at the immature stage of B cells [29].

3.2. *Zfp521* and pre-BCR pathway

The *Zfp521* gene was identified at the MLV integration site in the genomes of B-cell lymphomas in the AKXD mouse strain [30, 31]. This gene is also the most frequent integration site as well in the genome of pre–B-cell lymphoma in SL/Kh mice (**Figure 6**) and is related to immature B lymphomagenesis [11, 32]. *Zfp521* expression contributes to neural crest formation and the development of adipose cells, chondrocytes [33, 34], bone [34–36], and neural crest [35]. Recently, we reported that ZFP521 regulates and activates pre–B-cell receptor signal pathways, and it modulates the IL-7-signaling pathway [11].

The pre-BCR is expressed on large pre–B cells in which *Igh* recombination is completed. In the initiation of Igκ or Igλ gene rearrangement, signals of the IL-7 receptor gradually attenuate in pre–B cells, and B-cell maturation proceeds. Although both the IL-7R and the pre-BCR are required for murine B-cell lymphopoiesis, the orchestration of signal pathways has remained controversial. The responsiveness to IL-7 and stimulation through pre-BCR controls the development of pre–B cells into mature B cells [22, 23]. During the development of pro-B cells into pre–B cells, IL-7 signaling is the major mediator. The mature BCR replaces the pre-BCR. Zfp521 is expressed from professional pre–B cell of Fraction A (Fr. A) to Fr. B-C according to Hardy's classification. In this pre–B stage, Zfp521 may interact with adaptor molecules of Cd79a/b such as BANK1, Blnk, and Btk. Zfp521 may play as a transcriptional factor, because of a stimulation of this gene expression in a cell line, and the signal was located in the nucleus [30]. However, the binding motif on DNA is not clearly identified. The IL-7 receptor pathway interfered with Vpreb stimulation through the upregulation of BANK1 near or on *Bomb1* by *ZFP521*. BANK1 is disrupted by IL-7R signaling and interacts with phospholipase gamma 2 [37]. In fact, BANK1-PLCg2 binding is enhanced by B-lymphocyte kinase (BLK) [37]. Therefore, complicated per-BCR adaptors are hypothesized (**Figure 7**).

Cyclin D3 and Cyclin D2 are upregulated by overexpression of the *ZFP521* gene. Pre-BCR was shown to mediate Ras-MEK-extracellular signal-regulated kinase (ERK)-signaling pathway activation and light-chain recombination by silencing Cyclin D3 [38].

In humans, the fusion of the Pax5, which is essential for pre–B-cell development gene, exon 7 to ZFP521 exon 4, has been observed in pre–B-cell acute lymphocytic leukemia by genome-wide analysis of genetic alterations [39]. Dysregulation of *ZFP521* gene leads to pre–B-cell lymphomagenesis through the activation of pre–B-cell-specific molecular-signaling pathways [11]. Therefore, *ZFP521* could be considered as a target for molecular-targeted therapy.

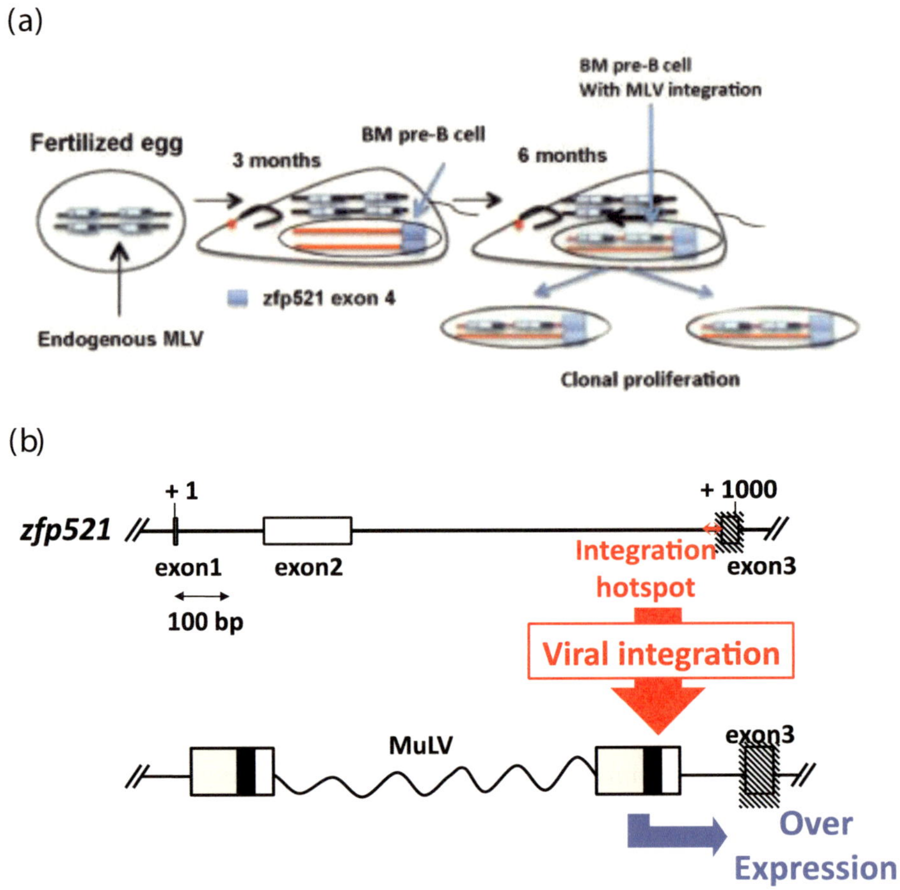

Figure 6. (a) Schematic representation of MLV integration in Zfp521 in SL/Kh mice. By the age of 2–3 months, the MLV host cell has grown in BM, and the endogenous MLV integrates into the genome of the host lymphocytes. The host cells clonally grow with higher expression of the *Zfp521* gene. The tandem box in the upper scheme represents long terminal repeat (LTR) of the provirus.

3.3. FLT3 signaling and LBL development via Fiz1

(a) Fms like tyrosine kinase 3 (FLT3) belongs to the immunoglobulin superfamily CD135 also known as fetal liver kinase-2 (Flk2). This protein is the receptor for the cytokine Flt3 ligand (FLT3L). FLT3 is a type III receptor tyrosine kinase with five immunoglobulin-like motifs in the extracellular region. In the intracellular region, a tyrosine kinase region (TK) and a C-terminal region composed of a juxtamembrane region (JM) and a kinase insert are contained. This protein is constitutively expressed in the hematopoietic stem and progenitor cells. On the other hand, the ligands that bind to the FLT3 receptor (FL) are produced in bone marrow stromal cells. FL directly stimulates hematopoietic stem cells or together with other cytokines and plays an important role in its survival, proliferation, and differentiation. FLT3 is also one of the critical developmental factors for B- and T-lymphocyte development [40].

http://dx.doi.org/10.5772/intechopen.68892

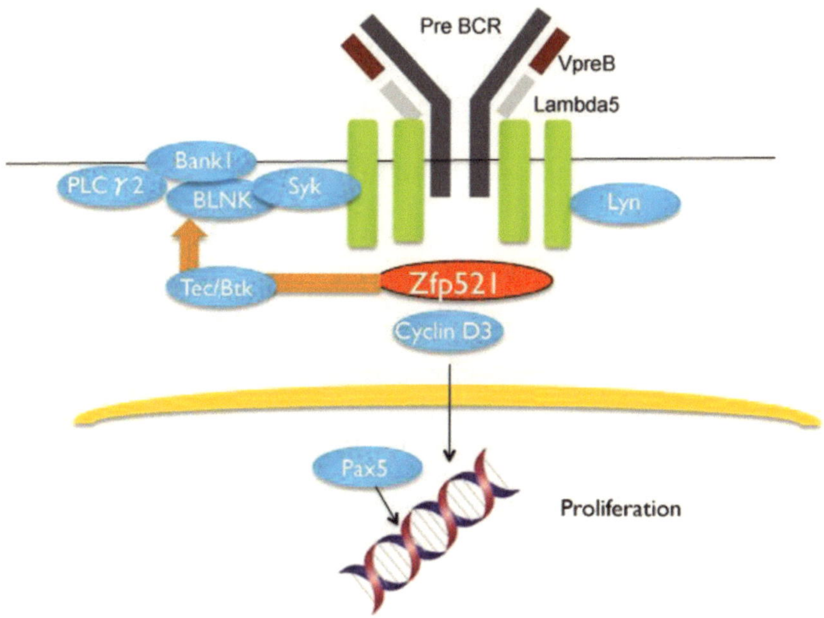

Figure 7. Pre-BCR pathway and Zfp521.

In the absence of FL, FLT3 remains in the inactivated monomeric form. When FLT3 binds to FL, a ternary complex is formed in which two FLT3 molecules are bridged by one (homodimeric) FLT3L. Ligand binding promotes conformational changes in FLT3 for dimerization, phosphorylation, and association with adaptor proteins such as Fiz1. The complex formation brings the intracellular domains close to each other, promoting initial phosphorylation of the kinase domain. Activated dimeric FLT3 transduces signals to the downstream effectors. In the pathogenesis analysis, FLT3 is expressed on the cell surface of most AML and ALL cells through proliferation activation and apoptosis suppression, which are caused by the stimulation of FL [41–43].

Internal tandem duplications (ITDs) occur in exon 14 or 15 of the JM, which are located directly between the transmembrane domain (TM) and tyrosine kinase region TK1 [44]. Insertions, deletions, and point mutations are frequently found in exon 20 of another tyrosine kinase region TK2.The functional kinase region is kept, and only the JM region is elongated. ITDs probably promote ligand-independent dimerization and activation of FLT3 by changing the conformation of the expressed receptor [44, 45]. In addition, another mutation was identified within the kinase activation loop, a part of the functional core. The conformational changes associated with ITDs might change the structure of the receptor such that unique adaptor proteins such as Fiz1 can now dock.

(b) Fiz 1: This gene encodes the zinc finger protein, which interacts with a receptor tyrosine kinase involved in the regulation of hematopoietic and lymphoid cells. This gene product also interacts with a transcription factor that regulates the expression of rod-specific genes in the retina. Fiz1 binds to the catalytic domain of Flt3 but not to c-Kit, Fms, or platelet-derived growth factor receptor [46, 47]. In a part of B-LBL in SL/Kh, Fiz1 is upregulated by MLV genome insertion and interaction with IL-7R pathway is observed. FLT3 stimulation enhances IL-7R signaling cascade by promotion of Stat5a phosphorylation [48]. Therefore, FLT3 and IL-7R signal pathways interact with each other in the development of B-LBL/ALL.

3.4. CD43 and Hipk2 in the development of B-LBL/ALL

HIPK2 is a conserved serine/threonine nuclear kinase that interacts with homeodomain transcription factors. This protein interacts with the cytoplasmic domain of CD43, which is expressed on immature pro- to pre–B cells, Fr. A-C in Hardy classification. In this immature stage, IL-7R is highly expressed and the CD43 pathway may interact with IL-7R pathway recruiting STAT5A. Hipk2 promotes Wnt signaling by stabilizing beta-catenin [49]. Hipk2 interacts with lymphoid-enhancing factor 1, which acts as a transcriptional factor, promoting c-Myc and cyclin D1 expression [50]. CD43 is an E-selectin counter-receptor highly expressed in human pre–B-cell leukemia NALL-1 cell line [51]. In our study, CD43 cross-linking resulted in an increase in STAT5A phosphorylation, when IL-7 was supplied. CD43 signaling may enhance the IL-7R signal pathway [48, 52].

4. Signaling pathway network responsible for pre–B lymphomagenesis

Probably, multiple genes are related to the activation of IL-7R-signaling pathway. Hipk2 and Fiz 1 are candidates of interaction with IL-7R pathway as well as Stat5. Considering the activation of FLT3 pathway in AML, B-LBL may share the activation pathway with AML [10]. We propose a scheme of interactions among the IL-7-, CD43-, and FLT3-signaling pathways (**Figure 8**) [48]. Thus, we hypothesize that these three pathways form an interacting network

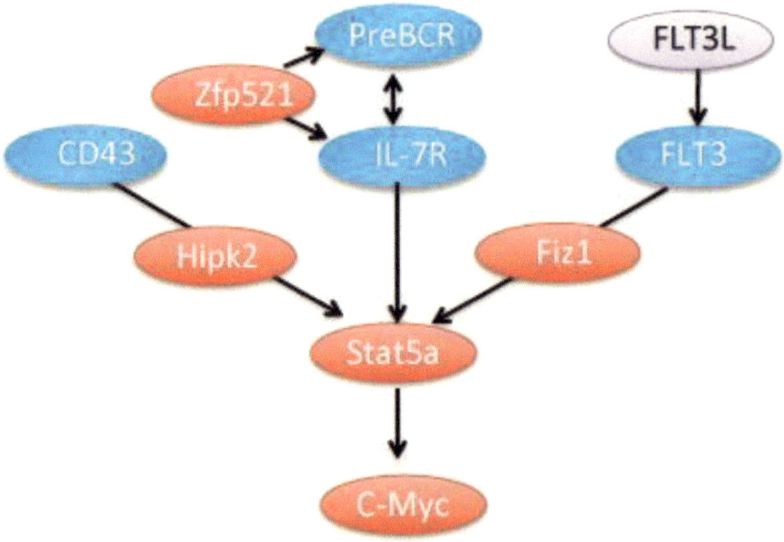

Figure 8. Signaling pathway network in association with IL-7R.

and affect B-LBL development. By contrast, pre-BCR pathway is activated by Zfp521 through the upregulation of BLNK [53, 54], BANK1 [37], Btk, and other pre–BCR-related molecules. Pre-BCR pathway has been considered to contribute to pre–B-cell development rather than to proliferation. Therefore, although stimulation of pre-BCR promotes pre-B cell proliferation, Zfp521 may not directly contribute to lymphomagenesis, but contribute to the stabilization of phenotype of B-LBL. Or interaction with IL-7R and pre-BCR may promote aberrant proliferation or development. Further research is required for precise understanding of the interaction between these two pathways in B-cell development.

Author details

Tatsuaki Tsuruyama* and Takuya Hiratsuka

*Address all correspondence to: tsuruyam@kuhp.kyoto-u.ac.jp

Department of Pathology, Graduate School of Medicine, Kyoto University, Kyoto, Kyoto Prefecture, Japan

References

[1] Arber DA, Orazi A, Hasserjian R, Thiele J, Borowitz MJ, Le Beau MM, et al. The 2016 revision to the World Health Organization classification of myeloid neoplasms and acute leukemia. Blood. 2016;**127**:2391–2405

[2] Swerdlow SH, Campo E, Pileri SA, Harris NL, Stein H, Siebert R, et al. The 2016 revision of the World Health Organization classification of lymphoid neoplasms. Blood. 2016;**127**:2375–2390

[3] Fugmann SD, Lee AI, Shockett PE, Villey IJ, Schatz DG. The RAG proteins and V(D)J recombination: Complexes, ends, and transposition. Annual Review of Immunology. 2000;**18**:495–527

[4] Geier JK, Schlissel MS. Pre-BCR signals and the control of Ig gene rearrangements. Seminars in Immunology. 2006;**18**:31–39

[5] Hendriks RW, Middendorp S. The pre-BCR checkpoint as a cell-autonomous proliferation switch. Trends in Immunology. 2004;**25**:249–256

[6] Berger A, Hoelbl-Kovacic A, Bourgeais J, Hoefling L, Warsch W, Grundschober E, et al. PAK-dependent STAT5 serine phosphorylation is required for BCR-ABL-induced leukemogenesis. Leukemia. 2014;**28**:629–641

[7] Berger A, Sexl V, Valent P, Moriggl R. Inhibition of STAT5: A therapeutic option in BCR-ABL1-driven leukemia. Oncotarget. 2014;**5**:9564–9576

[8] Guo Y, Fan BL, Chen YM, Hu Y, Zou Y, Chen XJ, et al. Analysis of cells in Tel/aml-1 positive childhood acute lymphoblastic leukemia by two-dimensional gel electrophoresis. Zhongguo Shi Yan Xue Ye Xue Za Zhi. 2009;**17**(5):1163–1167. PubMed PMID: 19840443

[9] Fronkova E, Madzo J, Zuna J, Reznickova L, Muzikova K, Hrusak O, et al. TEL/AML 1 real-time quantitative reverse transcriptase PCR can complement minimal residual disease assessment in childhood ALL. Leukemia. 2005;**19**:1296–1297

[10] Sazawal S, Bhatia K, Gutierrez MI, Saxena R, Arya LS, Bhargava M. Paucity of TEL-AML 1 translocation, by multiplex RT-PCR, in B-lineage acute lymphoblastic leukemia (ALL) in Indian patients. American Journal of Hematology. 2004;**76**:80–82

[11] Hiratsuka T, Takei Y, Ohmori R, Imai Y, Ozeki M, Tamaki K, et al. ZFP521 contributes to pre-B-cell lymphomagenesis through modulation of the pre-B-cell receptor signaling pathway. Oncogene. 2016;**35**:3227–3238

[12] Tsuruyama T, Hiratsuka T, Yamada N. Hotspots of MLV integration in the hematopoietic tumor genome. Oncogene. 2017;**36**:1169–1175

[13] Hiai H, Tsuruyama T, Yamada Y. Pre-B lymphomas in SL/Kh mice: A multifactorial disease model. Cancer Science. 2003;**94**:847–850

[14] Hiai H, Yamada Y, Abujiang P, Lu L, Kamoto T, Tsuruyama T. Genetic and epigenetic susceptibility to endogenous retrovirus-induced lymphomas in SL mice. Progress in Experimental Tumor Research. 1999;**35**:64–77

[15] Abujiang P, Yamada Y, Haller O, Kobayashi H, Kamoto T, Lu LM, et al. The origin of SL family mice. Laboratory Animal Science. 1996;**46**:410–417

[16] Akagi K, Suzuki T, Stephens RM, Jenkins NA, Copeland NG. RTCGD: Retroviral tagged cancer gene database. Nucleic Acids Research. 2004;**32**:D523–D527

[17] Kaszynski RH, Akatsuka S, Hiratsuka T, Jin G, Ozeki M, Okuno T, et al. A quantitative trait locus responsible for inducing B-cell lymphoblastic lymphoma is a hotspot for microsatellite instability. Cancer Science. 2010;**101**:800–805

[18] Bowman EP, Campbell JJ, Soler D, Dong Z, Manlongat N, Picarella D, et al. Developmental switches in chemokine response profiles during B cell differentiation and maturation. Journal of Experimental Medicine. 2000;**191**:1303–1318

[19] Hardy RR, Carmack CE, Shinton SA, Kemp JD, Hayakawa K. Resolution and characterization of pro-B and pre-pro-B cell stages in normal mouse bone marrow. Journal of Experimental Medicine. 1991;**173**:1213–1225

[20] Hiratsuka T, Tsuruyama T, Kaszynski R, Kometani K, Minato N, Nakamura T, et al. Bone marrow pre-B expansion by SL/Kh-Bomb1 locus: Not sufficient for lymphomagenesis. Leukemia Research. 2008;**32**:309–314

[21] Lu LM, Shimada R, Higashi S, Zeng Z, Hiai H. Bone marrow pre-B-1 (Bomb1): A quantitative trait locus inducing bone marrow pre-B-cell expansion in lymphoma-prone SL/Kh mice. Cancer Research. 1999;**59**:2593–2595

[22] Paige CJ, Marshall AJ, Fleming HE, Wu GE. Modulation of the IL-7 dose-response threshold during pro-B cell differentiation is dependent on pre-B cell receptor expression. Journal of Immunology. 1998;**161**:6038–6045

[23] Wei CJ, Zeff R, Goldschneider I. Murine pro-B cells require IL-7 and its receptor complex to up-regulate IL-7R alpha, terminal deoxynucleotidyltransferase, and c-mu expression. Journal of Immunology. 2000;**164**:1961–1970

[24] Ihle JN, Schwaller J, Parganas E, Wang DM, Cain D, Aster JC, et al. Stat5 is essential for the myelo- and lymphoproliferative disease induced by TEL/JAK2. Molecular Cell. 2000;**6**:693–704

[25] Valle-Mendiola A, Weiss-Steider B, Rocha-Zavaleta L, Soto-Cruz I. IL-2 enhances cervical cancer cells proliferation and JAK3/STAT5 phosphorylation at low doses, while at high doses IL-2 has opposite effects. Cancer Investigation. 2014;**32**:115–125

[26] Natarajan K, Xie Y, Burcu M, Linn DE, Qiu Y, Baer MR. Pim-1 kinase phosphorylates and stabilizes 130 kDa FLT3 and promotes aberrant STAT5 signaling in acute myeloid leukemia with FLT3 internal tandem duplication. PLoS One. 2013;**8**:e74653

[27] Matsumura I, Kitamura T, Wakao H, Tanaka H, Hashimoto K, Albanese C, et al. Transcriptional regulation of the cyclin D1 promoter by STAT5: Its involvement in cytokine-dependent growth of hematopoietic cells. EMBO Journal. 1999;**18**:1367–1377

[28] Nosaka T, Kawashima T, Misawa K, Ikuta K, Mui ALF, Kitamura T. STAT5 as a molecular regulator of proliferation, differentiation and apoptosis in hematopoietic cells. EMBO Journal. 1999;**18**:4754–4765

[29] Tsuruyama T, Hiratsuka T, Jin G, Imai Y, Takeuchi H, Maruyama Y, et al. Murine leukemia retrovirus integration induces the formation of transcription factor complexes on palindromic sequences in the signal transducer and activator of transcription factor 5a gene during the development of pre-B lymphomagenesis. American Journal of Pathology. 2011;**178**:1374–1386

[30] Copeland NG, Warming S, Liu P, Suzuki T, Akagi K, Lindtner S, et al. Evi3, a common retroviral integration site in murine B-cell lymphoma, encodes an EBFAZ-related Kruppel-like zinc finger protein. Blood. 2003;**101**:1934–1940

[31] Hentges KE, Weiser KC, Schountz T, Woodward LS, Morse HC, Justice MJ. Evi3, a zinc-finger protein related to EBFAZ, regulates EBF activity in B-cell leukemia. Oncogene. 2005;**24**:1220–1230

[32] Yamasaki N, Miyazaki K, Nagamachi A, Koller R, Oda H, Miyazaki M, et al. Identification of Zfp521/ZNF521 as a cooperative gene for E2A-HLF to develop acute B-lineage leukemia. Oncogene. 2010;**29**:1963–1975

[33] Correa D, Hesse E, Seriwatanachai D, Kiviranta R, Saito H, Yamana K, et al. Zfp521 is a target gene and key effector of parathyroid hormone-related peptide signaling in growth plate chondrocytes. Developmental Cell. 2010;**19**:533–546

[34] Seriwatanachai D, Densmore MJ, Sato T, Correa D, Neff L, Baron R, et al. Deletion of Zfp521 rescues the growth plate phenotype in a mouse model of Jansen metaphyseal chondrodysplasia. FASEB Journal. 2011;**25**:3057–3067

[35] Shen S, Pu J, Lang B, McCaig CD. A zinc finger protein Zfp521 directs neural differentiation and beyond. Stem Cell Research & Therapy. 2011;**2**:20

[36] Hesse E, Saito H, Kiviranta R, Correa D, Yamana K, Neff L, et al. Zfp521 controls bone mass by HDAC3-dependent attenuation of Runx2 activity. Journal of Cell Biology. 2010;**191**:1271–1283

[37] Bernal-Quiros M, Wu YY, Alarcon-Riquelme ME, Castillejo-Lopez C. BANK1 and BLK act through phospholipase C gamma 2 in B-cell signaling. PLoS One. 2013;**8**(3):e59842

[38] Rickert RC. New insights into pre-BCR and BCR signalling with relevance to B cell malignancies. Nature Review Immunology. 2013;**13**:578–591

[39] Mullighan CG, Goorha S, Radtke I, Miller CB, Coustan-Smith E, Dalton JD, et al. Genome-wide analysis of genetic alterations in acute lymphoblastic leukaemia. Nature. 2007;**446**:758–764

[40] Li LX, Goetz CA, Katerndahl CD, Sakaguchi N, Farrar MA. A Flt3- and Ras-dependent pathway primes B cell development by inducing a state of IL-7 responsiveness. Journal of Immunology. 2010;**184**:1728–1736

[41] Daver N, Strati P, Jabbour E, Kadia T, Luthra R, Wang S, et al. FLT3 mutations in myelodysplastic syndrome and chronic myelomonocytic leukemia. American Journal of Hematology. 2013;**88**:56–59

[42] Dicker F, Haferlach C, Sundermann J, Wendland N, Weiss T, Kern W, et al. Mutation analysis for RUNX1, MLL-PTD, FLT3-ITD, NPM1 and NRAS in 269 patients with MDS or secondary AML. Leukemia. 2010;**24**:1528–1532

[43] Georgiou G, Karali V, Zouvelou C, Kyriakou E, Dimou M, Chrisochoou S, et al. Serial determination of FLT3 mutations in myelodysplastic syndrome patients at diagnosis, follow up or acute myeloid leukaemia transformation: Incidence and their prognostic significance. British Journal of Haematology. 2006;**134**:302–306

[44] Gerloff D, Grundler R, Wurm AA, Brauer-Hartmann D, Katzerke C, Hartmann JU, et al. NF-kappaB/STAT5/miR-155 network targets PU.1 in FLT3-ITD driven acute myeloid leukemia. Leukemia. 2015;**29**:535–547

[45] Yoshimoto G, Miyamoto T, Jabbarzadeh-Tabrizi S, Iino T, Rocnik JL, Kikushige Y, et al. FLT3-ITD up-regulates MCL-1 to promote survival of stem cells in acute myeloid leukemia via FLT3-ITD-specific STAT5 activation. Blood. 2009;**114**:5034–5043

[46] Wolf I, Rohrschneider LR. Fiz1, a novel zinc finger protein interacting with the receptor tyrosine kinase Flt3. Journal of Biological Chemistry. 1999;**274**:21478–21484

[47] Vempati S, Reindl C, Wolf U, Kern R, Petropoulos K, Naidu VM, et al. Transformation by oncogenic mutants and ligand-dependent activation of FLT3 wild-type requires the tyrosine residues 589 and 591. Clinical Cancer Research. 2008;**14**:4437–4445

[48] Tsuruyama T, Imai Y, Takeuchi H, Hiratsuka T, Maruyama Y, Kanaya K, et al. Dual retrovirus integration tagging: Identification of new signaling molecules Fiz1 and Hipk2 that are involved in the IL-7 signaling pathway in B lymphoblastic lymphomas. Journal of Leukocyte Biology. 2010;**88**:107–116

[49] Tan M, Gong H, Zeng Y, Tao L, Wang J, Jiang J, et al. Downregulation of homeodomain-interacting protein kinase-2 contributes to bladder cancer metastasis by regulating Wnt signaling. Journal of Cell Biochemistry. 2014;**115**(10):1762–1767. DOI: 10.1002/jcb.24842. PubMed PMID: 24824041

[50] Wei G, Ku S, Ma GK, Saito S, Tang AA, Zhang J, et al. HIPK2 represses beta-catenin-mediated transcription, epidermal stem cell expansion, and skin tumorigenesis. Proceedings of the National Academy of Sciences United States of America. 2007;**104**:13040–13045

[51] Nonomura C, Kikuchi J, Kiyokawa N, Ozaki H, Mitsunaga K, Ando H, et al. CD43, but not P-selectin glycoprotein ligand-1, functions as an E-selectin counter-receptor in human pre-B-cell leukemia NALL-1. Cancer Research. 2008;**68**:790–799

[52] Mao JH, Wu D, Kim IJ, Kang HC, Wei G, Climent J, et al. Hipk2 cooperates with p53 to suppress gamma-ray radiation-induced mouse thymic lymphoma. Oncogene. 2012;**31**: 1176–1180

[53] Baba Y, Hashimoto S, Matsushita M, Watanabe D, Kishimoto T, Kurosaki T, et al. BLNK mediates Syk-dependent Btk activation. Proceedings of the National Academy of Sciences United States of America. 2001;**98**:2582–2586

[54] Imai C, Ross ME, Reid G, Coustan-Smith E, Schultz KR, Pui CH, et al. Expression of the adaptor protein BLNK/SLP-65 in childhood acute lymphoblastic leukemia. Leukemia. 2004;**18**:922–925

Chapter 3

Somatic Hypermutational Status and Gene Repertoire of Immunoglobulin Rearrangements in Chronic Lymphocytic Leukemia

Teodora Karan-Djurasevic and Sonja Pavlovic

Additional information is available at the end of the chapter

http://dx.doi.org/10.5772/intechopen.69110

Abstract

Immunoglobulin molecule is the key component of B cell receptor (BCR), which governs the survival, differentiation and function of normal B lymphocytes, but accumulating data suggest that, in the case of chronic lymphocytic leukaemia (CLL), it is also involved in the pathogenesis and clinical course of the disease. CLL is a malignancy of mature $CD5^+$ $CD19^+$ $CD23^+$ $sIgM^{low}$ B lymphocytes and is characterized by extremely heterogeneous clinical course, which varies from indolent to rapidly progressive. Somatic hypermutational status of immunoglobulin heavy chain variable genes (IGHV) defines two CLL subtypes, mutated (M-CLL) and unmutated (U-CLL). U-CLL patients suffer from more aggressive disease, characterized by shorter time to treatment, progression-free survival and overall survival in comparison to M-CLL patients. Since these correlations are not dependent on the clinical stage and since there is no interconversion between subtypes, IGHV mutational status is currently the most reliable prognostic marker in CLL. Several lines of evidence indicate that both M-CLL and U-CLL arise from an antigen-experienced cell of origin. Immunogenetic studies have revealed CLL-biased usage of immunoglobulin variable region genes, as well as the existence of highly homologous, 'stereotyped' BCRs in CLL clones, strongly implying the role of antigenic drive in the development and evolution of the disease.

Keywords: chronic lymphocytic leukaemia, B cell receptor, immunoglobulin rearrangements, gene repertoire, BCR stereotypy

1. Introduction

The central role that B lymphocytes play in immunity relies upon their capacity to produce a vast array of different immunoglobulin molecules which can recognize virtually limitless number of foreign and autoantigens. Immunoglobulins (IG) are expressed on the surface of B cells as antigen-binding component of B cell receptor (BCR), in complex with CD79A/79B heterodimer responsible for signal transduction. During the immune response, IG molecules are secreted as antibodies which exert different effector functions. BCR signalling is crucial for survival, proliferation and differentiation of normal B lymphocytes, but has also been implicated in the pathogenesis of several mature B cell malignancies, including chronic lymphocytic leukaemia.

Chronic lymphocytic leukaemia (CLL) manifests as clonal expansion of mature $CD5^+$ $CD19^+$ $CD23^+$ $sIgM^{low}$ B lymphocytes which gradually accumulate in blood, bone marrow and secondary lymphoid organs [1]. It is the most frequent type of leukaemia in Western countries, accounting for 30–40% of all adult leukaemia cases, while it is very rare in Asian and African countries [2]. CLL affects predominantly elderly individuals, aged approximately 67–72 years at diagnosis, men more frequently than women [1].

CLL is characterized by extremely heterogeneous clinical presentation, with diverse therapy requirements and overall survival. In some patients, rapid progression and need of treatment occur soon after diagnosis, while others may live for decades without developing any symptoms. The majority of cases, however, lie in between these extremes; the disease can follow an indolent course for years, but eventually turn into aggressive form.

Aetiology of CLL is still elusive. Familial clustering of CLL has been documented, implying a strong genetic basis of the disease. The relative risk of CLL has been estimated to be around eight-fold higher in first-degree relatives [3]. Genome-wide association studies have identified multiple CLL susceptibility loci mapping to genes involved in apoptosis, BCR signalling, immune response and maintenance of chromosome integrity [4, 5].

A growing body of evidence indicates that CLL development and evolution result from concerted action of intrinsic genetic abnormalities and extrinsic factors from the tissue microenvironment, including antigens [6]. The most common chromosomal aberrations in CLL are deletion 13q14, trisomy 12q, deletion 11q22-q23 and deletion 17p13, observed in approximately 80% of patients [7]. The genes localized within minimally deleted/gained regions in these aberrations include miR-15a and miR16-1 (del13q), CDK4, GLI and MDM2 (trisomy 12), ATM (del11q) and TP53 (del17p), which are involved in regulation of apoptosis and DNA repair [8–10]. The recent next-generation sequencing-based studies have identified a number of recurrently mutated genes in CLL (e.g. NOTCH1, SF3B1, MYD88, BIRC3, NFKBIE, TP53 and ATM), predominantly belonging to BCR, toll-like receptor, Notch1 and NF-κB signalling pathways [6, 11]. In addition, genetic alterations and aberrant expression of many apoptotic regulators involved in both mitochondrial and death receptor apoptotic pathways have been described in CLL, most notably overexpression of BCL2, detected in the majority of patients [12–14]. However, immunogenetic studies over the past few decades have pointed to the antigenic drive on the BCR of the cell of origin as the key player, and possibly an initiating event, in CLL pathogenesis [15, 16].

The diversity of mechanisms involved in pathobiology of CLL cells is likely the basis of the clinical heterogeneity, making the prognostication for individual patients very difficult. Currently, the most important prognostic markers, widely used in routine clinical practice, are clinical stage (Rai and Binet) and cytogenetic aberrations [17]. In an attempt to overcome the clinical variability and improve the prognosis assessment, particularly in early-stage disease, a number of cellular and molecular prognostic markers have been identified and validated. Among the novel markers that have entered clinical practice (e.g. CD38 and ZAP-70 expression, TP53 mutations), the most powerful one, in terms of prognosis definition, turned out to be the somatic hypermutational status of rearranged immunoglobulin heavy variable genes [17].

In this chapter, we will discuss the current concepts of immunoglobulin gene expression in chronic lymphocytic leukaemia, and its relevance for both the pathogenesis and clinical progression of the disease.

2. Immunoglobulin gene rearrangements and the development of B lymphocytes

2.1. Generation of immunoglobulin diversity

Immunoglobulin (IG) molecules are heterodimers composed of two identical heavy (H) chains and two identical light (L) chains (κ or λ), linked by disulphide bonds. Both heavy and light chains contain N-terminal variable (V) region and C-terminal constant (C) region (**Figure 1a**). Juxtaposed variable regions of H and L chains (VH and VL) form antigen-binding site, whose structure determines the specificity and the affinity of immunoglobulin molecules for antigens. Constant regions are not involved in antigen recognition. Heavy chain constant region (CH) defines IG isotypes (IgA, IgD, IgE, IgG and IgM) and mediates effector functions of antibodies. In addition, CH region is responsible for anchoring of membrane-bound IG in the plasma membrane of B cells. Variable region of each IG chain consists of four relatively conserved framework regions (FR1, FR2, FR3 and FR4) and three hypervariable complementarity-determining regions (CDR1, CDR2 and CDR3). The CDR regions of H and L chains form six loops which create a surface that directly interacts with antigens. Heavy chain CDR3 region (VH CDR3) exerts the highest variability and is the key determinant of antibody specificity [18].

IG molecules are encoded by a multitude of tandemly arranged gene segments that constitute IGH (heavy chain) locus, IGK and IGL locus (κ and λ light chains). Human IGH locus, located on chromosome 14q32.33, consists of four types of gene segments: V (variable), D (diversity), J (joining) and C (constant), in 5′–3′ orientation. There are 38–46 functional IGHV gene segments, which can be divided into 6–7 subgroups based on sequence homology, 23 functional IGHD gene segments, 6 functional IGHJ gene segments and 9 functional IGHC

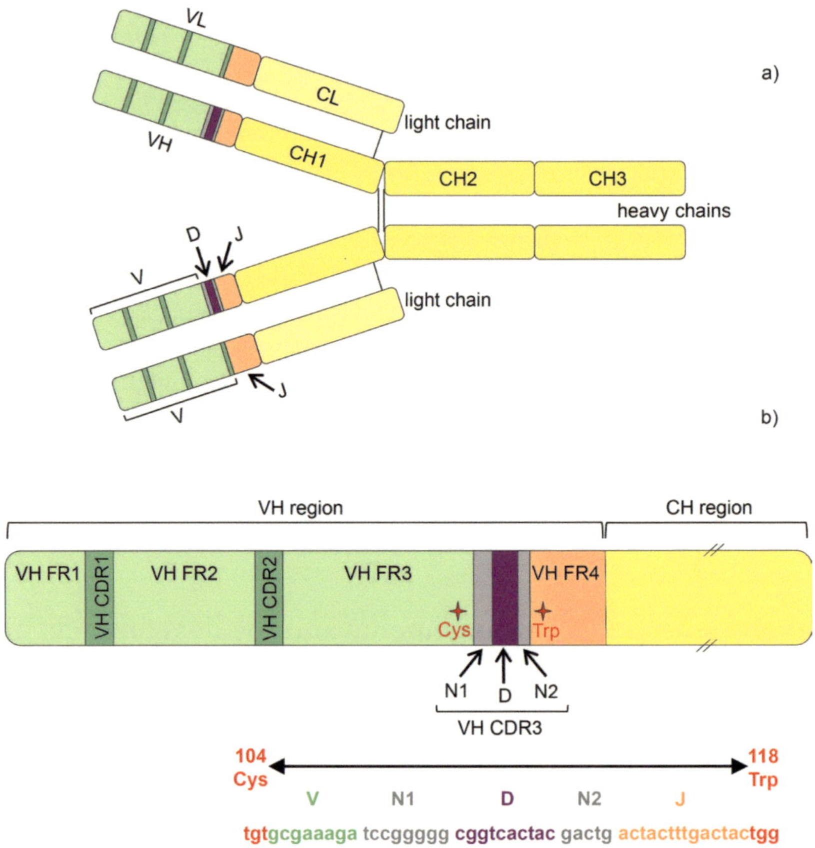

Figure 1. Schematic representation of an immunoglobulin molecule. (a) IG molecules consist of two identical heavy (H) chains and two identical light (L) chains. Both H and L chains contain variable region (VH and VL, respectively) and constant region (CH and CL, respectively). VH region is encoded by rearranged V, D and J gene segments, while VL is encoded by rearranged V and J gene segments. (b) VH region consists of four framework regions (VH FR1, VH FR2, VH FR3 and VH FR4) and three hypervariable complementarity-determining regions (VH CDR1, VH CDR2 and VH CDR3). VH FR1-3, VH CDR1 and VH CDR2 are encoded entirely by IGHV gene segment; VH FR4 is encoded by IGHJ gene segment. VH CDR3 is positioned at the IGHV-IGHD-IGHJ junction, and comprises amino acids between conserved cysteine (codon 104) in FR3 and conserved tryptophan (codon 118) in FR4 [19]. N1 and N2 regions are being created via random addition and deletion of nucleotides during IGHV-IGHD and IGHD-IGHJ joining.

gene segments (**Figure 2**). Light chain loci, on the other hand, lack D segments. Human IGK locus (chromosome 2p11.2) contains a cluster of 34–38 functional IGKV gene segments which belong to 5 subgroups, followed by 5 IGKJ gene segments and a single C gene segment. Human IGL locus (chromosome 22q11.2) is composed of 29–33 functional IGLV gene segments, divided into 10 subgroups, and 4–5 functional IGLJ-IGLC tandems [20]. Allelic variants of many gene segments exist, particularly in the IGH locus. It should be noted that the actual number of gene segments in all three loci is much higher, due to the presence of pseudogenes and ORFs (open reading frames). In addition, the number of functional gene segments in a locus depends on the haplotype, since some genes can be inserted or deleted, or can be functional or pseudogene, depending on the allele.

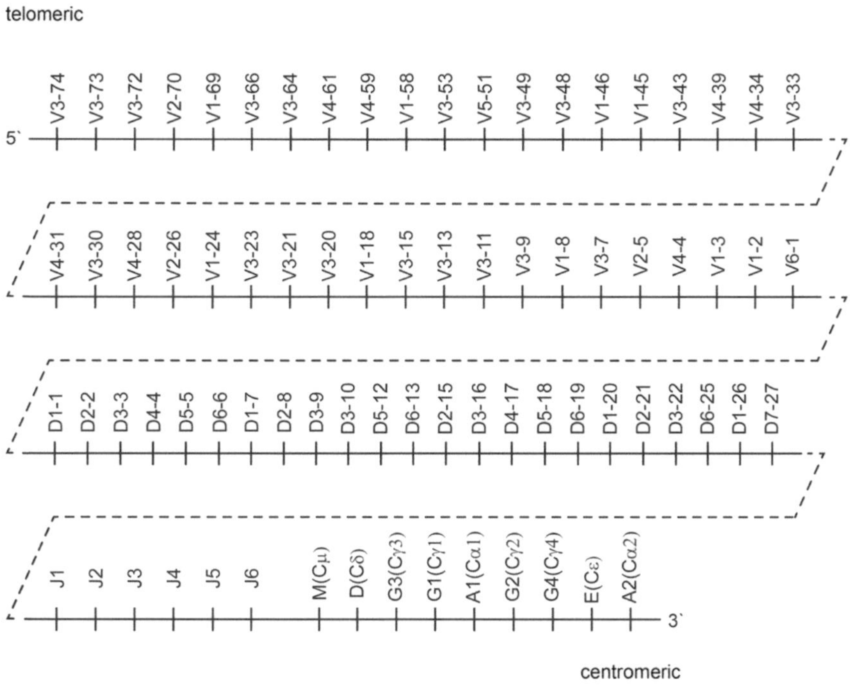

Figure 2. Schematic representation of the human IGH locus (not to scale). Human IGH locus contains 38–46 functional IGHV gene segments, 23 functional IGHD gene segments, 6 functional IGHJ gene segments and 9 functional IGHC gene segments. IGHV gene segments are designated by a number for the subgroup, followed by an hyphen and a number for the localization in the locus, in the 3′–5′ direction; IGHD and IGHJ gene segments are numbered in the opposite direction (5′–3′) [21]. Only functional genes are depicted.

Immunoglobulin variable region is being generated by somatic recombination between V, D and J gene segments (H chains) and V and J gene segments (L chains), which occur during differentiation of B lymphocytes. At the IGH locus, which rearranges before IGL loci, the first recombination event joins one of the IGHD gene segments to one of the IGHJ gene segments, and the sequence between the rearranged genes is being deleted. The obtained IGHD-IGHJ rearrangement then recombines with one of the IGHV gene segments, leading to the formation of complete IGHV-IGHD-IGHJ rearrangement which will be fused to an IGHC gene (Cμ or Cδ) during RNA splicing and, ultimately, expressed at the cell surface as IgM or IgD. Productive rearrangement of one IGH locus inhibits the rearrangement of IGH locus on the other chromosome (allelic exclusion), thus ensuring the monospecificity of B lymphocyte [22]. However, if the rearrangement of one allele is unproductive, the other one will undergo recombination and, if the second rearrangement fails, the cell will die by apoptosis. Similar recombination process occurs between V and J gene segments at the light chain loci. IGK locus rearranges before IGL; successful recombination at one IGK allele inhibits the rearrangement of the other one (allelic exclusion), as well as the rearrangement of IGL loci (isotypic exclusion). Alternatively, unproductive rearrangement of one IGK locus leads to recombination of the other allele and, if unsuccessful, the IGL locus will rearrange. Once again, if neither of the attempts results in productive light chain rearrangement, the cell will undergo apoptosis.

Given the number of germline gene segments that can recombine at IG loci, as well as random pairing of heavy and light chains, it is clear that B lymphocytes can produce a vast number of different antibodies ('combinatorial diversity'). However, the actual number of combinations is lower than the theoretical estimate of $\sim 1.6 \times 10^6$, since not all gene segment recombinations occur with the same frequencies and not all IGH-IGL pairs are functional. In addition, it has been shown that V(D)J recombinations are not a stochastic process, but are determined by genetic factors and are regulated during ontogeny [23].

The diversity of the primary antibody repertoire (the repertoire of naïve B cells) is further increased by 'junctional diversity'. The process of somatic recombination is catalysed by several enzymes jointly called V(D)J recombinase and, although very precise, their action introduces variability at the junctions of V, (D) and J gene segments. Recombination is enabled by the presence of conserved recombination signal (RS) sequences which flank 3′ end of V genes, 5′ end of J genes and both ends of D genes. RS sequences, recognized by recombination activating gene 1 and 2 (RAG1 and RAG2) enzymes, ensure that light chain V genes can rearrange only with J genes, while IGHV genes can rearrange only with IGHD, and IGHD only with IGHJ genes. During this process, trimming of the ends of recombining gene segments by exonucleases occurs, as well as the addition of short palindromic sequences and non-templated nucleotides (the latter catalysed by terminal deoxynucleotidyl transferase, TdT) [24]. The random addition and deletion of nucleotides during IGHV-IGHD and IGHD-IGHJ ligation creates two N regions (N1 and N2), and is the source of the extreme variability of VH CDR3, which is positioned at the VDJ junction (**Figure 1b**). Diversity of VH CDR3 in both length and amino acid sequence results in the production of much larger IG repertoire than it would be generated solely by combining germline gene segments (up to 10^{11} different IGs).

Diversification of immunoglobulins continues after antigen encounter (secondary antibody repertoire) via somatic hypermutations and class-switch recombination, generating B lymphocytes with enormously wide range of specificities (see next section).

2.2. B cell differentiation

B cell differentiation is a multi-step process which can be divided into two phases: antigen-independent phase, taking place in bone marrow (and fetal liver), followed by antigen-dependent phase in secondary lymphoid organs.

The first stage of B cell development in bone marrow is early pro-B cell, defined by the beginning of IGHD-IGHJ recombinations. Joining of IGHV gene to IGHD-IGHJ rearrangement occurs in late pro-B cells and leads to transcription and synthesis of μ heavy chain, which contains IGHV-IGHD-IGHJ complex attached to Cμ. The expression of μ heavy chain defines the large pre-B cell stage. The μ chain is predominantly cytoplasmic, but it can associate with surrogate light chains and, in complex with CD79A/CD79B, is transiently expressed at the cell surface as the pre-BCR. Subsequently, the cell enters the small pre-B stage in which rearrangements of light chain loci occur, enabling pairing of previously synthesized μ chain with IGK or IGL and, thus, assembly of IgM. Expression of surface IgM, as a part of BCR, marks the immature B cell. At this stage, self-reacting clones are being eliminated, or their specificities may be changed via receptor editing and IGHV replacement [25]. Immature B cells migrate to the spleen where they become mature naïve B cells. As a result of alternative splicing of IGH transcripts, which joins IGHV-IGHD-IGHJ gene to either Cμ or Cδ, these cells coexpress membrane-bound IgM and IgD with the same antigen specificity.

Naïve B lymphocytes reside in secondary lymphoid organs (spleen, lymph nodes and mucosal lymphoid tissues) where they encounter various antigens. Engagement of BCR with a specific antigen gives rise to a cascade of signalling events that activate B cell, leading to proliferation of antigen-specific clone and, ultimately, differentiation into antibody-secreting plasma cells and memory cells. Based on the requirement for T cell help in activation of B lymphocytes, two types of response to antigen stimulation exist. Bacterial polysaccharides and lipopolysaccharides can directly activate B cells (T cell-independent response), resulting in rapid IgM production. In contrast, the response to protein antigens is T cell-dependent and requires the interaction of B cells with $CD4^+$ T cells and antigen-presenting cells. Upon T cell-mediated activation, proliferating B cells migrate deep into lymphoid follicle, forming the structure called germinal centre. In a highly specialized microenvironment of germinal centres, B cells start to proliferate at high rate and undergo somatic hypermutations and class-switch recombination [26].

The process of somatic hypermutation (SHM), mediated by activation-induced cytidine deaminase (AID), introduces point mutations into the rearranged immunoglobulin loci at a rate 10^6 times higher than the spontaneous mutation rate of other genes. The single base substitutions are localized in the variable region of heavy and light chains, while the constant region remains unaffected. They are preferentially targeted to specific hotspot motifs (RGYW and its inverse repeat WRCY), with transitions predominating over transversions, and accumulate in both FRs and CDRs [27]. Replacement mutations tend to be clustered in CDRs, since they alter the affinity of IGs to antigens. In FRs, on the other hand, replacement mutations, which could disrupt the basic IG architecture, are counter-selected, and silent mutations are more frequent. The somatic hypermutation process can also introduce small insertions or deletions, although this is a rare event created by a mechanism different than AID-mediated SHM.

Accumulation of somatic hypermutations generates clonal progeny of activated B cell with diversified IG rearrangements and, hence, different affinity for antigen. These cells are subsequently subjected to selection by antigen: B cells that efficiently recognize antigen presented by follicular dendritic cells receive survival signals, provided by BCR engagement and T cell co-stimulation, and continue to proliferate, while B cells that do not bind antigen or bind it with low affinity die by apoptosis. Multiple rounds of proliferation, somatic hypermutation and selection result in affinity maturation, i.e. production of B lymphocytes with increasing specificity and affinity for antigen. Along with affinity maturation, the cells undergo class-switch recombination (also mediated by AID), which leads to fusion of IGHV-IGHD-IGHJ rearrangement to a downstream constant gene segment. This enables production of isotypes other than IgM and IgD, but with the same antigen specificity [28]. Antigen-selected B cells ultimately exit the germinal centre and finalize their differentiation into high-affinity antigen-specific plasma cells and memory cells, with specific effector functions.

Somatic hypermutations and class-switch recombination further enhance immunoglobulin variability and, in combination with other sources of diversity (combinatorial and junctional diversity), enable formation of up to 10^{12} possible antibody specificities [20]. The potential of B cells to create such a huge IG repertoire, however, comes at a high cost since it causes a considerable wastage of cells along the pathway of their differentiation. The mechanisms responsible for variability of immunoglobulin rearrangements can also render them unproductive due to recombination of non-functional pseudogenes, out-of-frame junctions, generation of stop codons at the junctions, as well as introduction of frameshifts and stop codons by SHM. In addition, replacement mutations induced by SHM process can impair the structure of immunoglobulin molecule or lower its affinity for antigen. As mentioned above, B cells that fail to generate productive heavy- and light chain rearrangements and produce functional antibodies undergo apoptotic cell death.

3. Immunoglobulin gene rearrangements in CLL

3.1. IGHV mutational status

The extreme clinical heterogeneity of chronic lymphocytic leukaemia has inspired an extensive search for molecular and cellular markers with the prognostic and predictive value. Immunoglobulin rearrangements of CLL clones were brought into the spotlight upon the findings that, in around 50% of CLL patients, heavy chain rearrangements carry somatic hypermutations, and that SHM status of rearranged IGHV genes significantly correlates with the clinical course of the disease. Patients with unmutated IGHV-IGHD-IGHJ rearrangements are usually in advanced clinical stages, have progressive disease, atypical morphology and require chemotherapy soon after diagnosis. In contrast, patients with mutated IGHV-IGHD-IGHJ rearrangements predominantly present with non-progressive disease, typical morphology, require no or minimal chemotherapy and have significantly longer time to first treatment, progression-free survival and overall survival [29–33]. These correlations have been confirmed in multiple studies, and today, it is widely accepted that CLL can be divided into two subtypes, mutated (M-CLL) and unmutated (U-CLL), with different clinical outcome. The IGHV mutational status turned out to be the strongest independent prognostic marker whose value, *inter alia,* lies in the fact that it does not change over time and that it can predict the clinical behaviour of CLL at the time of diagnosis as well as at any stage of the disease (i.e. regardless of the tumour burden).

The cut-off level that is being in use for distinguishing M-CLL from U-CLL is 98% of identity between the rearranged IGHV gene and its germline counterpart (calculated from codon 1 to codon 104); cases with ≥98% identity are considered unmutated, while those with <98% identity are considered mutated [34, 35]. This cut-off has originally been chosen in order to eliminate the possibility of interpreting allelic polymorphisms as somatic mutations. Although in some studies other cut-off values (97% and 95%) allowed better separation of the two prognostic groups, 2% of somatic mutations are generally accepted as the best discriminator between mutated and unmutated cases [36–38]. However, since this level of mutations is an arbitrary cut-off, the caution is recommended when interpreting the prognostic implications in cases with the borderline mutational status [34]. Indeed, it has been demonstrated that the group of patients with the borderline mutated rearrangements (97–97.9% identity) comprised cases with both poor and good prognosis [38, 39]. In addition, sequencing of the unrearranged IGH genes in patients with high percentage of identity (98–99.6%) revealed that the divergence of rearranged IGHV gene from the closest germline gene, even in this group, is actually due to somatic hypermutation, further underscoring the statistical, rather than biological rationale for the 98% cut-off [40]. However, the fact that median survival does not differ between patients with 100% and those with 99% or 98%, but is significantly shorter in comparison to survival of patients with <98% identity, justifies the application of 98% cut-off in clinical practice [39]. Finally, it should be noted that the absence of correlation between IGHV mutational status and the prognosis in a proportion of patients can be attributed, at least in some cases, to other factors that influence the clinical outcome (see below).

Besides the borderline cases, clinical prognostication can be challenging in cases carrying double IGHV-IGHD-IGHJ rearrangements. In the majority of these cases only one rearrangement is productive, but in rare instances (up to 5% of cases), double productive rearrangements can be detected [41, 42]. Expression of double productive rearrangements may be the result of the lack of allelic exclusion, which has been described in CLL B cells or, alternatively, double (or multiple) productive rearrangements originate from different CLL clones [41, 43]. If both rearrangements are of the same mutational status, prognostic interpretation is straightforward regardless of whether both or just one rearrangement is productive. The cases with productive mutated and unproductive unmutated IGHV-IGHD-IGHJ rearrangements are considered mutated, since the productive rearrangement is relevant for the biology of CLL cells. However, if double productive rearrangements are of discordant mutational status or if unmutated rearrangement is productive while the mutated rearrangement is unproductive (implying that the cell has undergone the SHM process), the clinical implications currently cannot be predicted [44].

The association of IGHV mutational status with other prognostic markers in CLL has been extensively studied. Besides the contribution to better understanding of the disease biology, the research also aimed at finding a potential surrogate marker that could substitute the effortful IGHV mutational analysis in clinical practice. The four most frequent clonal chromosomal aberrations (del13q, del11q, trisomy 12q and del17p) represent strong independent prognostic markers and are differentially distributed between M-CLL and U-CLL [7, 45, 46]. The aberrations with adverse prognostic impact (del11q, trisomy 12q and del17p) are associated predominantly with unmutated IGHV-IGHD-IGHJ rearrangements, while favourable del13q is more frequent in mutated cases [36, 37, 47–49]. Furthermore, unmutated CLL subtype is characterized by high risk of acquiring adverse chromosomal aberrations during the disease course [50]. In contrast to cytogenetic abnormalities, the association of CD38 and ZAP-70 with IGHV mutational status is less consistent. The expression of CD38 on the surface of >30% of leukemic cells is an independent negative prognostic factor associated with the progressive disease, shorter time to first treatment and shorter overall survival, although the level of expression may vary over time [29, 51–53]. In some studies, CD38 positivity was strongly correlated to unmutated IGHV status, while others failed to detect any association, regardless of the cut-off level used for defining CD38 status [29, 36, 49, 54]. Similarly to CD38, the expression of zeta-chain-associated protein kinase 70 (ZAP-70) is also independent negative prognostic marker associated with adverse clinical characteristics and poor prognosis [55–59]. Initially, in many studies, ZAP-70 was found to be expressed predominantly in unmutated CLL and was suggested as a surrogate marker for IGHV mutational status; however, subsequent research revealed a substantial discordance between these two markers [49, 55, 57, 60–63].

The expression of several other genes has been reported to exert a strong prognostic value, qualifying them as potential biomarkers. Among those RNA-based markers, lipoprotein lipase (LPL) emerged as the most powerful one, whose high expression level correlates with advanced clinical stage, shorter time to first treatment and overall survival, as well as with other adverse prognostic parameters (short lymphocyte doubling time, ZAP-70 and CD38 positivity, poor-risk cytogenetics) [64–70]. Moreover, LPL expression turned out to be a potent predictor of IGHV mutational status, as high levels of LPL were found to be strongly associated with unmutated IGHV-IGHD-IGHJ rearrangements [55, 60, 64–67, 71].

To conclude, despite certain limitations, IGHV mutational status analysis is currently the golden standard for CLL prognostication, which has been introduced into clinical practice in many centres. It is integrated into the most advanced prognostic scoring systems suggested for risk stratification of CLL patients [72–75].

3.2. Immunoglobulin variable region gene repertoire in CLL

The analyses of immunoglobulin heavy chain rearrangements in CLL revealed that not only IGHV, IGHD and IGHJ gene usage in CLL B lymphocytes is distinct from that of normal peripheral blood B cells, but also the gene repertoires of U-CLL and M-CLL clones significantly differ.

The most commonly used IGHV subgroup in CLL rearrangements is IGHV3 (as is the case with normal B cells), followed by IGHV1 and IGHV4. However, the comparison of IGHV subgroup usage between CLL and normal B cells showed that there is a significant over-representation of IGHV1 subgroup, as well as underrepresentation of IGHV3 subgroup in CLL [33, 76–80]. In addition, the frequencies of IGHV subgroups are different in the two CLL subtypes: IGHV1 genes are present predominantly in the rearrangements of U-CLL clones, in contrast to IGHV3 and IGHV4 genes that predominate in M-CLL clones. Moreover, a hierarchy in the SHM level among IGHV subgroups has been documented: IGHV3 and IGHV4 genes show a high mutational load while IGHV1 genes carry very few mutations (IGHV3 > IGHV4 > IGHV1) [30, 33, 80].

A strong bias in usage of individual IGHV genes has also been detected. In most studies, only 6–7 IGHV genes were utilized in more than 50% of CLL IGHV-IGHD-IGHJ rearrangements. The most frequently used IGHV genes were IGHV1-69, IGHV3-23, IGHV3-7 and IGHV4-34, followed by several others (IGHV3-30, IGHV3-30.3, IGHV3-48, IGHV1-2, IGHV1-3, IGHV1-18, IGHV4-39 and IGHV4-59), depending on the cohort [30, 33, 79–82]. It should be noted, though, that normal B cell repertoire is not random, and that certain genes (such as

IGHV3-23, IGHV3-7 and IGHV3-30.3) are overused [76]. Hence, some of the most common IGHV genes in CLL are represented with frequencies similar to those of normal B cells [33, 76, 79]. However, CLL-related over-representation of IGHV1-69 has been consistently reported, as well as its predominance in unmutated rearrangements. On the other hand, IGHV3-23, IGHV3-7, IGHV4-34 and IGHV3-48 are the most frequently used genes in mutated rearrangements. The differences in the mutational load, observed for IGHV subgroups, are even more evident when individual genes are considered. For example, IGHV1-69 gene usually harbours no or just a few somatic mutations, whereas IGHV3-7, IGHV3-23 and IGHV4-34 genes are highly mutated [30, 33, 78–80, 82].

The majority of CLL IGHV-IGHD-IGHJ rearrangements contain IGHJ4 and IGHJ6 genes; IGHJ6 gene is predominantly used in unmutated rearrangements, in contrast to IGHJ4, which is over-represented in mutated rearrangements. Since IGHJ6 is the longest IGHJ gene, this results in significantly longer median VH CDR3 lengths of unmutated vs. mutated rearrangements [30, 33, 80].

Besides the biased usage of IGH subgroups and individual genes in CLL, early studies of CLL immunoglobulin repertoire have also revealed the over-representation of certain IGHV-IGHD-IGHJ combinations. For example, IGHV1-69 was frequently found in combination with IGHJ6 and IGHD3-3 or IGHD2-2, creating VH CDR3 longer than the average, which is not common in rearrangements of normal B cells [33, 83, 84]. In contrast, the majority of IGHV3-7 genes were found to be combined with IGHJ4 and IGHD3 yielding shorter VH CDR3, while IGHV4-34 was associated with both IGHJ4 and IGHJ6 genes [33]. These findings pointed to the CLL-biased VH CDR3 features and laid the foundations of the stereotyped B cell receptor concept (see below).

Geographical and ethnical differences in IGHV gene usage in CLL rearrangements have also been reported [79, 82, 85–89]. For example, IGHV3-21 gene has been detected in IGHV-IGHD-IGHJ rearrangements of more than 11% of Scandinavian patients, while it was less frequent in the UK (7.9%) and very rare in Mediterranean cohorts (less than 3% of cases) [79, 90–93]. In addition, IGHV1 genes have been shown to be represented with lower and IGHV4 genes with higher frequencies in CLL clones of patients from Asian countries in comparison to patients from Western populations [94–96].

The light chain variable region gene repertoire in CLL has been substantially less studied but, nevertheless, some similarities with the repertoire of heavy chains have been observed. The ratio of expressed κ and λ light chains in CLL B lymphocytes mirrors that of normal B cells (2:1) [97]. As is the case with IGH rearrangements, roughly 50% of IGK/IGL rearrangements belong to the mutated subtype and, in most cases, IGH and IGK/IGL rearrangements are of the same mutational status [98]. A skewed usage of IGKV/IGLV and IGKJ/IGLJ subgroups and individual genes has been reported, but the interpretations of whether their relative frequencies differ from those of normal B cells are discrepant, probably due to different normal control datasets used for comparison. Similar to IGHV, the distribution of individual IGKV and IGLV genes between mutated and unmutated rearrangements is asymmetrical and, for some genes, CLL-biased. In addition, certain IGKV-IGKJ and IGLV-IGLJ combinations are over-represented and CLL-related [97–99]. Importantly, non-stochastic pairing of heavy and light chains has been detected and shown to depend on VH CDR3 motifs [100]. Since preferential pairing of specific IGHV and IGKV or IGLV genes has not been observed in normal B cell repertoire, biased usage of certain VH CDR3/VL CDR3 associations strongly implies that the expression of BCRs with specific antigen-binding characteristics is favoured in CLL [101, 102].

The usage of particular IGHV genes has been found to correlate with clinical course of CLL. The most striking example is IGHV3-21 gene, which emerged as an adverse prognostic factor regardless of the IGHV mutational status. IGHV3-21 is expressed in both CLL subtypes, but predominantly in M-CLL. However, median overall survival of patients expressing mutated IGHV3-21 rearrangements was found to be significantly shorter than median survival of non-IGHV3-21 mutated patients, and comparable to the survival of unmutated cases [90, 91, 103, 104]. Other IGHV genes also exhibited association with certain clinical characteristics; for example, IGHV3-23 has been indicated as a marker of worse prognosis within M-CLL subtype, IGHV3-72 is over-represented in highly stable CLL, and IGHV3-30 has been linked to spontaneous regression [105–107]. The associations of IG repertoire with clinicobiological features of CLL will be further discussed in the next section, in the context of BCR stereotypy.

3.3. BCR stereotypy

The discovery that CLL includes patients with both mutated and unmutated IGHV-IGHD-IGHJ rearrangements was the first evidence pointing towards the role of antigens in the pathogenesis of the disease. The presence of somatic hypermutations and higher replacement/silent mutations (R/S) ratio in VH CDRs than in FRs indicate that M-CLL cells have undergone germinal centre reactions and been selected by T cell-dependent antigen [33]. Consequently, due to the lack of SHM in IGH rearrangements, U-CLL cells have initially been thought to originate from naïve B lymphocytes. However, further studies revealed that both U-CLL and M-CLL cells express highly restricted, non-random immunoglobulin repertoire. CLL-biased representation of certain IGHV genes and IGHV-IGHD-IGHJ combinations, as well as VH CDR3 characteristics, implies the recognition of limited set of antigens, suggesting that CLL clones, both mutated and unmutated, derive from activated B cells. In the case of U-CLL, the cell of origin could have been activated either by T cell-independent antigens and autoantigens outside germinal centres or by antigens that select against SHM [108]. High R/S ratio in VH CDR3 of minimally mutated U-CLL rearrangements (<2% mutations) further argues in favour of an antigen-driven process, since even a single mutation can significantly enhance antigen-binding affinity of BCR and, hence, be selected for. In keeping with these observations, studies of gene expression profiles and surface phenotypes showed that both M-CLL and U-CLL cells exhibit characteristics of antigen-experienced B lymphocytes [60, 109, 110]. Finally, the most compelling evidence for the involvement of antigen in the development of CLL comes from the discovery of 'stereotyped' B cell receptors.

Following the initial findings on IG gene repertoire and VH CDR3 restrictions, it has been observed in multiple studies that a proportion of unrelated CLL patients expresses highly homologous, almost identical BCRs (stereotyped BCRs) [42, 79, 82, 85, 111–115]. Stereotyped BCRs have been detected in both CLL subtypes, although with higher frequency in U-CLL.

Closely related BCRs have been clustered into stereotyped subsets. With the increase in the number of cases investigated in these studies, the number of identified stereotyped subsets grew larger, reaching several hundreds. However, the proportion of cases which could be assigned to stereotyped subsets did not exceed ~30%, regardless of the cohort size [116]. In the largest study conducted by now, which included >7000 CLL patients, 19 subsets accounted for 41% of the stereotyped cases (major subsets) and 12% of the total cohort; other stereotyped subsets accounted for 18% of cases, while the remaining 70% of cases were heterogeneous, i.e. did not belong to any of the stereotypes [115].

The required criteria initially adopted for stereotyped subset definition included the usage of the same IGHV, IGHD and IGHJ gene and IGHD reading frame, as well as identity of VH CDR3 amino acid sequence ≥60% [111, 113]. However, it soon became apparent that different IGHV genes (although with substantial sequence similarity) could generate highly homologous VH CDR3s if recombined with the same IGHD and IGHJ genes. In addition, introduction of somatic hypermutations could lead to convergence of VH CDR3 sequences encoded by different IGHV genes [115, 117]. Therefore, a revised set of criteria for clustering of IGH rearrangements into stereotyped subsets has been developed, which included additional parameters: (1) the presence of IGHV genes of the same phylogenetic clan, (2) identical VH CDR3 length and a unique amino acid motif at the exact position within VH CDR3, (3) VH CDR3 amino acid identity >50% and similarity > 70% [115]. Conserved amino acid motifs which define a subset can encompass almost the entire VH CDR3 sequence (e.g. subset #6 and #10) or, alternatively, can involve just a few, or even just one, critical amino acid residue (e.g. subset #2). Furthermore, in some subsets, the conserved motifs are encoded solely by specific IGHD-IGHJ combinations (e.g. subsets #3, #5 and #8), while in others, conserved amino acids are located in junctional N1 and N2 regions (e.g. subsets #4, #16, #77 and #201) [115]. The strong bias in usage of individual IGHV genes in stereotyped BCRs has been detected, since only a few genes (IGHV1-69, IGHV1-2, IGHV1-3, IGHV3-21, IGHV4-34 and IGHV4-39) are expressed in around 80% of clustered cases, while IGHV3-7, IGHV3-23, IGHV3-30 and IGHV3-33, though frequent in CLL, are virtually absent from stereotyped subsets [117]. In addition, the majority of subsets exhibit restricted light chain usage with subset-biased κ and λ CDR3 motifs, thus evidencing the significant role of light chains in antigen-binding specificities of stereotyped BCRs [118]. Most of the major subsets are characterized by exclusively mutated or unmutated rearrangements, while several of them (e.g. subset #1, #2 and #99) can be detected among both M-CLL and U-CLL clones [115, 117]. Characteristics of the most frequent among major stereotyped subsets are depicted in **Table 1**.

Extensive research on BCR stereotypy revealed the consistent association of certain stereotyped subsets with clinicobiological features of patients. It is well known that proliferation and survival of CLL cells rely on BCR signalling, along with signalling via other surface receptors which transduce signals from the microenvironment, since they rapidly undergo apoptosis when cultivated *in vitro* [16, 119]. The differences in aggressiveness of M-CLL and U-CLL clones have been attributed, at least in part, to their different BCR signalling capacity; CLL cells with unmutated BCRs have been shown to respond more avidly to sIgM cross-linking and express higher levels of BCR target genes than M-CLL cells, which are more

Subset	Mutational status	IGHV	IGHD	IGHD RF	IGHJ	VH CDR3 length	VH CDR3 pattern*	IGKV/IGLV
#1	mostly U	V1/5/7	D6-19	3	J4	13	AR.[NQ]W[AVLI]....FD.	KV1-39 KV1D-39
#2	mostly M	V3-21	no D		J6	9	[AVLI].[DE]...M[DE].	LV3-21
#3	U	V1-69	D2-2	3	J6	22	A.....[AVLI][AVLI]V..A....YYGMD.	Variable
#4	M	V4-34	D5-5 D4-17 D3-10	1 3 3	J6	20	[AVLI]RG.......[KRH]RYYYYG.[DE].	KV2-30
#5	U	V1-69	D3-10	3	J6	20	AR......[AVLI]...YYYY.MD.	Variable
#6	U	V1-69	D6-13	2	J3	21	ARGG.YDY[AVLI]WGSYR..[DE][AVLI]FD.	KV3-20
#8	U	V4-39	D6-13	1	J5	19	A....YSSSW....NWFDP	KV1-39 KV1D-39

Subset #2 is the most frequent stereotyped subset, followed by subset #1, #4, #6, #5, #3 and #8 [115].

*A dot represents any amino acid at a given position; a pair of square brackets represents one amino acid position and any of the enclosed amino acids can be found at that position. Abbreviations: M = mutated; U = unmutated; and RF = reading frame.

Table 1. The most common major stereotyped subsets.

anergic [120–123]. However, it has been observed that patients belonging to specific stereotyped subsets follow different clinical course from patients assigned to other subsets, even if expressing the same IGHV gene and having the same IGHV mutational status [82, 93, 124, 125]. The culprit for these subset-related clinical distinctions could be the stereotyped BCR itself, since differences in antigen reactivity and signalling capacity of BCRs belonging to certain subsets have been detected. For example, it has been demonstrated that subset #1 and #2 primary B cells were significantly less responsive to antigenic stimulations *in vitro* in comparison to subset #8 cells [126]. Additionally, subset-specific distribution of prognostically significant chromosomal aberrations (del13q, del11q, trisomy 12q and del17p), as well as recurrent mutations in frequently mutated genes in CLL (TP53, BIRC3, MYD88, NOTCH1 and SF3B1) has been reported, further underscoring the differences between stereotyped subsets [127, 128].

As mentioned in the previous section, the usage of IGHV3-21 gene has been identified as a factor of poor prognosis independent of IGHV mutational status in several studies. However, subsequent research revealed that this was only true for a proportion of cases, which turned out to belong to subset #2. Subset #2 (IGHV3-21/IGLV3-21) is the largest among stereotyped subsets, detected in both U-CLL and M-CLL, and associated with del11q, del13q, CD38 expression and SF3B1 mutations [124, 127, 128]. It has been found that IGHV3-21-utilizing cases assigned to subset #2, whether mutated or not, follow an aggressive clinical course, while cases carrying IGHV3-21 in heterogeneous BCRs have variable clinical course which correlates to IGHV mutational status [79, 85, 129].

Subset #1 (IGHV1/5/7/IGKV1(D)-39) is the second largest stereotyped subset, mostly unmutated, and also associated with aggressive disease and adverse prognosis. Recent studies revealed a significant enrichment for TP53 defects (del17p and/or TP53 mutations), trisomy 12q and NOTCH1 mutations [128, 130]. In addition, subset #1 B cells exhibited higher proliferation rate following *in vitro* BCR ligation with anti-IgM antibodies than non-subset #1 unmutated B cells [130]. Similarly to subset #2, cases assigned to subset #1 have worse prognosis when compared to unclustered cases using the same IGHV genes [82, 85, 130].

The aforementioned subset #8 (IGHV4-39/IGKV1(D)-39) is associated with the highest risk of Richter's transformation among all CLL [131]. In addition to broad polyreactivity and higher capacity for BCR signalling compared to subsets #1 and #2, the observed association with trisomy 12q and enrichment for NOTCH1 mutations likely contribute to the aggressiveness of subset #8 clones [124, 128].

In contrast to clinically aggressive subsets #1, #2 and #8, subset #4 (IGHV4-34/IGKV2-30), the largest within M-CLL subtype, is associated with younger age at diagnosis and remarkably indolent clinical course in comparison to non-subset #4 IGHV4-34 cases, as well as to all other M-CLL cases [42, 82]. Subset #4 is characterized by CD38 negativity, the lack of recurrent gene mutations and the presence of favourable deletion 13q14 as the only recurrent chromosomal abnormality [127, 128]. Gene expression profiling and *in vitro* antigenic stimulation of subset #4 leukemic cells revealed diminished response to BCR-mediated signalling and the resemblance with anergic B cells, which probably underlie the indolent phenotype of subset #4 patients [132, 133].

Given that mathematical probability of two independent B cells creating identical IG rearrangements is virtually negligible, the existence of stereotyped BCRs is considered to be the strongest evidence for recognition of common antigens leading to selection of the CLL clones. This implies that BCR reactivity and intensity of response to antigenic stimulation, as well as the frequency of exposure to antigens, could determine the behaviour of CLL clones and, hence, the course of the disease. Similar clinical characteristics of cases belonging to the same stereotyped subset corroborate this notion. Therefore, BCR stereotypy could potentially become a reliable prognostic marker for at least a proportion of patients. However, most of the clinical variability in CLL is confined to cases with heterogeneous BCRs, for whom the prognosis definition remains dependent on IGHV mutational status and other molecular markers.

4. Concluding remarks

Although the cellular origin of CLL is still a controversial issue, immunogenetic studies of BCR gene repertoire have provided unequivocal evidence that CLL precursor, in both M-CLL and U-CLL subtype, is an antigen-experienced B lymphocyte [134]. Studies of antigen reactivity have revealed that U-CLL cells generally express low-affinity polyreactive BCRs that recognize microbial antigens and autoantigens present on the surface of apoptotic cells (single- and double-stranded DNA, cytoskeletal proteins, oxidized LDL and lipopolysaccharides) [135–139]. B cell receptors of M-CLL cells, on the other hand, exhibit more restricted antigen specificities and are mainly oligo and monoreactive. Auto-reactivity has been demonstrated for several stereotyped subsets. For example, it has been observed that subset #6 (IGHV1-69/IGHD3-16/IGHJ3) antibodies bind non-muscle myosin heavy chain IIA, exposed on apoptotic cells, while subset #1(IGHV1/5/7/IGKV1(D)-39) recognizes oxidized LDL, as well as vimentin and calreticulin on stromal cells [137, 140, 141]. Furthermore, analysis of IGHV-IGHD-IGHJ sequence of subset #4 (IGHV4-34/IGKV2-30) has indicated similarities with anti-DNA antibodies, as well as the binding of N-acetyllactosamine, which is a common epitope present on various autoantigens (I/i blood group antigen, B cell isoform of CD45) and microorganisms [142]. The recognition of bacterial and viral antigens by CLL BCRs is further supported by the association of persistent infections with Epstein-Barr virus and cytomegalovirus with subset #4, and hepatitis C virus with subset #13 (IGHV4-59/IGKV3-20), the latter exhibiting rheumatoid factor activity [143, 144]. The unmutated IGHV1-69-utilizing BCRs have been shown to react with hepatitis C, HIV-1 and intestinal commensal bacteria antigens [145]. In addition, reactivity against the capsular polysaccharides of *Streptococcus pneumoniae* has been detected, which is in agreement with the observed association of respiratory tract infections with elevated risk of CLL [137, 146]. Fungal antigens have also been implicated in CLL, after the notion that mutated IGHV3-7/IGKV2-24 BCRs recognize β-(1,6)-glucan, antigenic determinant of yeast and filamentous fungi [147].

Whatever the antigens might be, they clearly play a key role in the natural history of CLL. However, the major unanswered questions concern the moment in the disease development at which BCR-antigen interaction occurs, and to what extent the nature of this interaction influences the disease progression. Stimulation by auto- and/or exo-antigen may be limited to phases prior to or during malignant transformation, leading to the selection and clonal expansion of precursor cell with the distinctive BCR, during which it acquires the oncogenic hit and becomes CLL cell [148]. Yet, it is still unclear whether antigenic stimulation continues after transformation. Several studies have investigated if CLL cells accumulate somatic hypermutations post-transformation, and have detected extensive intraclonal diversification in cases assigned to stereotyped subset #4 (but not in subsets #2, #8 and #16 and heterogeneous BCRs), implying an on-going antigenic triggering in this subset [149, 150]. In addition, gene expression profiling of CLL cells from lymph nodes has revealed up-regulation of BCR target genes, thus indicating continual antigenic stimulation [122]. The fundamental role of BCRs in CLL is underscored by the success of newly developed therapeutic strategies targeting BCR signalling pathways (BTK, PI3K and SYK inhibitors) [151–154].

The configuration of BCR expressed on the surface of the CLL clone represents its specific molecular signature which does not change during the disease course. Hence, it is reasonable to believe that, in addition to IGHV mutational status, the informations about the clonotypic BCR will in future become important for individual patient prognostication and, ultimately, will contribute to tailoring of patient-specific treatment modalities.

Acknowledgements

This work was supported by Ministry of Education, Science and Technological Development, Republic of Serbia (Grant No. III41004).

Author details

Teodora Karan-Djurasevic* and Sonja Pavlovic

*Address all correspondence to: dora_karan@yahoo.com

Institute of Molecular Genetics and Genetic Engineering, University of Belgrade, Belgrade, Serbia

References

[1] Hallek M. Chronic lymphocytic leukemia: 2015 Update on diagnosis, risk stratification, and treatment. American Journal of Hematology. 2015;**90**(5):446-460

[2] Dores GM, Anderson WF, Curtis RE, Landgren O, Ostroumova E, Bluhm EC, et al. Chronic lymphocytic leukaemia and small lymphocytic lymphoma: Overview of the descriptive epidemiology. British Journal of Haematology. 2007;**139**(5):809-819

[3] Goldin LR, Bjorkholm M, Kristinsson SY, Turesson I, Landgren O. Elevated risk of chronic lymphocytic leukemia and other indolent non-Hodgkin's lymphomas among relatives of patients with chronic lymphocytic leukemia. Haematologica. 2009;**94**(5):647-653

[4] Berndt SI, Camp NJ, Skibola CF, Vijai J, Wang Z, Gu J, et al. Meta-analysis of genome-wide association studies discovers multiple loci for chronic lymphocytic leukemia. Nature Communications. 2016;**7**:10933

[5] Law PJ, Berndt SI, Speedy HE, Camp NJ, Sava GP, Skibola CF, et al. Genome-wide association analysis implicates dysregulation of immunity genes in chronic lymphocytic leukaemia. Nature Communications. 2017;**8**:14175

[6] Sutton LA, Rosenquist R. The complex interplay between cell-intrinsic and cell-extrinsic factors driving the evolution of chronic lymphocytic leukemia. Seminars in Cancer Biology. 2015;**34**:22-35

[7] Dohner H, Stilgenbauer S, Benner A, Leupolt E, Krober A, Bullinger L, et al. Genomic aberrations and survival in chronic lymphocytic leukemia. The New England Journal of Medicine. 2000;**343**(26):1910-1916

[8] Austen B, Skowronska A, Baker C, Powell JE, Gardiner A, Oscier D, et al. Mutation status of the residual ATM allele is an important determinant of the cellular response to chemotherapy and survival in patients with chronic lymphocytic leukemia containing an 11q deletion. Journal of Clinical Oncology. 2007;**25**(34):5448-5457

[9] Calin GA, Dumitru CD, Shimizu M, Bichi R, Zupo S, Noch E, et al. Frequent deletions and down-regulation of micro- RNA genes miR15 and miR16 at 13q14 in chronic lymphocytic leukemia. Proceedings of the National Academy of Sciences of the United States of America. 2002;**99**(24):15524-15529

[10] Zenz T, Habe S, Denzel T, Mohr J, Winkler D, Buhler A, et al. Detailed analysis of p53 pathway defects in fludarabine-refractory chronic lymphocytic leukemia (CLL): Dissecting the contribution of 17p deletion, TP53 mutation, p53-p21 dysfunction, and miR34a in a prospective clinical trial. Blood. 2009;**114**(13):2589-2597

[11] Rossi D, Rasi S, Spina V, Bruscaggin A, Monti S, Ciardullo C, et al. Integrated mutational and cytogenetic analysis identifies new prognostic subgroups in chronic lymphocytic leukemia. Blood. 2013;**121**(8):1403-1412

[12] Packham G, Stevenson FK. Bodyguards and assassins: Bcl-2 family proteins and apoptosis control in chronic lymphocytic leukaemia. Immunology. 2005;**114**(4):441-449

[13] Karan-Djurasevic T, Palibrk V, Zukic B, Spasovski V, Glumac I, Colovic M, et al. Expression of Bcl2L12 in chronic lymphocytic leukemia patients: Association with clinical and molecular prognostic markers. Medical Oncology. 2013;**30**(1):405

[14] Vucicevic K, Jakovljevic V, Colovic N, Tosic N, Kostic T, Glumac I, et al. Association of bax expression and BCL2/BAX ratio with clinical and molecular prognostic markers in chronic lymphocytic leukemia. The Journal of Biochemistry. 2016;**35**(2):150-157

[15] Niemann CU, Wiestner A. B-cell receptor signaling as a driver of lymphoma development and evolution. Seminars in Cancer Biology. 2013;**23**(6):410-421

[16] Stevenson FK, Forconi F, Packham G. The meaning and relevance of B-cell receptor structure and function in chronic lymphocytic leukemia. Seminars in Hematology. 2014;**51**(3):158-167

[17] Hallek M, Cheson BD, Catovsky D, Caligaris-Cappio F, Dighiero G, Dohner H, et al. Guidelines for the diagnosis and treatment of chronic lymphocytic leukemia: A report from the International Workshop on Chronic Lymphocytic Leukemia updating the National Cancer Institute-Working Group 1996 guidelines. Blood. 2008;**111**(12):5446-5456

[18] Xu JL, Davis MM. Diversity in the CDR3 region of V(H) is sufficient for most antibody specificities. Immunity. 2000;**13**(1):37-45

[19] Lefranc MP, Pommie C, Ruiz M, Giudicelli V, Foulquier E, Truong L, et al. IMGT unique numbering for immunoglobulin and T cell receptor variable domains and Ig superfamily V-like domains. Developmental & Comparative Immunology. 2003;**27**(1):55-77

[20] Lefranc M-P, Lefranc G. The immunoglobulin FactsBook. London, UK: Academic Press; 2001

[21] Lefranc MP. Nomenclature of the human immunoglobulin heavy (IGH) genes. Experimental and Clinical Immunogenetics. 2001;**18**(2):100-116

[22] Brady BL, Steinel NC, Bassing CH. Antigen receptor allelic exclusion: An update and reappraisal. Journal of Immunology. 2010;**185**(7):3801-3808

[23] Glanville J, Kuo TC, von Budingen HC, Guey L, Berka J, Sundar PD, et al. Naive antibody gene-segment frequencies are heritable and unaltered by chronic lymphocyte ablation. Proceedings of the National Academy of Sciences of the United States of America. 2011;**108**(50):20066-20071

[24] Schatz DG, Spanopoulou E. Biochemistry of V(D)J recombination. Current Topics in Microbiology and Immunology. 2005;**290**:49-85

[25] Luning Prak ET, Monestier M, Eisenberg RA. B cell receptor editing in tolerance and autoimmunity. Annals of the New York Academy of Sciences. 2011;**1217**:96-121

[26] De Silva NS, Klein U. Dynamics of B cells in germinal centres. Nature Reviews Immunology. 2015;**15**(3):137-148

[27] Peled JU, Kuang FL, Iglesias-Ussel MD, Roa S, Kalis SL, Goodman MF, et al. The biochemistry of somatic hypermutation. Annual Review of Immunology. 2008;**26**:481-511

[28] Stavnezer J, Guikema JE, Schrader CE. Mechanism and regulation of class switch recombination. Annual Review of Immunology. 2008;**26**:261-292

[29] Damle RN, Wasil T, Fais F, Ghiotto F, Valetto A, Allen SL, et al. Ig V gene mutation status and CD38 expression as novel prognostic indicators in chronic lymphocytic leukemia. Blood. 1999;**94**(6):1840-1847

[30] Hamblin TJ, Davis Z, Gardiner A, Oscier DG, Stevenson FK. Unmutated Ig V(H) genes are associated with a more aggressive form of chronic lymphocytic leukemia. Blood. 1999;**94**(6):1848-1854

[31] Maloum K, Davi F, Merle-Beral H, Pritsch O, Magnac C, Vuillier F, et al. Expression of unmutated VH genes is a detrimental prognostic factor in chronic lymphocytic leukemia. Blood. 2000;**96**(1):377-379

[32] Thompson PA, Tam CS, O'Brien SM, Wierda WG, Stingo F, Plunkett W, et al. Fludarabine, cyclophosphamide, and rituximab treatment achieves long-term disease-free survival in IGHV-mutated chronic lymphocytic leukemia. Blood. 2016;**127**(3):303-309

[33] Fais F, Ghiotto F, Hashimoto S, Sellars B, Valetto A, Allen SL, et al. Chronic lymphocytic leukemia B cells express restricted sets of mutated and unmutated antigen receptors. The Journal of Clinical Investigation. 1998;**102**(8):1515-1525

[34] Ghia P, Stamatopoulos K, Belessi C, Moreno C, Stilgenbauer S, Stevenson F, et al. ERIC recommendations on IGHV gene mutational status analysis in chronic lymphocytic leukemia. Leukemia. 2007;**21**(1):1-3

[35] Giudicelli V, Brochet X, Lefranc MP. IMGT/V-QUEST: IMGT standardized analysis of the immunoglobulin (IG) and T cell receptor (TR) nucleotide sequences. Cold Spring Harbor Protocols. 2011;**2011**(6):695-715

[36] Krober A, Seiler T, Benner A, Bullinger L, Bruckle E, Lichter P, et al. V(H) mutation status, CD38 expression level, genomic aberrations, and survival in chronic lymphocytic leukemia. Blood. 2002;**100**(4):1410-1416

[37] Lin K, Sherrington PD, Dennis M, Matrai Z, Cawley JC, Pettitt AR. Relationship between p53 dysfunction, CD38 expression, and IgV(H) mutation in chronic lymphocytic leukemia. Blood. 2002;**100**(4):1404-1409

[38] Tobin G, Thunberg U, Laurell A, Karlsson K, Aleskog A, Willander K, et al. Patients with chronic lymphocytic leukemia with mutated VH genes presenting with Binet stage B or C form a subgroup with a poor outcome. Haematologica. 2005;**90**(4):465-469

[39] Hamblin TJ, Davis ZA, Oscier DG. Determination of how many immunoglobulin variable region heavy chain mutations are allowable in unmutated chronic lymphocytic leukaemia—Long-term follow up of patients with different percentages of mutations. British Journal of Haematology. 2008;**140**(3):320-323

[40] Davis ZA, Orchard JA, Corcoran MM, Oscier DG. Divergence from the germ-line sequence in unmutated chronic lymphocytic leukemia is due to somatic mutation rather than polymorphisms. Blood. 2003;**102**(8):3075

[41] Rassenti LZ, Kipps TJ. Lack of allelic exclusion in B cell chronic lymphocytic leukemia. The Journal of Experimental Medicine. 1997;**185**(8):1435-1445

[42] Murray F, Darzentas N, Hadzidimitriou A, Tobin G, Boudjogra M, Scielzo C, et al. Stereotyped patterns of somatic hypermutation in subsets of patients with chronic

lymphocytic leukemia: Implications for the role of antigen selection in leukemogenesis. Blood. 2008;**111**(3):1524-1533

[43] Plevova K, Francova HS, Burckova K, Brychtova Y, Doubek M, Pavlova S, et al. Multiple productive immunoglobulin heavy chain gene rearrangements in chronic lymphocytic leukemia are mostly derived from independent clones. Haematologica. 2014;**99**(2):329-338

[44] Langerak AW, Davi F, Ghia P, Hadzidimitriou A, Murray F, Potter KN, et al. Immunoglobulin sequence analysis and prognostication in CLL: Guidelines from the ERIC review board for reliable interpretation of problematic cases. Leukemia. 2011;**25**(6):979-984

[45] Grever MR, Lucas DM, Dewald GW, Neuberg DS, Reed JC, Kitada S, et al. Comprehensive assessment of genetic and molecular features predicting outcome in patients with chronic lymphocytic leukemia: Results from the US Intergroup Phase III Trial E2997. Journal of Clinical Oncology. 2007;**25**(7):799-804

[46] Parikh SA, Strati P, Tsang M, West CP, Shanafelt TD. Should IGHV status and FISH testing be performed in all CLL patients at diagnosis? A systematic review and meta-analysis. Blood. 2016;**127**(14):1752-1760

[47] Oscier DG, Gardiner AC, Mould SJ, Glide S, Davis ZA, Ibbotson RE, et al. Multivariate analysis of prognostic factors in CLL: Clinical stage, IGVH gene mutational status, and loss or mutation of the p53 gene are independent prognostic factors. Blood. 2002;**100**(4):1177-1184

[48] Stilgenbauer S, Bullinger L, Lichter P, Dohner H. Genetics of chronic lymphocytic leukemia: Genomic aberrations and V(H) gene mutation status in pathogenesis and clinical course. Leukemia. 2002;**16**(6):993-1007

[49] Haferlach C, Dicker F, Schnittger S, Kern W, Haferlach T. Comprehensive genetic characterization of CLL: A study on 506 cases analysed with chromosome banding analysis, interphase FISH, IgV(H) status and immunophenotyping. Leukemia. 2007;**21**(12):2442-2451

[50] Stilgenbauer S, Sander S, Bullinger L, Benner A, Leupolt E, Winkler D, et al. Clonal evolution in chronic lymphocytic leukemia: Acquisition of high-risk genomic aberrations associated with unmutated VH, resistance to therapy, and short survival. Haematologica. 2007;**92**(9):1242-1245

[51] Ghia P, Guida G, Stella S, Gottardi D, Geuna M, Strola G, et al. The pattern of CD38 expression defines a distinct subset of chronic lymphocytic leukemia (CLL) patients at risk of disease progression. Blood. 2003;**101**(4):1262-1269

[52] Hamblin TJ, Orchard JA, Ibbotson RE, Davis Z, Thomas PW, Stevenson FK, et al. CD38 expression and immunoglobulin variable region mutations are independent prognostic variables in chronic lymphocytic leukemia, but CD38 expression may vary during the course of the disease. Blood. 2002;**99**(3):1023-1029

[53] Dürig J, Naschar M, Schmücker U, Renzing-Köhler K, Hölter T, Hüttmann A, et al. CD38 expression is an important prognostic marker in chronic lymphocytic leukaemia. Leukemia. 2002;**16**(1):30-35

[54] Jelinek DF, Tschumper RC, Geyer SM, Bone ND, Dewald GW, Hanson CA, et al. Analysis of clonal B-cell CD38 and immunoglobulin variable region sequence status in relation to clinical outcome for B-chronic lymphocytic leukaemia. British Journal of Haematology. 2001;**115**(4):854-861

[55] Crespo M, Bosch F, Villamor N, Bellosillo B, Colomer D, Rozman M, et al. ZAP-70 expression as a surrogate for immunoglobulin-variable-region mutations in chronic lymphocytic leukemia. The New England Journal of Medicine. 2003;**348**(18):1764-1775

[56] Rassenti LZ, Jain S, Keating MJ, Wierda WG, Grever MR, Byrd JC, et al. Relative value of ZAP-70, CD38, and immunoglobulin mutation status in predicting aggressive disease in chronic lymphocytic leukemia. Blood. 2008;**112**(5):1923-1930

[57] Rassenti LZ, Huynh L, Toy TL, Chen L, Keating MJ, Gribben JG, et al. ZAP-70 compared with immunoglobulin heavy-chain gene mutation status as a predictor of disease progression in chronic lymphocytic leukemia. The New England Journal of Medicine. 2004;**351**(9):893-901

[58] Orchard JA, Ibbotson RE, Davis Z, Wiestner A, Rosenwald A, Thomas PW, et al. ZAP-70 expression and prognosis in chronic lymphocytic leukaemia. Lancet. 2004;**363**(9403):105-111

[59] Stamatopoulos B, Meuleman N, Haibe-Kains B, Duvillier H, Massy M, Martiat P, et al. Quantification of ZAP70 mRNA in B cells by real-time PCR is a powerful prognostic factor in chronic lymphocytic leukemia. Clinical Chemistry. 2007;**53**(10):1757-1766

[60] Rosenwald A, Alizadeh AA, Widhopf G, Simon R, Davis RE, Yu X, et al. Relation of gene expression phenotype to immunoglobulin mutation genotype in B cell chronic lymphocytic leukemia. The Journal of Experimental Medicine. 2001;**194**(11):1639-1647

[61] Catherwood MA, Matthews C, Niblock R, Dobbin E, Morris TC, Alexander HD. ZAP-70 mRNA quantification in B-cell chronic lymphocytic leukaemia. European Journal of Haematology. 2006;**76**(4):294-298

[62] Krober A, Bloehdorn J, Hafner S, Buhler A, Seiler T, Kienle D, et al. Additional genetic high-risk features such as 11q deletion, 17p deletion, and V3-21 usage characterize discordance of ZAP-70 and VH mutation status in chronic lymphocytic leukemia. Journal of Clinical Oncology. 2006;**24**(6):969-975

[63] Wiestner A, Rosenwald A, Barry TS, Wright G, Davis RE, Henrickson SE, et al. ZAP-70 expression identifies a chronic lymphocytic leukemia subtype with unmutated immunoglobulin genes, inferior clinical outcome, and distinct gene expression profile. Blood. 2003;**101**(12):4944-4951

[64] Heintel D, Kienle D, Shehata M, Krober A, Kroemer E, Schwarzinger I, et al. High expression of lipoprotein lipase in poor risk B-cell chronic lymphocytic leukemia. Leukemia. 2005;**19**(7):1216-1223

[65] Nikitin EA, Malakho SG, Biderman BV, Baranova AV, Lorie YY, Shevelev AY, et al. Expression level of lipoprotein lipase and dystrophin genes predict survival in B-cell chronic lymphocytic leukemia. Leukemia & Lymphoma. 2007;**48**(5):912-922

[66] Van Bockstaele F, Pede V, Janssens A, Callewaert F, Offner F, Verhasselt B, et al. Lipoprotein lipase mRNA expression in whole blood is a prognostic marker in B cell chronic lymphocytic leukemia. Clinical Chemistry. 2007;**53**(2):204-212

[67] Mansouri M, Sevov M, Fahlgren E, Tobin G, Jondal M, Osorio L, et al. Lipoprotein lipase is differentially expressed in prognostic subsets of chronic lymphocytic leukemia but displays invariably low catalytical activity. Leukemia Research. 2010;**34**(3):301-306

[68] Nuckel H, Huttmann A, Klein-Hitpass L, Schroers R, Fuhrer A, Sellmann L, et al. Lipoprotein lipase expression is a novel prognostic factor in B-cell chronic lymphocytic leukemia. Leuk Lymphoma. 2006;**47**(6):1053-1061

[69] Kaderi MA, Kanduri M, Buhl AM, Sevov M, Cahill N, Gunnarsson R, et al. LPL is the strongest prognostic factor in a comparative analysis of RNA-based markers in early chronic lymphocytic leukemia. Haematologica. 2011;**96**(8):1153-1160

[70] Antic D, Mihaljevic B, Cokic V, Fekete MD, Djurasevic TK, Pavlovic S, et al. Patients with early stage chronic lymphocytic leukemia: New risk stratification based on molecular profiling. Leuk Lymphoma. 2011;**52**(7):1394-1397

[71] van't Veer MB, Brooijmans AM, Langerak AW, Verhaaf B, Goudswaard CS, Graveland WJ, et al. The predictive value of lipoprotein lipase for survival in chronic lymphocytic leukemia. Haematologica. 2006;**91**(1):56-63

[72] International CLL-IPI working group. An international prognostic index for patients with chronic lymphocytic leukaemia (CLL-IPI): a meta-analysis of individual patient data. The Lancet Oncology. 2016;**17**(6):779-790

[73] Delgado J, Doubek M, Baumann T, Kotaskova J, Molica S, Mozas P, et al. Chronic lymphocytic leukemia: A prognostic model comprising only two biomarkers (IGHV mutational status and FISH cytogenetics) separates patients with different outcome and simplifies the CLL-IPI. American Journal of Hematology. 2017;**92**(4):375-380.

[74] Pflug N, Bahlo J, Shanafelt TD, Eichhorst BF, Bergmann MA, Elter T, et al. Development of a comprehensive prognostic index for patients with chronic lymphocytic leukemia. Blood. 2014;**124**(1):49-62

[75] Visentin A, Frezzato F, Imbergamo S, Trimarco V, Martini V, Severin F, et al. Evaluation of Integrated CLL Scoring System (ICSS) in 420 Patients with Chronic Lymphocytic Leukemia. Blood. 2016;**128**(22):5563-5563

[76] Brezinschek HP, Foster SJ, Brezinschek RI, Dorner T, Domiati-Saad R, Lipsky PE. Analysis of the human VH gene repertoire. Differential effects of selection and somatic hypermutation on human peripheral CD5(+)/IgM+ and CD5(-)/IgM+ B cells. The Journal of Clinical Investigation. 1997;**99**(10):2488-2501

[77] Schroeder Jr. HW, Dighiero G. The pathogenesis of chronic lymphocytic leukemia: Analysis of the antibody repertoire. Immunology Today. 1994;**15**(6):288-294

[78] Duke VM, Gandini D, Sherrington PD, Lin K, Heelan B, Amlot P, et al. V(H) gene usage differs in germline and mutated B-cell chronic lymphocytic leukemia. Haematologica. 2003;**88**(11):1259-1271

[79] Ghia P, Stamatopoulos K, Belessi C, Moreno C, Stella S, Guida G, et al. Geographic patterns and pathogenetic implications of IGHV gene usage in chronic lymphocytic leukemia: The lesson of the IGHV3-21 gene. Blood. 2005;**105**(4):1678-1685

[80] Mauerer K, Zahrieh D, Gorgun G, Li A, Zhou J, Ansen S, et al. Immunoglobulin gene segment usage, location and immunogenicity in mutated and unmutated chronic lymphocytic leukaemia. British journal of Haematology. 2005;**129**(4):499-510

[81] Messmer BT, Albesiano E, Messmer D, Chiorazzi N. The pattern and distribution of immunoglobulin VH gene mutations in chronic lymphocytic leukemia B cells are consistent with the canonical somatic hypermutation process. Blood. 2004;**103**(9):3490-3495

[82] Stamatopoulos K, Belessi C, Moreno C, Boudjograh M, Guida G, Smilevska T, et al. Over 20% of patients with chronic lymphocytic leukemia carry stereotyped receptors: Pathogenetic implications and clinical correlations. Blood. 2007;**109**(1):259-270

[83] Widhopf 2nd GF, Kipps TJ. Normal B cells express 51p1-encoded Ig heavy chains that are distinct from those expressed by chronic lymphocytic leukemia B cells. Journal of Immunology. 2001;**166**(1):95-102

[84] Potter KN, Orchard J, Critchley E, Mockridge CI, Jose A, Stevenson FK. Features of the overexpressed V1-69 genes in the unmutated subset of chronic lymphocytic leukemia are distinct from those in the healthy elderly repertoire. Blood. 2003;**101**(8):3082-3084

[85] Bomben R, Dal Bo M, Capello D, Forconi F, Maffei R, Laurenti L, et al. Molecular and clinical features of chronic lymphocytic leukaemia with stereotyped B cell receptors: Results from an Italian multicentre study. British Journal of Haematology. 2009;**144**(4):492-506

[86] Bilous N, Bomben R, Dal Bo M, Capello D, Forconi F, Laurenti L, et al. Molecular and clinical features of chronic lymphocytic leukemia with stereotyped B-cell receptors in a Ukrainian cohort. Leuk Lymphoma. 2010;**51**(5):822-838

[87] Karan-Djurasevic T, Palibrk V, Kostic T, Spasovski V, Nikcevic G, Srzentic S, et al. Mutational status and gene repertoire of IGHV-IGHD-IGHJ rearrangements in Serbian patients with chronic lymphocytic leukemia. Clinical Lymphoma, Myeloma & Leukemia. 2012;**12**(4):252-260

[88] Bianchi S, Moreno P, Landoni AI, Naya H, Oppezzo P, Dighiero G, et al. Immunoglobulin heavy chain V-D-J gene rearrangement and mutational status in Uruguayan patients with chronic lymphocytic leukemia. Leuk Lymphoma. 2010;**51**(11):2070-2078

[89] Gonzalez-Gascon YMI, Hernandez JA, Martin A, Alcoceba M, Sarasquete ME, Rodriguez-Vicente A, et al. Mutation status and immunoglobulin gene rearrangements in patients from northwest and central region of Spain with chronic lymphocytic leukemia. BioMed Research International. 2014;**2014**:257517

[90] Tobin G, Thunberg U, Johnson A, Thorn I, Soderberg O, Hultdin M, et al. Somatically mutated Ig V(H)3-21 genes characterize a new subset of chronic lymphocytic leukemia. Blood. 2002;**99**(6):2262-2264

[91] Tobin G, Thunberg U, Johnson A, Eriksson I, Soderberg O, Karlsson K, et al. Chronic lymphocytic leukemias utilizing the VH3-21 gene display highly restricted Vlambda2-14 gene use and homologous CDR3s: Implicating recognition of a common antigen epitope. Blood. 2003;**101**(12):4952-4957

[92] Matthews C, Catherwood MA, Morris TC, Alexander HD. V(H)3-48 and V(H)3-53, as well as V(H)3-21, gene rearrangements define unique subgroups in CLL and are associated with biased lambda light chain restriction, homologous LCDR3 sequences and poor prognosis. Leukemia Research. 2007;**31**(2):231-234

[93] Bomben R, Dal Bo M, Capello D, Benedetti D, Marconi D, Zucchetto A, et al. Comprehensive characterization of IGHV3-21-expressing B-cell chronic lymphocytic leukemia: An Italian multicenter study. Blood. 2007;**109**(7):2989-2998

[94] Hojjat-Farsangi M, Jeddi-Tehrani M, Razavi SM, Sharifian RA, Mellstedt H, Shokri F, et al. Immunoglobulin heavy chain variable region gene usage and mutational status of the leukemic B cells in Iranian patients with chronic lymphocytic leukemia. Cancer Science. 2009;**100**(12):2346-2353

[95] Chen L, Zhang Y, Zheng W, Wu Y, Qiao C, Fan L, et al. Distinctive IgVH gene segments usage and mutation status in Chinese patients with chronic lymphocytic leukemia. Leukemia Research. 2008;**32**(10):1491-1498

[96] Koiso H, Yamane A, Mitsui T, Matsushima T, Tsukamoto N, Murakami H, et al. Distinctive immunoglobulin VH gene usage in Japanese patients with chronic lymphocytic leukemia. Leukemia Research. 2006;**30**(3):272-276

[97] Ghiotto F, Fais F, Albesiano E, Sison C, Valetto A, Gaidano G, et al. Similarities and differences between the light and heavy chain Ig variable region gene repertoires in chronic lymphocytic leukemia. Molecular Medicine. 2006;**12**(11-12):300-308

[98] Stamatopoulos K, Belessi C, Hadzidimitriou A, Smilevska T, Kalagiakou E, Hatzi K, et al. Immunoglobulin light chain repertoire in chronic lymphocytic leukemia. Blood. 2005;**106**(10):3575-3583

[99] Belessi C, Stamatopoulos K, Hadzidimitriou A, Hatzi K, Smilevska T, Stavroyianni N, et al. Analysis of expressed and non-expressed IGK locus rearrangements in chronic lymphocytic leukemia. Molecular Medicine. 2005;**11**(1-12):52-58

[100] Widhopf GF, 2nd, Goldberg CJ, Toy TL, Rassenti LZ, Wierda WG, Byrd JC, et al. Nonstochastic pairing of immunoglobulin heavy and light chains expressed by chronic lymphocytic leukemia B cells is predicated on the heavy chain CDR3. Blood. 2008;**111**(6):3137-3144

[101] Brezinschek HP, Foster SJ, Dorner T, Brezinschek RI, Lipsky PE. Pairing of variable heavy and variable kappa chains in individual naive and memory B cells. Journal of Immunology. 1998;**160**(10):4762-4767

[102] de Wildt RM, Hoet RM, van Venrooij WJ, Tomlinson IM, Winter G. Analysis of heavy and light chain pairings indicates that receptor editing shapes the human antibody repertoire. Journal of Molecular Biology. 1999;**285**(3):895-901

[103] Lin K, Manocha S, Harris RJ, Matrai Z, Sherrington PD, Pettitt AR. High frequency of p53 dysfunction and low level of VH mutation in chronic lymphocytic leukemia patients using the VH3-21 gene segment. Blood. 2003;**102**(3):1145-1146

[104] Thorselius M, Krober A, Murray F, Thunberg U, Tobin G, Buhler A, et al. Strikingly homologous immunoglobulin gene rearrangements and poor outcome in VH3-21-using chronic lymphocytic leukemia patients independent of geographic origin and mutational status. Blood. 2006;**107**(7):2889-2894

[105] Bomben R, Dal-Bo M, Benedetti D, Capello D, Forconi F, Marconi D, et al. Expression of mutated IGHV3-23 genes in chronic lymphocytic leukemia identifies a disease subset with peculiar clinical and biological features. Clinical Cancer Research. 2010;**16**(2):620-628

[106] Capello D, Guarini A, Berra E, Mauro FR, Rossi D, Ghia E, et al. Evidence of biased immunoglobulin variable gene usage in highly stable B-cell chronic lymphocytic leukemia. Leukemia. 2004;**18**(12):1941-1947

[107] Del Giudice I, Chiaretti S, Tavolaro S, De Propris MS, Maggio R, Mancini F, et al. Spontaneous regression of chronic lymphocytic leukemia: Clinical and biologic features of 9 cases. Blood. 2009;**114**(3):638-646

[108] Weill JC, Weller S, Reynaud CA. Human marginal zone B cells. Annual Review of Immunology. 2009;**27**:267-285

[109] Damle RN, Ghiotto F, Valetto A, Albesiano E, Fais F, Yan XJ, et al. B-cell chronic lymphocytic leukemia cells express a surface membrane phenotype of activated, antigen-experienced B lymphocytes. Blood. 2002;**99**(11):4087-4093

[110] Klein U, Tu Y, Stolovitzky GA, Mattioli M, Cattoretti G, Husson H, et al. Gene expression profiling of B cell chronic lymphocytic leukemia reveals a homogeneous phenotype related to memory B cells. The Journal of Experimental Medicine. 2001; **194**(11):1625-1638

[111] Messmer BT, Albesiano E, Efremov DG, Ghiotto F, Allen SL, Kolitz J, et al. Multiple distinct sets of stereotyped antigen receptors indicate a role for antigen in promoting chronic lymphocytic leukemia. The Journal of Experimental Medicine. 2004;**200**(4):519-525

[112] Ghiotto F, Fais F, Valetto A, Albesiano E, Hashimoto S, Dono M, et al. Remarkably similar antigen receptors among a subset of patients with chronic lymphocytic leukemia. The Journal of Clinical Investigation. 2004;**113**(7):1008-1016

[113] Tobin G, Thunberg U, Karlsson K, Murray F, Laurell A, Willander K, et al. Subsets with restricted immunoglobulin gene rearrangement features indicate a role for antigen selection in the development of chronic lymphocytic leukemia. Blood. 2004;**104**(9):2879-2885

[114] Widhopf GF, 2nd, Rassenti LZ, Toy TL, Gribben JG, Wierda WG, Kipps TJ. Chronic lymphocytic leukemia B cells of more than 1% of patients express virtually identical immunoglobulins. Blood. 2004;**104**(8):2499-2504

[115] Agathangelidis A, Darzentas N, Hadzidimitriou A, Brochet X, Murray F, Yan XJ, et al. Stereotyped B-cell receptors in one-third of chronic lymphocytic leukemia: A molecular classification with implications for targeted therapies. Blood. 2012;**119**(19):4467-4475

[116] Stamatopoulos K, Agathangelidis A, Rosenquist R, Ghia P. Antigen receptor stereotypy in chronic lymphocytic leukemia. Leukemia. 2017;**31**(2):282-291

[117] Darzentas N, Hadzidimitriou A, Murray F, Hatzi K, Josefsson P, Laoutaris N, et al. A different ontogenesis for chronic lymphocytic leukemia cases carrying stereotyped antigen receptors: Molecular and computational evidence. Leukemia. 2010;**24**(1):125-132

[118] Hadzidimitriou A, Darzentas N, Murray F, Smilevska T, Arvaniti E, Tresoldi C, et al. Evidence for the significant role of immunoglobulin light chains in antigen recognition and selection in chronic lymphocytic leukemia. Blood. 2009;**113**(2):403-411

[119] Caligaris-Cappio F, Bertilaccio MT, Scielzo C. How the microenvironment wires the natural history of chronic lymphocytic leukemia. Seminars in Cancer Biology. 2014;**24**:43-48

[120] Chen L, Widhopf G, Huynh L, Rassenti L, Rai KR, Weiss A, et al. Expression of ZAP-70 is associated with increased B-cell receptor signaling in chronic lymphocytic leukemia. Blood. 2002;**100**(13):4609-4614

[121] Lanham S, Hamblin T, Oscier D, Ibbotson R, Stevenson F, Packham G. Differential signaling via surface IgM is associated with VH gene mutational status and CD38 expression in chronic lymphocytic leukemia. Blood. 2003;**101**(3):1087-1093

[122] Herishanu Y, Perez-Galan P, Liu D, Biancotto A, Pittaluga S, Vire B, et al. The lymph node microenvironment promotes B-cell receptor signaling, NF-kappaB activation, and tumor proliferation in chronic lymphocytic leukemia. Blood. 2011;**117**(2):563-574

[123] Guarini A, Chiaretti S, Tavolaro S, Maggio R, Peragine N, Citarella F, et al. BCR ligation induced by IgM stimulation results in gene expression and functional changes only in IgV H unmutated chronic lymphocytic leukemia (CLL) cells. Blood. 2008;**112**(3):782-792

[124] Baliakas P, Hadzidimitriou A, Sutton LA, Minga E, Agathangelidis A, Nichelatti M, et al. Clinical effect of stereotyped B-cell receptor immunoglobulins in chronic lymphocytic leukaemia: A retrospective multicentre study. The Lancet Haematology. 2014;**1**(2):e74-e84

[125] Maura F, Cutrona G, Fabris S, Colombo M, Tuana G, Agnelli L, et al. Relevance of stereotyped B-cell receptors in the context of the molecular, cytogenetic and clinical features of chronic lymphocytic leukemia. PLoS One. 2011;**6**(8):e24313

[126] Gounari M, Ntoufa S, Apollonio B, Papakonstantinou N, Ponzoni M, Chu CC, et al. Excessive antigen reactivity may underlie the clinical aggressiveness of chronic lymphocytic leukemia stereotyped subset #8. Blood. 2015;**125**(23):3580-3587

[127] Marincevic M, Cahill N, Gunnarsson R, Isaksson A, Mansouri M, Goransson H, et al. High-density screening reveals a different spectrum of genomic aberrations in chronic lymphocytic leukemia patients with 'stereotyped' IGHV3-21 and IGHV4-34 B-cell receptors. Haematologica. 2010;**95**(9):1519-1525

[128] Sutton LA, Young E, Baliakas P, Hadzidimitriou A, Moysiadis T, Plevova K, et al. Different spectra of recurrent gene mutations in subsets of chronic lymphocytic leukemia harboring stereotyped B-cell receptors. Haematologica. 2016;**101**(8):959-967

[129] Baliakas P, Agathangelidis A, Hadzidimitriou A, Sutton LA, Minga E, Tsanousa A, et al. Not all IGHV3-21 chronic lymphocytic leukemias are equal: Prognostic considerations. Blood. 2015;**125**(5):856-859

[130] Del Giudice I, Chiaretti S, Santangelo S, Tavolaro S, Peragine N, Marinelli M, et al. Stereotyped subset #1 chronic lymphocytic leukemia: A direct link between B-cell receptor structure, function, and patients' prognosis. American Journal of Hematology. 2014;**89**(1):74-82

[131] Rossi D, Spina V, Cerri M, Rasi S, Deambrogi C, De Paoli L, et al. Stereotyped B-cell receptor is an independent risk factor of chronic lymphocytic leukemia transformation to Richter syndrome. Clinical Cancer Research. 2009;**15**(13):4415-4422

[132] Marincevic M, Mansouri M, Kanduri M, Isaksson A, Goransson H, Smedby KE, et al. Distinct gene expression profiles in subsets of chronic lymphocytic leukemia expressing stereotyped IGHV4-34 B-cell receptors. Haematologica. 2010;**95**(12):2072-2079

[133] Ntoufa S, Papakonstantinou N, Apollonio B, Gounari M, Galigalidou C, Fonte E, et al. B cell anergy modulated by TLR1/2 and the miR-17 approximately 92 cluster underlies the indolent clinical course of chronic lymphocytic leukemia stereotyped subset #4. Journal of Immunology. 2016;**196**(10):4410-4417

[134] Chiorazzi N, Ferrarini M. Cellular origin(s) of chronic lymphocytic leukemia: Cautionary notes and additional considerations and possibilities. Blood. 2011;**117**(6):1781-1791

[135] Herve M, Xu K, Ng YS, Wardemann H, Albesiano E, Messmer BT, et al. Unmutated and mutated chronic lymphocytic leukemias derive from self-reactive B cell precursors despite expressing different antibody reactivity. The Journal of Clinical Investigation. 2005;**115**(6):1636-1643

[136] Catera R, Silverman GJ, Hatzi K, Seiler T, Didier S, Zhang L, et al. Chronic lymphocytic leukemia cells recognize conserved epitopes associated with apoptosis and oxidation. Molecular Medicine. 2008;**14**(11-12):665-674

[137] Lanemo Myhrinder A, Hellqvist E, Sidorova E, Soderberg A, Baxendale H, Dahle C, et al. A new perspective: Molecular motifs on oxidized LDL, apoptotic cells, and bacteria are targets for chronic lymphocytic leukemia antibodies. Blood. 2008;**111**(7):3838-3848

[138] Zwick C, Fadle N, Regitz E, Kemele M, Stilgenbauer S, Buhler A, et al. Autoantigenic targets of B-cell receptors derived from chronic lymphocytic leukemias bind to and induce proliferation of leukemic cells. Blood. 2013;**121**(23):4708-4717

[139] Seiler T, Woelfle M, Yancopoulos S, Catera R, Li W, Hatzi K, et al. Characterization of structurally defined epitopes recognized by monoclonal antibodies produced by chronic lymphocytic leukemia B cells. Blood. 2009;**114**(17):3615-3624

[140] Binder M, Lechenne B, Ummanni R, Scharf C, Balabanov S, Trusch M, et al. Stereotypical chronic lymphocytic leukemia B-cell receptors recognize survival promoting antigens on stromal cells. PLoS One. 2010;**5**(12):e15992

[141] Chu CC, Catera R, Hatzi K, Yan XJ, Zhang L, Wang XB, et al. Chronic lymphocytic leukemia antibodies with a common stereotypic rearrangement recognize nonmuscle myosin heavy chain IIA. Blood. 2008;**112**(13):5122-5129

[142] Potter KN, Hobby P, Klijn S, Stevenson FK, Sutton BJ. Evidence for involvement of a hydrophobic patch in framework region 1 of human V4-34-encoded Igs in recognition of the red blood cell I antigen. Journal of Immunology. 2002;**169**(7):3777-3782

[143] Kostareli E, Hadzidimitriou A, Stavroyianni N, Darzentas N, Athanasiadou A, Gounari M, et al. Molecular evidence for EBV and CMV persistence in a subset of patients with chronic lymphocytic leukemia expressing stereotyped IGHV4-34 B-cell receptors. Leukemia. 2009;**23**(5):919-924

[144] Kostareli E, Gounari M, Janus A, Murray F, Brochet X, Giudicelli V, et al. Antigen receptor stereotypy across B-cell lymphoproliferations: The case of IGHV4-59/IGKV3-20 receptors with rheumatoid factor activity. Leukemia. 2012;**26**(5):1127-1131

[145] Hwang KK, Trama AM, Kozink DM, Chen X, Wiehe K, Cooper AJ, et al. IGHV1-69 B cell chronic lymphocytic leukemia antibodies cross-react with HIV-1 and hepatitis C virus antigens as well as intestinal commensal bacteria. PLoS One. 2014;**9**(3):e90725

[146] Landgren O, Rapkin JS, Caporaso NE, Mellemkjaer L, Gridley G, Goldin LR, et al. Respiratory tract infections and subsequent risk of chronic lymphocytic leukemia. Blood. 2007;**109**(5):2198-2201

[147] Hoogeboom R, van Kessel KP, Hochstenbach F, Wormhoudt TA, Reinten RJ, Wagner K, et al. A mutated B cell chronic lymphocytic leukemia subset that recognizes and responds to fungi. The Journal of Experimental Medicine. 2013;**210**(1):59-70

[148] Rosen A, Murray F, Evaldsson C, Rosenquist R. Antigens in chronic lymphocytic leukemia—Implications for cell origin and leukemogenesis. Seminars in Cancer Biology. 2010;**20**(6):400-409

[149] Sutton LA, Kostareli E, Hadzidimitriou A, Darzentas N, Tsaftaris A, Anagnostopoulos A, et al. Extensive intraclonal diversification in a subgroup of chronic lymphocytic

leukemia patients with stereotyped IGHV4-34 receptors: Implications for ongoing interactions with antigen. Blood. 2009;**114**(20):4460-4468

[150] Kostareli E, Sutton LA, Hadzidimitriou A, Darzentas N, Kouvatsi A, Tsaftaris A, et al. Intraclonal diversification of immunoglobulin light chains in a subset of chronic lymphocytic leukemia alludes to antigen-driven clonal evolution. Leukemia. 2010;**24**(7):1317-1324

[151] Woyach JA, Smucker K, Smith LL, Lozanski A, Zhong Y, Ruppert AS, et al. Prolonged lymphocytosis during ibrutinib therapy is associated with distinct molecular characteristics and does not indicate a suboptimal response to therapy. Blood. 2014;**123**(12):1810-1817

[152] Byrd JC, Furman RR, Coutre SE, Flinn IW, Burger JA, Blum KA, et al. Targeting BTK with ibrutinib in relapsed chronic lymphocytic leukemia. The New England Journal of Medicine. 2013;**369**(1):32-42

[153] Furman RR, Sharman JP, Coutre SE, Cheson BD, Pagel JM, Hillmen P, et al. Idelalisib and rituximab in relapsed chronic lymphocytic leukemia. The New England Journal of Medicine. 2014;**370**(11):997-1007

[154] Herman SE, Barr PM, McAuley EM, Liu D, Wiestner A, Friedberg JW. Fostamatinib inhibits B-cell receptor signaling, cellular activation and tumor proliferation in patients with relapsed and refractory chronic lymphocytic leukemia. Leukemia. 2013;**27**(8):1769-1773

Chapter 4

Malignant Interaction between B Cells and T Helper Cells

Simone Bürgler

Additional information is available at the end of the chapter

http://dx.doi.org/10.5772/intechopen.68731

Abstract

Collaboration of T helper (T_h) cells with B cells is central for the generation of high-affinity antibodies with distinct effector function and thus for the establishment of effective immune responses. Physiological T cell help for B cells takes place in germinal centers (GC) in peripheral lymphoid organs, where follicular T helper (T_{fh}) cells interact with mature, antigen-stimulated B cells. Occasionally, B cells undergo malignant transformation, which may lead to the development of leukemia or lymphoma. Over the past decades, it has become increasingly clear that cancer cells depend on interactions with the tumor microenvironment for growth and survival. Since many B cell malignancies develop in GC—the place of physiological T_h cell-B cell interaction—T_h cells are a central part of the tumor microenvironment of B cell leukemia and lymphoma. Thus, while the interaction between T_h cells and normal B cells is crucial for the development of an effective immune response, this interaction also contributes to the development and pathogenesis of malignancies. The present chapter discusses the mechanisms underlying T_h cell-mediated support of malignant B cells contributing to the pathogenesis of leukemia and lymphoma. Research efforts aiming to elucidate such mechanisms are of high importance as therapeutic targeting of these malignant interactions may increase treatment efficiency and reduce disease relapse.

Keywords: T helper cells, B cells, leukemia, lymphoma, B cell malignancies, T_h cell-B cell interaction, tumor microenvironment

1. Introduction

The human immune system is made up of two branches: the innate immune system consisting of dendritic cells, macrophages, granulocytes and natural killer (NK) cells mounts a fast but nonspecific response against invading pathogens. The adaptive immune system, in contrast, raises a delayed but highly specific response. In this response, T cells and B cells use their greatly diverse receptors—T cell receptors (TCRs) and B cell receptors (BCRs), respectively—to recognize antigenic epitopes of invading pathogens [1]. Antigenic stimulation of the receptors on the B cell's and T cell's surface induces intracellular signaling cascades that lead to the activation, proliferation and differentiation of the cell. The BCR is also synthesized in a soluble form and can be secreted by B cells as antibody, also known as immunoglobulin (Ig). Antibodies recognize pathogens and neutralize them by various mechanisms. In order to generate high-affinity antibodies with distinct effector functions, B cells need the help of T cells. Thus, the establishment of a specific and efficient immune response requires a close collaboration of T cells and B cells.

1.1. Physiological T_h cell-B cell interaction

T cells arise in the bone marrow (BM) and mature in the thymus. Two T cell populations can be distinguished: the $CD8^+$ T cytotoxic (T_c) cells and the $CD4^+$ T_h cells. T_c cells can kill infected cells through release of molecules like granzymes or perforin, while T_h cells have the task to activate other immune cells and to instruct them to raise an appropriate immune response.

Naïve T_h cells leave the thymus and migrate to the periphery, where they encounter antigenic peptides presented by antigen-presenting cells (APCs) such as macrophages, B cells and dendritic cells (DCs). APC secrete a distinct set of cytokines, the composition of which depends on the pathogen encountered. Upon stimulation, the activated T_h cells rapidly divide and differentiate into one of several different effector subsets that are characterized by the expression of distinct transcription factors, surface markers and cytokines. This differentiation is governed by the cytokines that are secreted by the APC and the surrounding cells at the time point of naïve T_h cell activation. Thereby, APC not only activates naïve T_h cells but also tailors their properties according to the pathogens to be defeated.

The first T_h cell subsets that have been described were T_h1 cells, characterized by expression interferon (IFN)-γ, and T_h2 cells, producing interleukin (IL)-4, IL-5 and IL-13 [2]. Later, further effector lineages such as T_h17, T_h9 or T_h22 have been described. In addition, several T_h cell subsets with regulatory or suppressive functions, so-called regulatory T (T_{reg}) cells, exist [3].

Follicular helper T (T_{fh}) cells are a unique population of T_h cells distinct from extrafollicular and peripheral T_h cells. T_{fh} cells are characterized by the expression of the inducible T cell costimulator (ICOS) receptor, the chemokine receptor CXCR5, the programmed cell death-1 (PD-1) inhibitory receptor and the transcription factor BCL6 that controls their development and function [4–6].

B cells develop and mature in the BM and then migrate to the secondary lymphoid organs, where the antigen-dependent phase of their development takes place. While this process can be independent of T cell help, conventional B cells predominantly undergo T cell-dependent (TD) responses. Upon BCR stimulation by an antigen presented by follicular dendritic cells (FDCs), B cells migrate to the boundary between the follicle and the outer T cell zone, where they interact with T_{fh} cells [7]. Cognate interaction of B cells and T_{fh} cells involves internalization and presentation of an antigen via the BCR, ligation of CD40 on the B cell by its ligand

http://dx.doi.org/10.5772/intechopen.68731

CD40L on the T_{fh} cell, as well as the cytokines IL-4 and IL-21. B cells then develop either into short-lived plasma cells that secrete low-affinity antibodies or they differentiate into GC B cells that further give rise to long-lived memory B cells and plasma cells producing high-affinity antibodies. While memory B cells enter the circulation, plasma cells migrate and home to the BM.

The activating signals from T_{fh} cells induce upregulation of activation-induced cytidine deaminase (AID), a DNA-editing enzyme that initiates somatic hypermutation (SHM) and class-switch recombination (CSR) [8]. Introduction of point mutation by AID into the variable region of the *IG* genes during SHM leads to highly variable Ig proteins that build the base for high-affinity antibodies [9]. During CSR, the constant parts of IgM and IgD (C_μ and C_δ, respectively) are replaced by C_γ, C_α or C_ε, giving rise to IgG, IgA or IgE. Thereby, CSR creates antibodies with diverse effector functions while retaining the antigen specificity [10]. B cells then differentiate into highly proliferating GC B cells called centroblasts before developing into centrocytes. As centrocytes, they screen antigens on the surface of FDC using their newly mutated BCR. High-affinity interaction with antigen results in survival and thus selection of centrocytes with high-affinity BCR, leading to recycling of centrocytes into centroblasts and to the differentiation of centrocytes into memory B cells and plasma cells.

During B cell development, however, B cells or their precursors occasionally undergo malignant transformation, which may result in the development of leukemia or lymphoma (**Figure 1**). Such transformations are frequently initiated by genetic events leading to aberrantly expressed proteins. Nevertheless, these chromosomal abnormalities alone are usually not sufficient for

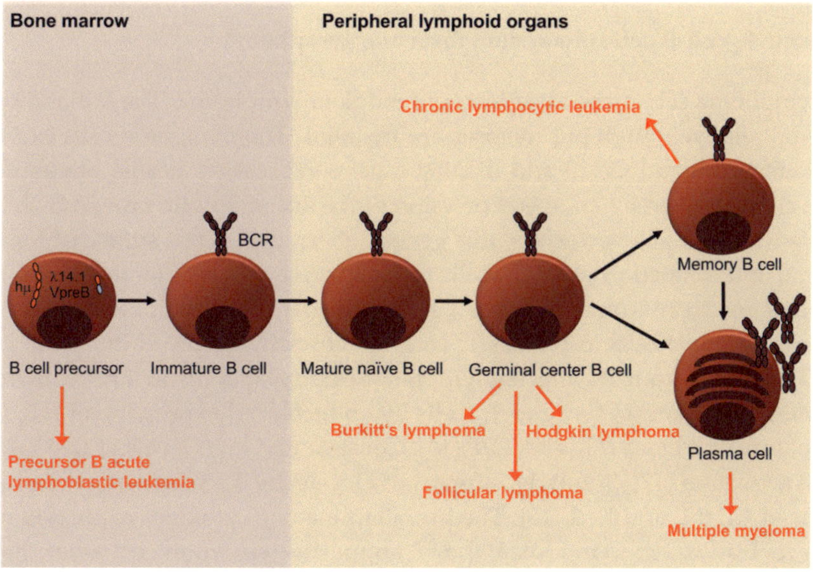

Figure 1. Schematic overview over the B cell development in the BM and GC with the most important developmental stages (black) and the B cell malignancies covered in this chapter (red). Red arrows indicate the presumed cell of origin of the malignant cells.

cancer development, and the transformed cells are not able to survive and outgrow when isolated and cultured *in vitro*. Thus, while mutations may trigger malignant transformation, interactions with the tumor microenvironment seem to be essential for the development and pathogenesis of most B cell malignancies.

2. Main body

2.1. Malignant T_h cell-B cell interaction

The tumor microenvironment plays a key role in supporting survival and expansion of cancer cells in virtually all known malignancies [11–13]. Malignancies of B cell origin often arise from GC B cells. Consequently, the cells of the GC microenvironment represent key collaboration partners of cancer cells during pathogenesis, progression and relapse of leukemia and lymphoma. The supportive tumor microenvironment in GC is made up by nonhematopoetic as well as lymphoid cells such as mesenchymal stromal cells, fibroblasts, macrophages, FDC and T_{fh} cells, which build a complex network and mutually regulate their activation differentiation, migration and expansion. Thus, while cells of the microenvironment support the tumor cells, the tumor cells in turn support and shape the cells that surround them in a way that maximizes their own benefit.

Generally, malignantly transformed B cells seem to retain their ability to interact with T_h cells, and thus remain capable of profiting from T_h cell help. Hence, while the support of normal mature B cells by T_h cells plays a central role in the generation of an adaptive immune response, the support of malignant B cells by T_h cells may promote lymphoma or leukemia.

2.2. Malignant T_h cell-B cell interaction: follicular lymphoma

Follicular lymphoma (FL) is the most frequent indolent lymphoma. The initial response rates to therapy are relatively high but relapses are frequent. The malignant cells express the GC B cell markers BCL6 and CD10 and display a gene expression profile of centrocytes [14]. FL cells are characterized by an overexpression of the antiapoptotic protein BCL2 caused by a t(14;18) translocation. Nevertheless, this genetic aberration is not sufficient for lymphoma development, and isolated primary FL cells fail to survive and proliferate *in vitro*, suggesting that the tumor microenvironment plays a major role in FL development and progression. Both nonhematopoietic cells as well as T_h cells are crucially involved in FL cell growth and survival [15]. T_{fh} cells from FL-affected lymph nodes display a distinct gene expression profile that differs from normal tonsillar T_{fh} cells by an increased expression of *IL2, IL4* and the proinflammatory cytokines *IFN* and *TNF* [16]. Consistently, high levels of IL-4 are associated with FL cell activation [17]. Similarly, support of FL cells by T_h cells seems to be mediated by T_{fh} cell-derived CD40L and IL-4 [18]. The proinflammatory cytokines expressed by T_{fh} of FL patients, in contrast, seem to modulate the FL supportive environment rather than having a direct effect on FL cells. TNF, e.g., has been suggested to sustain differentiation and survival of the lymphoid stroma network in FL [19].

Besides cytokines, the membrane-bound molecule CD40L is important for T_h cell-mediated FL cell support, since FL cells showed an increased survival when stimulated by CD40 cross-linking *in vitro* [20] as well as upon cognate interaction with T_h cells [21], and it has been suggested that CD40L stimulation protects FL cells from TRAIL-mediated apoptosis in an NF-κB-dependent manner [22].

About 70% of FL patients display BM infiltration at diagnosis. Interestingly, the affected BM is characterized by an overrepresentation of T_h cells [23]. This further supports the importance of T_{fh} cells in FL disease pathogenesis.

2.3. Malignant T_h cell-B cell interaction: Burkitt's lymphoma

Burkitt's lymphoma (BL) is an aggressive B cell cancer, probably arising from GC B cells [24]. Three main subtypes of BL are currently identified epidemiologically, though histologically the tumors are indistinguishable. Endemic BL (eBL), the classical BL, is found in malaria-endemic regions, while sporadic BL (sBL) is relatively rare and most commonly found outside malaria-affected areas. HIV-associated BL is often described as separate subtype as well [25]. eBL is strongly associated with the Epstein-Barr Virus (EBV), even though the pathogenic mechanism is not clear [26, 27]. The role of T_h cells in BL development and progression is highly controversial. Several studies showed that EBV-specific T_h cells can kill BL cell lines or EBV-transformed B cells [28–35] or limit their proliferation [36]. Most of these studies, however, used a nonphysiologically high effector to target ratio and thus require careful interpretation. Other researchers, in contrast, have reported that EBV-specific T_h cells induced B cell proliferation [37], and in several mouse models EBV-specific T_h cells were even required for lymphomagenesis [38–40]. Finally, two studies found that virus and autoantigen-specific T_h cells can both kill and support EBV-transformed B cells [41, 42], suggesting that the role of T_h cells in BL and other EBV-associated malignancies is likely to be context dependent. Interestingly, the chance of BL development in HIV patients is associated with $CD4^+$ T cell count, as the incident of BL development decreases with reduced $CD4^+$ T cell numbers [43], supporting a BL-promoting role for T_h cells.

2.4. Malignant T_h cell-B cell interaction: Hodgkin lymphoma

In Hodgkin lymphoma (HL), the malignant B cells—called Reed-Sternberg (RS) cells—constitute only a minor fraction of the tumor. The remainder consists of eosinophils, fibroblasts, macrophages, plasma cells and T_c as well as T_h cells. Infiltration of certain T_h cell subsets has been correlated with reduced overall patient survival, even though the exact function of these infiltrating T_h cells is not fully clear [44, 45]. Several cytokines seem to have a stimulatory effect on RS cells, one of which is the T_h2 cytokine IL-13 [46]. Nevertheless, IL-13 can also be produced by RS cells themselves and act in an autocrine manner. Thus, a direct role of T_h cells remains to be demonstrated. The complexity of the tumor microenvironment in HL, where a wide range of cells mutually influence each other, makes it intricate to discern the roles of the individual components.

2.5. Malignant T_h cell-B cell interaction: chronic lymphocytic leukemia

Chronic lymphocytic leukemia (CLL) is a malignancy of mature clonal $CD5^+$ B cells, although the precise cell of origin is still debated [47]. CLL cells proliferate in pseudofollicles in secondary lymphoid organs and in the BM, where they receive support from cells of the stromal microenvironment [48]. CLL cells were found to interact with endothelial cells, stroma cells and monocyte-derived nurse-like cells, and to receive antiapoptotic signals via cytokines and chemokines. In addition, T_h cells infiltrate such CLL pseudofollicles [49]. The infiltrating T_h cells were shown to have an activated phenotype and to be actively recruited to these niches by CLL cells via chemokines [50]. Furthermore, they were able to activate CLL cells and to induce an upregulation of the surface molecule CD38, which is associated with poor prognosis [51].

We hypothesized that proliferation of CLL cells in patients was driven by a cognate interaction of T_h cells with CLL cells, comparable to the physiological interaction between T_h cells and GC B cells [52]. According to this hypothesis, CLL cells would present antigen to antigen-specific T_h cells and in turn receive stimuli for their survival. Such an antigen could either be endogenous or it could be derived from an external pathogen. A key premise for this mechanism of CLL expansion in patients is the ability of resting CLL cells to efficiently activate T_h cells. Thus, to study the antigen-presentation capacity of CLL cells, we used a human T_h cell clone that is specific for a peptide derived from the mouse Ig kappa (Igκ) light chain [53], and human leukocyte antigen (HLA)-matched CLL cells from CLL patients, which allowed us to study antigen-dependent cognate interaction of CLL cells and T_h cells (**Figure 2**). Using this model, we found that CLL cells were able to endocytose antigen through endocytic receptors such as the Fc receptors CD32 and CD23 and through their BCR. Furthermore, CLL cells were surprisingly potent stimulators of T_h cell proliferation. With the exception of one patient, the

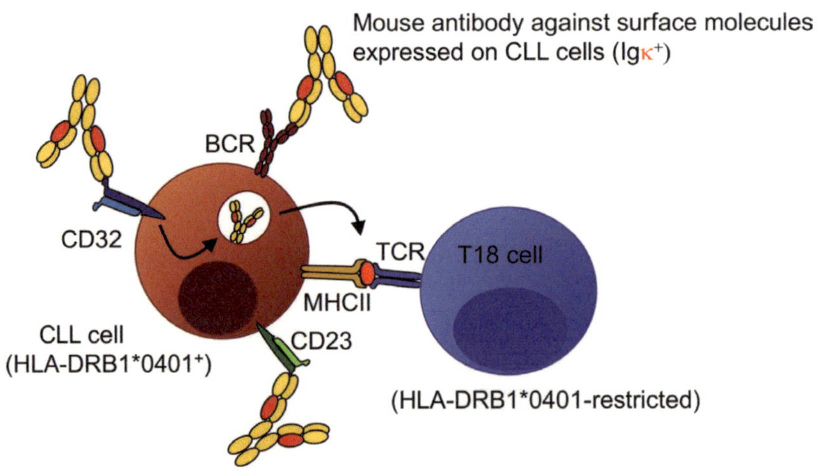

Figure 2. Model system to assess the antigen-presentation capacity of CLL cells: HLA-DRB1*0401⁺ CLL cells are cocultured with a human T_h cell clone (T18) that is specific for an epitope in mouse Igκ chain, when presented on HLA-DRB1*0401. Mouse $Ig\kappa^+$ antibodies against various surface molecules on the CLL cells such as CD23, CD32 or BCR are added. T18 cell proliferation is assessed as a read out for the capacity of CLL cells to endocytose and process these antibodies and to present Igκ peptides to the T18 cells together with provision of costimulatory signals.

function of CLL cells was comparable to that of normal B cells. Reciprocally, CLL cells were activated by antigen-activated T_h cells. They upregulated the activation markers CD38 and CD69, and molecules involved in the interaction with T_h cells such as HLA-DR, the costimulatory molecule CD86, the adhesion molecule CD54 and receptors for T_h cell help such as CD40 and CD25. Surface expression of CD27 and CD275 (ICOS-ligand) was reduced, in line with activation-induced shedding. In addition, CLL cells proliferated upon interaction with T_h cells, which was dependent on antigen and cell-cell contacts, as well as on CD40-CD40L interaction. Furthermore, the T_h cell-stimulated CLL cells had a gene expression profile similar to CLL cells within CLL proliferation centers, suggesting that *in vitro* interactions with T_h cells reflected interactions with the lymph node microenvironment in patients.

While the results obtained using this model system demonstrated that CLL cells had the ability to activate T_h cells and receive help for their survival and proliferation, it remained to be elucidated whether such interaction actually occurred in CLL patients. Indeed, we found that CLL patients harbored T_h cells that proliferated in response to both autologous CLL cells as well as autologous CLL cell lysate presented by peripheral blood mononuclear cells (PBMCs) from HLA-matched donors. Similar to the results obtained using the model system, CLL-specific T_h cells stimulated CLL cell activation and proliferation in an antigen- and CD40L-dependent manner. In *in vivo* xenograft experiments, the T_h cell-induced CLL proliferation was even more pronounced, suggesting that stromal factors may act synergistically during the T_h cell-CLL cell collaboration.

The remaining unresolved point was the identification of the antigenic source of the cognate interaction between T_h cells and CLL cells. The hypervariable regions of the CLL cells' BCR represent good candidate for endogenous antigens, since peptides derived from these regions are presented on major histocompatibility complex class II (MHCII), and are likely to be recognized as foreign by autologous T_h cells.

To test this hypothesis, we used monoclonal antibodies derived from CLL cell hybridoma as source of antigen and HLA-matched donor PBMC as antigen-presenting cells, and assessed proliferation of autologous T_h cells. Indeed, a significant fraction of T_h cells proliferated upon stimulation with CLL-BCR-derived antigen, demonstrating that effector T_h cells specific for endogenous CLL antigens are present in CLL patients and that they can support CLL cell activation and expansion.

Interestingly, the patient-derived CLL-specific T_h cells had a T_h1-like phenotype, characterized by IFN-γ secretion as well as expression of the IFN-γ-associated transcription factor T-bet and the surface markers CXCR3 and CCR5. In contrast, they lacked typical T_{fh} markers such as CXCR5, ICOS, PD-1, or IL-21 and BCL-6. These findings are in agreement with the observation that IFN-γ levels in CLL patients as well as IFN-γR expression on CLL cells correlated with disease severity [54–56]. Even though the exact mechanisms remain to be elucidated, IFN-γ seems to confer resistance to apoptosis and to increase CLL migration. We further demonstrated that IFN-γ secretion was a major mechanism by which CLL-specific T_h cells increased CD38 expression on CLL cells [57]. CD38 levels on CLL cells are an indicator of poor prognosis, even though a mechanistic involvement of CD38 in CLL pathogenesis is still debated [58]. Within a patient, proliferating CLL cells are more frequently found in the population that has a higher CD38 expression, and CD38 has been linked to CLL cell migration and survival. In our studies, we found that expression of the IFN-γ-inducible transcription factor T-bet in peripheral blood CLL cells is significantly correlated with CD38 expression [57]. Furthermore, T_h cell-derived IFN-γ upregulated CD38 in a mechanism that involved binding of the transcription factor T-bet to two consensus sites in 5′-regulatory regions of intron 1 of the *CD38* gene. Thus, it seems that T_h cell promote the development of a more aggressive CLL subset through secretion of IFN-γ.

CLL cells seem to express polyreactive and/or autoreactive BCR that provide a certain level of constant signaling [59, 60]. However, sustained BCR signaling can induce anergy and apoptosis. Our studies are in agreement with the view that CLL cells are autoreactive B cells that are rescued from anergy by combined BCR and CD40L activation [50–52, 57, 61, 62]. BCR signaling components such as the kinase Syk are promising drug targets in CLL [63–65]. Thus, we studied how BCR pathway inhibitors may impact the T_h cell help of CLL cells [66]. Interestingly, we found that stimulation by CD40L activated the BCR pathway in CLL cells, including Syk and the downstream components Akt, BLNK, Btk/Itk and pErk1/2. This activation—indicated by blastogenesis and proliferation—was significantly higher in CLL cells compared to normal B cells and could be blocked by Syk inhibition in CLL cells but not in normal B cells.

2.6. Malignant T_h cell-B cell interaction: multiple myeloma

Multiple myeloma (MM) is a malignancy characterized by the expansion of plasma cell-derived myeloma cells in the BM. The BM of MM patients and patients with monoclonal gammopathy of undetermined significance (MGUS) display increased numbers of T cells [67], but their role in MM disease development is not fully understood. Primary human MM cells express MHCII molecules as well as the costimulatory molecules CD80 and CD86 and have been shown to be good antigen-presenting cells for T_h cells [68, 69]. In addition to the fact that they express high levels of CD40, this suggests that they can participate in cognate interactions with T_h cells and benefit from their support. Indeed, CD40 stimulation induced MM cell migration, which is associated with MM disease progression [70]. CD40 stimulation also triggered secretion of IL-6 by myeloma cells, which may mediate MM cell proliferation in an autocrine and/or paracrine mechanism [71]. In addition to CD40L-mediated stimulation, myeloma-specific T_h cells can also support MM cells by secreting cytokines [72]. T_h17 cytokines such as IL-17 enhanced proliferation of MM cell lines *in vitro* and *in vivo*, and supported colony formation of primary human MM cells.

Very recently, we demonstrated that polyclonally activated allogeneic as well as autologous T_h cells stimulated blastogenesis and proliferation of MM cells in a CD40L-dependent manner [73]. MM cells increased their cell size, became more granular, reduced their cell surface Ig expression and upregulated the expression of HLA-DR. Proliferation of MM cells was even more pronounced when the T_h cell growth factors IL-2 and IL-15 were added. The T_h cells from MM patients expressed the chemokine receptors CXCR3 and CCR6 and the transcription factor T-bet as well as low levels of ROR-γt, thus displayed a T_h1/17 phenotype. Compared to T_h cells from healthy controls, the MM patient-derived T_h cells produced lower amounts of IL-4,

IL-10, IL-13, and IFN-γ and TNF-α, but higher levels of IL-1β, IL-2, IL-6 and IL-17. Together, our recent study and the previous reports by others suggest that CD40L stimulations is a key mechanism in T_h cell-mediated MM cell support, but cytokines such as IL-6 and IL-17 are important components as well.

2.7. Malignant T_h cell-B cell interaction: precursor B cell acute lymphoblastic leukemia

The B cell malignancies described in this chapter so far all originate from mature B cells. In contrast, precursor B acute lymphoblastic leukemia (BCP-ALL) derives from B cells of precursor stages during B cell development in the BM. As in most malignancies, the tumor microenvironment plays a key role in BCP-ALL development and progression [12]. Mesenchymal stromal cells, BM endothelial cells, osteoblasts as well as adipocytes have been described to support survival and proliferation of BCP-ALL cells and to confer drug resistance in mechanisms involving both soluble factors and cell membrane-bound molecules.

Memory T_h cells generated in the periphery during an immune response migrate to the BM in order to provide long-term memory [74–77]. These BM T_h cells seem to play a crucial role in normal hematopoiesis [78], but the knowledge about the physiological interactions between BM T_h cells and normal precursor B cells is very limited. Both normal precursor B cells and BCP-ALL cells express CD40 [79], MHCII, molecules for adhesion and costimulation [80], receptors for cytokines such as IL-2 and IL-6 [81–85] and receptors for BAFF [86, 87]. Thus, they possess all molecules required for cognate interaction with T_h cells and therefore seem to be capable of receiving support through the conventional T_h cell-B cells interaction pathways. BCP-ALL cells are indeed able to respond to CD40L stimulation with proliferation [88] and with upregulation of the surface molecule CD70 [89]. Furthermore, they upregulate the receptor for IL-3 [90], a cytokine that induces BCP-ALL cell proliferation. Stimulation with CD40L also induces the secretion of chemoattractants [91] and upregulates components of the antigen-processing machinery [92], suggesting that BCP-ALL cells are able to attract T_h cells and activate them, thereby inducing a positive feedback loop. T_h cell-derived *cytokines* can act on BCP-ALL cells as well, albeit with diverse effects. IL-2, IL-17 and IL-21, e.g., have been found to stimulate proliferation [83, 93], while IL-4 and IL-13 inhibited BCP-ALL cell growth [88, 94–96], and IL-4 as well as TGF-β-induced apoptosis [97, 98]. Cell-cell contact of BCP-ALL cells and activated allogenic T_h cells induced activation and maturation of BCP-ALL cells [99]. Further support of an involvement of T_h cell in BCP-ALL development comes from the observation that BCP-ALL is associated with certain MHCII haplotypes, suggesting that antigen-presentation to T_h cells is involved in the pathogenic mechanisms contributing to BCP-ALL development [100, 101]. In summary, there is evidence that BCP-ALL possess the capacity to exploit microenvironmental T_h cells, but whether such leukemia supportive T_h cell-BCP-ALL cell interactions actually taking place in patients remains to be determined.

2.8. Concluding remarks

The tumor microenvironment plays a key role in supporting malignant cells. In B cell leukemia and lymphoma, the malignant B cells seem to have retained their ability to receive help from their physiological interaction partners, the T_h cells. Consistently, current research supports a contribution of T_h cells to the development and progression of various types of B cell malignancies. Effective anticancer therapies should include targeting the cells of the tumor microenvironment. Thus, research efforts leading to the identification and characterization of malignant collaboration between T_h cells and malignant B cells may provide novel strategies for therapies aiming to target the tumor microenvironment.

Author details

Simone Bürgler

Address all correspondence to: simone.buergler@kispi.uzh.ch

Experimental Infectious Diseases and Cancer Research, University Children's Hospital Zurich, Zurich, Switzerland

References

[1] Cooper MD, Alder MN. The evolution of adaptive immune systems. Cell. 2006;**124**(4): 815-822

[2] Mosmann TR, Cherwinski H, Bond MW, Giedlin MA, Coffman RL. Two types of murine helper T cell clone. I. Definition according to profiles of lymphokine activities and secreted proteins. 1986. Journal of Immunology. 2005;**175**(1):5-14

[3] Liston A, Gray DH. Homeostatic control of regulatory T cell diversity. Nature Reviews Immunology. 2014;**14**(3):154-165

[4] Schaerli P, Willimann K, Lang AB, Lipp M, Loetscher P, Moser B. CXC chemokine receptor 5 expression defines follicular homing T cells with B cell helper function. The Journal of Experimental Medicine. 2000;**192**(11):1553-1562

[5] Johnston RJ, Poholek AC, DiToro D, Yusuf I, Eto D, Barnett B, et al. Bcl6 and Blimp-1 are reciprocal and antagonistic regulators of T follicular helper cell differentiation. Science. 2009;**325**(5943):1006-1010

[6] Bauquet AT, Jin H, Paterson AM, Mitsdoerffer M, Ho IC, Sharpe AH, et al. The costimulatory molecule ICOS regulates the expression of c-Maf and IL-21 in the development of follicular T helper cells and TH-17 cells. Nature Immunology. 2009;**10**(2):167-175

[7] MacLennan IC. Germinal centers. Annual Review of Immunology. 1994;**12**:117-139

[8] Muramatsu M, Kinoshita K, Fagarasan S, Yamada S, Shinkai Y, Honjo T. Class switch recombination and hypermutation require activation-induced cytidine deaminase (AID), a potential RNA editing enzyme. Cell. 2000;**102**(5):553-563

[9] Papavasiliou FN, Schatz DG. Somatic hypermutation of immunoglobulin genes: Merging mechanisms for genetic diversity. Cell. 2002;**109**(Suppl):S35-S44

[10] Chaudhuri J, Alt FW. Class-switch recombination: Interplay of transcription, DNA deamination and DNA repair. Nature Reviews Immunology. 2004;**4**(7):541-552

[11] Sison EA, Brown P. The bone marrow microenvironment and leukemia: Biology and therapeutic targeting. Expert Review of Hematology. 2011;**4**(3):271-283

[12] Purizaca J, Meza I, Pelayo R. Early lymphoid development and microenvironmental cues in B-cell acute lymphoblastic leukemia. Archives of Medical Research. 2012;**43**(2):89-101

[13] Ayala F, Dewar R, Kieran M, Kalluri R. Contribution of bone microenvironment to leukemogenesis and leukemia progression. Leukemia. 2009;**23**(12):2233-2241

[14] Shaffer AL, 3rd, Young RM, Staudt LM. Pathogenesis of human B cell lymphomas. Annual Review of Immunology. 2012;**30**:565-610

[15] Ame-Thomas P, Tarte K. The yin and the yang of follicular lymphoma cell niches: Role of microenvironment heterogeneity and plasticity. Seminars in Cancer Biology. 2014;**24**:23-32

[16] Ame-Thomas P, Le Priol J, Yssel H, Caron G, Pangault C, Jean R, et al. Characterization of intratumoral follicular helper T cells in follicular lymphoma: Role in the survival of malignant B cells. Leukemia. 2012;**26**(5):1053-1063

[17] Calvo KR, Dabir B, Kovach A, Devor C, Bandle R, Bond A, et al. IL-4 protein expression and basal activation of Erk *in vivo* in follicular lymphoma. Blood. 2008;**112**(9):3818-3826

[18] Pangault C, Ame-Thomas P, Ruminy P, Rossille D, Caron G, Baia M, et al. Follicular lymphoma cell niche: Identification of a preeminent IL-4-dependent T(FH)-B cell axis. Leukemia. 2010;**24**(12):2080-2089

[19] Ame-Thomas P, Maby-El Hajjami H, Monvoisin C, Jean R, Monnier D, Caulet-Maugendre S, et al. Human mesenchymal stem cells isolated from bone marrow and lymphoid organs support tumor B-cell growth: Role of stromal cells in follicular lymphoma pathogenesis. Blood. 2007;**109**(2):693-702

[20] Johnson PW, Watt SM, Betts DR, Davies D, Jordan S, Norton AJ, et al. Isolated follicular lymphoma cells are resistant to apoptosis and can be grown *in vitro* in the CD40/stromal cell system. Blood. 1993;**82**(6):1848-1857

[21] Umetsu DT, Esserman L, Donlon TA, DeKruyff RH, Levy R. Induction of proliferation of human follicular (B type) lymphoma cells by cognate interaction with CD4+T cell clones. Journal of Immunology. 1990;**144**(7):2550-2557

[22] Travert M, Ame-Thomas P, Pangault C, Morizot A, Micheau O, Semana G, et al. CD40 ligand protects from TRAIL-induced apoptosis in follicular lymphomas through NF-kappaB activation and up-regulation of c-FLIP and Bcl-xL. Journal of Immunology. 2008;**181**(2):1001-1011

[23] Wahlin BE, Sander B, Christensson B, Ostenstad B, Holte H, Brown PD, et al. Entourage: The immune microenvironment following follicular lymphoma. Blood Cancer Journal. 2012;**2**(1):e52

[24] Jaffe ES, Pittaluga S. Aggressive B-cell lymphomas: A review of new and old entities in the WHO classification. Hematology/The Education Program of the American Society of Hematology. 2011;**2011**:506-514

[25] Young LS, Rickinson AB. Epstein-Barr virus: 40 years on. Nature Reviews Cancer. 2004;**4**(10):757-768

[26] Magrath I. The pathogenesis of Burkitt's lymphoma. Advances in Cancer Research. 1990;**55**:133-270

[27] Bornkamm GW. Epstein-Barr virus and the pathogenesis of Burkitt's lymphoma: More questions than answers. The International Journal of Cancer. 2009;**124**(8):1745-1755

[28] Sun Q, Burton RL, Lucas KG. Cytokine production and cytolytic mechanism of CD4(+) cytotoxic T lymphocytes in ex vivo expanded therapeutic Epstein-Barr virus-specific T-cell cultures. Blood. 2002;**99**(9):3302-3309

[29] Adhikary D, Behrends U, Moosmann A, Witter K, Bornkamm GW, Mautner J. Control of Epstein-Barr virus infection *in vitro* by T helper cells specific for virion glycoproteins. The Journal of Experimental Medicine. 2006;**203**(4):995-1006

[30] Landais E, Saulquin X, Scotet E, Trautmann L, Peyrat MA, Yates JL, et al. Direct killing of Epstein-Barr virus (EBV)-infected B cells by CD4 T cells directed against the EBV lytic protein BHRF1. Blood. 2004;**103**(4):1408-1416

[31] Khanolkar A, Yagita H, Cannon MJ. Preferential utilization of the perforin/granzyme pathway for lysis of Epstein-Barr virus-transformed lymphoblastoid cells by virus-specific CD4+T cells. Virology. 2001;**287**(1):79-88

[32] Freeman ML, Burkum CE, Cookenham T, Roberts AD, Lanzer KG, Huston GE, et al. CD4 T cells specific for a latency-associated gamma-herpesvirus epitope are polyfunctional and cytotoxic. Journal of Immunology. 2014;**193**(12):5827-5834

[33] von Gegerfelt A, Valentin A, Alicea C, Van Rompay KK, Marthas ML, Montefiori DC, et al. Emergence of simian immunodeficiency virus-specific cytotoxic CD4+T cells and increased humoral responses correlate with control of rebounding viremia in CD8-depleted macaques infected with Rev-independent live-attenuated simian immunodeficiency virus. Journal of Immunology. 2010;**185**(6):3348-3358

[34] Fu T, Voo KS, Wang RF. Critical role of EBNA1-specific CD4+T cells in the control of mouse Burkitt lymphoma *in vivo*. The Journal of Clinical Investigation. 2004;**114**(4):542-550

[35] Paludan C, Bickham K, Nikiforow S, Tsang ML, Goodman K, Hanekom WA, et al. Epstein-Barr nuclear antigen 1-specific CD4(+) Th1 cells kill Burkitt's lymphoma cells. Journal of Immunology. 2002;**169**(3):1593-1603

[36] Nikiforow S, Bottomly K, Miller G. CD4+T-cell effectors inhibit Epstein-Barr virus-induced B-cell proliferation. Journal of Virology. 2001;**75**(8):3740-3752

[37] Fu Z, Cannon MJ. Functional analysis of the CD4(+) T-cell response to Epstein-Barr virus: T-cell-mediated activation of resting B cells and induction of viral BZLF1 expression. Journal of Virology. 2000;**74**(14):6675-6679

[38] Coles RE, Boyle TJ, DiMaio JM, Berend KR, Via DF, Lyerly HK. T cells or active Epstein-Barr virus infection in the development of lymphoproliferative disease in human B cell-injected severe combined immunodeficient mice. The Annals of Surgical Oncology. 1994;**1**(5):405-410

[39] Ma SD, Xu X, Plowshay J, Ranheim EA, Burlingham WJ, Jensen JL, et al. LMP1-deficient Epstein-Barr virus mutant requires T cells for lymphomagenesis. The Journal of Clinical Investigation. 2015;**125**(1):304-315

[40] Veronese ML, Veronesi A, D'Andrea E, Del Mistro A, Indraccolo S, Mazza MR, et al. Lymphoproliferative disease in human peripheral blood mononuclear cell-injected SCID mice. I. T lymphocyte requirement for B cell tumor generation. The Journal of Experimental Medicine. 1992;**176**(6):1763-1767

[41] Linnerbauer S, Behrends U, Adhikary D, Witter K, Bornkamm GW, Mautner J. Virus and autoantigen-specific CD4+T cells are key effectors in a SCID mouse model of EBV-associated post-transplant lymphoproliferative disorders. PLOS Pathogens. 2014;**10**(5):e1004068

[42] MacArthur GJ, Wilson AD, Birchall MA, Morgan AJ. Primary CD4+T-cell responses provide both helper and cytotoxic functions during Epstein-Barr virus infection and transformation of fetal cord blood B cells. Journal of Virology. 2007;**81**(9):4766-4775

[43] Guech-Ongey M, Simard EP, Anderson WF, Engels EA, Bhatia K, Devesa SS, et al. AIDS-related Burkitt lymphoma in the United States: What do age and CD4 lymphocyte patterns tell us about etiology and/or biology? Blood. 2010;**116**(25):5600-5604

[44] Alvaro T, Lejeune M, Salvado MT, Bosch R, Garcia JF, Jaen J, et al. Outcome in Hodgkin's lymphoma can be predicted from the presence of accompanying cytotoxic and regulatory T cells. Clinical Cancer Research. 2005;**11**(4):1467-1473

[45] Muenst S, Hoeller S, Dirnhofer S, Tzankov A. Increased programmed death-1+tumor-infiltrating lymphocytes in classical Hodgkin lymphoma substantiate reduced overall survival. Human Pathology. 2009;**40**(12):1715-1722

[46] Skinnider BF, Mak TW. The role of cytokines in classical Hodgkin lymphoma. Blood. 2002;**99**(12):4283-4297

[47] Chiorazzi N, Ferrarini M. Cellular origin(s) of chronic lymphocytic leukemia: Cautionary notes and additional considerations and possibilities. Blood. 2011;**117**(6):1781-1791

[48] Burger JA, Ghia P, Rosenwald A, Caligaris-Cappio F. The microenvironment in mature B-cell malignancies: A target for new treatment strategies. Blood. 2009;**114**(16):3367-3375

[49] Pizzolo G, Chilosi M, Ambrosetti A, Semenzato G, Fiore-Donati L, Perona G. Immunohistologic study of bone marrow involvement in B-chronic lymphocytic leukemia. Blood. 1983;**62**(6):1289-1296

[50] Ghia P, Strola G, Granziero L, Geuna M, Guida G, Sallusto F, et al. Chronic lymphocytic leukemia B cells are endowed with the capacity to attract CD4+, CD40L+T cells by producing CCL22. The European Journal of Immunology. 2002;**32**(5):1403-1413

[51] Patten PE, Buggins AG, Richards J, Wotherspoon A, Salisbury J, Mufti GJ, et al. CD38 expression in chronic lymphocytic leukemia is regulated by the tumor microenvironment. Blood. 2008;**111**(10):5173-5181

[52] Os A, Burgler S, Ribes AP, Funderud A, Wang D, Thompson KM, et al. Chronic lymphocytic leukemia cells are activated and proliferate in response to specific T helper cells. Cell Reports. 2013;**4**(3):566-577

[53] Schjetne KW, Thompson KM, Aarvak T, Fleckenstein B, Sollid LM, Bogen B. A mouse C kappa-specific T cell clone indicates that DC-SIGN is an efficient target for antibody-mediated delivery of T cell epitopes for MHC class II presentation. International Immunology. 2002;**14**(12):1423-1430

[54] Buschle M, Campana D, Carding SR, Richard C, Hoffbrand AV, Brenner MK. Interferon gamma inhibits apoptotic cell death in B cell chronic lymphocytic leukemia. The Journal of Experimental Medicine. 1993;**177**(1):213-218

[55] Wilkinson PC, Islam LN. Recombinant IL-4 and IFN-gamma activate locomotor capacity in human B lymphocytes. Immunology. 1989;**67**(2):237-243

[56] Cordingley FT, Bianchi A, Hoffbrand AV, Reittie JE, Heslop HE, Vyakarnam A, et al. Tumour necrosis factor as an autocrine tumour growth factor for chronic B-cell malignancies. Lancet. 1988;**1**(8592):969-971

[57] Burgler S, Gimeno A, Parente-Ribes A, Wang D, Os A, Devereux S, et al. Chronic lymphocytic leukemia cells express CD38 in response to Th1 cell-derived IFN-gamma by a T-bet-dependent mechanism. Journal of Immunology. 2015;**194**(2):827-835

[58] Burgler S. Role of CD38 expression in diagnosis and pathogenesis of chronic lymphocytic leukemia and its potential as therapeutic target. Critical Reviews in Immunology. 2015;**35**(5):417-432

[59] Stevenson FK, Krysov S, Davies AJ, Steele AJ, Packham G. B-cell receptor signaling in chronic lymphocytic leukemia. Blood. 2011;**118**(16):4313-4320

[60] Duhren-von Minden M, Ubelhart R, Schneider D, Wossning T, Bach MP, Buchner M, et al. Chronic lymphocytic leukaemia is driven by antigen-independent cell-autonomous signalling. Nature. 2012;**489**(7415):309-312

[61] Caligaris-Cappio F. B-chronic lymphocytic leukemia: A malignancy of anti-self B cells. Blood. 1996;**87**(7):2615-2620

[62] Muzio M, Apollonio B, Scielzo C, Frenquelli M, Vandoni I, Boussiotis V, et al. Constitutive activation of distinct BCR-signaling pathways in a subset of CLL patients: A molecular signature of anergy. Blood. 2008;**112**(1):188-195

[63] Friedberg JW, Sharman J, Sweetenham J, Johnston PB, Vose JM, Lacasce A, et al. Inhibition of Syk with fostamatinib disodium has significant clinical activity in non-Hodgkin lymphoma and chronic lymphocytic leukemia. Blood. 2010;**115**(13):2578-2585

[64] Spurgeon SE, Coffey G, Fletcher LB, Burke R, Tyner JW, Druker BJ, et al. The selective SYK inhibitor P505-15 (PRT062607) inhibits B cell signaling and function *in vitro* and *in vivo* and augments the activity of fludarabine in chronic lymphocytic leukemia. The Journal of Pharmacology and Experimental Therapeutics. 2013;**344**(2):378-387

[65] Sharman J, Hawkins M, Kolibaba K, Boxer M, Klein L, Wu M, et al. An open-label phase 2 trial of entospletinib (GS-9973), a selective spleen tyrosine kinase inhibitor, in chronic lymphocytic leukemia. Blood. 2015;**125**(15):2336-2343

[66] Parente-Ribes A, Skanland SS, Burgler S, Os A, Wang D, Bogen B, et al. Spleen tyrosine kinase inhibitors reduce CD40L-induced proliferation of chronic lymphocytic leukemia cells but not normal B cells. Haematologica. 2016;**101**(2):e59-e62

[67] Perez-Andres M, Almeida J, Martin-Ayuso M, Moro MJ, Martin-Nunez G, Galende J, et al. Characterization of bone marrow T cells in monoclonal gammopathy of undetermined significance, multiple myeloma, and plasma cell leukemia demonstrates increased infiltration by cytotoxic/Th1 T cells demonstrating a squed TCR-Vbeta repertoire. Cancer. 2006;**106**(6):1296-1305

[68] Yi Q, Dabadghao S, Osterborg A, Bergenbrant S, Holm G. Myeloma bone marrow plasma cells: Evidence for their capacity as antigen-presenting cells. Blood. 1997;**90**(5):1960-1967

[69] Walz S, Stickel JS, Kowalewski DJ, Schuster H, Weisel K, Backert L, et al. The antigenic landscape of multiple myeloma: Mass spectrometry (re)defines targets for T-cell-based immunotherapy. Blood. 2015;**126**(10):1203-1213

[70] Tai YT, Podar K, Mitsiades N, Lin B, Mitsiades C, Gupta D, et al. CD40 induces human multiple myeloma cell migration via phosphatidylinositol 3-kinase/AKT/NF-kappa B signaling. Blood. 2003;**101**(7):2762-2769

[71] Urashima M, Chauhan D, Uchiyama H, Freeman GJ, Anderson KC. CD40 ligand triggered interleukin-6 secretion in multiple myeloma. Blood. 1995;**85**(7):1903-1912

[72] Prabhala RH, Pelluru D, Fulciniti M, Prabhala HK, Nanjappa P, Song W, et al. Elevated IL-17 produced by TH17 cells promotes myeloma cell growth and inhibits immune function in multiple myeloma. Blood. 2010;**115**(26):5385-5392

[73] Wang D, Fløisand Y, Myklebust CV, Bürgler S, Parente-Ribes A, Hofgaard PO, et al. Autologous bone marrow Th cells can support multiple myeloma cell proliferation in vitro and in xenografted mice. Leukemia, 2017 Mar 28. doi: 10.1038/leu.2017.69

[74] Dhodapkar MV, Krasovsky J, Osman K, Geller MD. Vigorous premalignancy-specific effector T cell response in the bone marrow of patients with monoclonal gammopathy. The Journal of Experimental Medicine. 2003;**198**(11):1753-1757

[75] Herndler-Brandstetter D, Landgraf K, Jenewein B, Tzankov A, Brunauer R, Brunner S, et al. Human bone marrow hosts polyfunctional memory CD4+ and CD8+ T cells with close contact to IL-15-producing cells. Journal of Immunology. 2011;**186**(12):6965-6971

[76] Tokoyoda K, Zehentmeier S, Hegazy AN, Albrecht I, Grun JR, Lohning M, et al. Professional memory CD4+T lymphocytes preferentially reside and rest in the bone marrow. Immunity. 2009;**30**(5):721-730

[77] Okhrimenko A, Grun JR, Westendorf K, Fang Z, Reinke S, von Roth P, et al. Human memory T cells from the bone marrow are resting and maintain long-lasting systemic memory. Proceedings of the National Academy of Sciences of the United States of America. 2014;**111**(25):9229-9234

[78] Monteiro JP, Benjamin A, Costa ES, Barcinski MA, Bonomo A. Normal hematopoiesis is maintained by activated bone marrow CD4+T cells. Blood. 2005;**105**(4):1484-1491

[79] Law CL, Wormann B, LeBien TW. Analysis of expression and function of CD40 on normal and leukemic human B cell precursors. Leukemia. 1990;**4**(11):732-738

[80] Mirkowska P, Hofmann A, Sedek L, Slamova L, Mejstrikova E, Szczepanski T, et al. Leukemia surfaceome analysis reveals new disease-associated features. Blood. 2013; **121**(25):e149-e159

[81] Wormann B, Anderson JM, Ling ZD, LeBien TW. Structure/function analyses of IL-2 binding proteins on human B cell precursor acute lymphoblastic leukemias. Leukemia. 1987;**1**(9):660-666

[82] Inoue K, Sugiyama H, Ogawa H, Yamagami T, Azuma T, Oka Y, et al. Expression of the interleukin-6 (IL-6), IL-6 receptor, and gp130 genes in acute leukemia. Blood. 1994;**84**(8):2672-2680

[83] Touw I, Delwel R, Bolhuis R, van Zanen G, Lowenberg B. Common and pre-B acute lymphoblastic leukemia cells express interleukin 2 receptors, and interleukin 2 stimulates *in vitro* colony formation. Blood. 1985;**66**(3):556-561

[84] Kebelmann-Betzing C, Korner G, Badiali L, Buchwald D, Moricke A, Korte A, et al. Characterization of cytokine, growth factor receptor, costimulatory and adhesion molecule expression patterns of bone marrow blasts in relapsed childhood B cell precursor all. Cytokine. 2001;**13**(1):39-50

[85] Nakase K, Kita K, Miwa H, Nishii K, Shikami M, Tanaka I, et al. Clinical and prognostic significance of cytokine receptor expression in adult acute lymphoblastic leukemia: Interleukin-2 receptor alpha-chain predicts a poor prognosis. Leukemia. 2007;**21**(2):326-332

[86] Parameswaran R, Muschen M, Kim YM, Groffen J, Heisterkamp N. A functional receptor for B-cell-activating factor is expressed on human acute lymphoblastic leukemias. Cancer Research. 2010;**70**(11):4346-4356

[87] Maia S, Pelletier M, Ding J, Hsu YM, Sallan SE, Rao SP, et al. Aberrant expression of functional BAFF-system receptors by malignant B-cell precursors impacts leukemia cell survival. PLoS One. 2011;**6**(6):e20787

[88] Planken EV, Dijkstra NH, Bakkus M, Willemze R, Kluin-Nelemans JC. Proliferation of precursor B-lineage acute lymphoblastic leukaemia by activating the CD40 antigen. The British Journal of Haematology. 1996;**95**(2):319-326

[89] Troeger A, Glouchkova L, Ackermann B, Escherich G, Hanenberg H, Janka G, et al. Significantly increased CD70 up regulation on TEL-AML positive B cell precursor acute lymphoblastic leukemia cells following CD40 stimulation. Klinische Pädiatrie, 2014; 226(06/07): 332-337

[90] Zhou M, Gu L, Holden J, Yeager AM, Findley HW. CD40 ligand upregulates expression of the IL-3 receptor and stimulates proliferation of B-lineage acute lymphoblastic leukemia cells in the presence of IL-3. Leukemia. 2000;**14**(3):403-411

[91] Ghia P, Transidico P, Veiga JP, Schaniel C, Sallusto F, Matsushima K, et al. Chemoattractants MDC and TARC are secreted by malignant B-cell precursors following CD40 ligation and support the migration of leukemia-specific T cells. Blood. 2001;**98** (3):533-540

[92] Luczynski W, Kowalczuk O, Ilendo E, Stasiak-Barmuta A, Krawczuk-Rybak M. Upregulation of antigen-processing machinery components at mRNA level in acute lymphoblastic leukemia cells after CD40 stimulation. Annals of Hematology. 2007;**86**(5):339-345

[93] Bi L, Wu J, Ye A, Wu J, Yu K, Zhang S, et al. Increased Th17 cells and IL-17A exist in patients with B cell acute lymphoblastic leukemia and promote proliferation and resistance to daunorubicin through activation of Akt signaling. The Journal of Translational Medicine. 2016;**14**(1):132

[94] Okabe M, Kuni-eda Y, Sugiwura T, Tanaka M, Miyagishima T, Saiki I, et al. Inhibitory effect of interleukin-4 on the *in vitro* growth of Ph1-positive acute lymphoblastic leukemia cells. Blood. 1991;**78**(6):1574-1580

[95] Consolini R, Legitimo A, Cattani M, Simi P, Mattii L, Petrini M, et al. The effect of cytokines, including IL4, IL7, stem cell factor, insulin-like growth factor on childhood acute lymphoblastic leukemia. Leukemia Research. 1997;**21**(8):753-761

[96] Renard N, Duvert V, Banchereau J, Saeland S. Interleukin-13 inhibits the proliferation of normal and leukemic human B-cell precursors. Blood. 1994;**84**(7):2253-2260

[97] Manabe A, Coustan-Smith E, Kumagai M, Behm FG, Raimondi SC, Pui CH, et al. Interleukin-4 induces programmed cell death (apoptosis) in cases of high-risk acute lymphoblastic leukemia. Blood. 1994;**83**(7):1731-1737

[98] Buske C, Becker D, Feuring-Buske M, Hannig H, Wulf G, Schafer C, et al. TGF-beta inhibits growth and induces apoptosis in leukemic B cell precursors. Leukemia. 1997;**11**(3):386-392

[99] Renard N, Lafage-Pochitaloff M, Durand I, Duvert V, Coignet L, Banchereau J, et al. Demonstration of functional CD40 in B-lineage acute lymphoblastic leukemia cells in response to T-cell CD40 ligand. Blood. 1996;**87**(12):5162-5170

[100] Thompson P, Urayama K, Zheng J, Yang P, Ford M, Buffler P, et al. Differences in meiotic recombination rates in childhood acute lymphoblastic leukemia at an MHC class II hotspot close to disease associated haplotypes. PLoS One. 2014;**9**(6):e100480

[101] Taylor GM, Hussain A, Verhage V, Thompson PD, Fergusson WD, Watkins G, et al. Strong association of the HLA-DP6 supertype with childhood leukaemia is due to a single allele, DPB1*0601. Leukemia. 2009;**23**(5):863-869

Chapter 5

Multiple Players in the Mechanical Control of T Cell Quiescence

Ahmed Fadhil Neama, Chung Yeng Looi and
Won Fen Wong

Additional information is available at the end of the chapter

http://dx.doi.org/10.5772/intechopen.68869

Abstract

Naive T cells are kept in a quiescence state, characterized by small cell size, with low proliferative and metabolic activities, until antigen engagement. T lymphocyte quiescence is a tightly controlled mechanism regulated by multiple quiescence-associated factors. Loss or impaired functions of these factors regularly result in spontaneous activation of T cells that is ensured by fatal autoimmune diseases. Elucidating the mechanism to facilitate the switch on or off of T cells could be beneficial to ameliorate pathology triggered by T cell hyperactivation or dysfunction. In this chapter, we discuss multiple quiescence-associated factors along with the mechanisms utilized to promote lymphocyte quiescence and longevity.

Keywords: T cell quiescence, Foxo, KLF2

1. Introduction

T lymphocytes are important players in adaptive immune responses to invading pathogens. In an individual, T lymphocyte repertoires are principally generated through a somatic recombinant process named as VDJ rearrangement in the thymus. Upon maturation, these T cells exit thymus to reside in the secondary lymph organs and patrol in the circulation. It is crucial to maintain T cell repertoires as standby for future assault by diverse types of antigens that might come from the massive array of microbes. Eventually, most of the lymphocyte reservoirs do not encounter their cognate (or specific) antigens throughout their lifetime. These virgin or naïve T cells must be kept in a state known as quiescence to prevent immune activation that is often ensued by activation-induced cell exhaustion or death. At quiescence state, cells are sustained through homeostatic cell renewal without activation or expansion to maintain the size of the peripheral lymphocyte pool. Loss control of T cell quiescence has been associated with autoimmune diseases; hence, this stage is imperative to render an immune tolerance. In this chapter, we discuss the intricate transcriptional mechanism of T lymphocytes at quiescence stage to attain a long-term standby status until they encounter the cognate antigens.

Lymphocyte quiescence refers to a state of inaction of cells characterized by small cell size with limited cytoplasmic region, low rates of cell metabolism, proliferation, transcription, and translation activities. Quiescence suppresses cell activation and prevents the unnecessary use of energy resources that will be consumed by the huge T lymphocyte repertoires in an individual. In addition, cells at quiescence state can reduce genetic damage due to repetitive replication therefore preventing development of malignancy [1] because constant replication of lymphocytes may increase the risk of leukemia and lymphoma [2]. Upon identification of a specific antigen, activation of a T cell beyond the cell signaling threshold triggers cells to exit quiescence state in a non-reversible manner, thus, the T cell undergoes robust clonal expansion followed by cell cytotoxicity and cytokine-secreting activities.

A quiescence state of lymphocytes was previously regarded as a default stage of cells in the absence of antigen recognition activation [3]. However, recent evidences accumulated suggest that quiescence is a steadily regulated stage by functionally diverse mechanisms [4], which include intrinsic control by gene expression programs as well as extrinsic suppression by regulatory T cells (Treg). Evidence derived from the microarray study demonstrates strikingly distinct expression patterns of diverse molecules in the quiescence versus stimulated T lymphocytes [5, 6]. Following T cell activation, the major change in gene expression profile is not limited to only increased expression of genes that promote growth and differentiation but also suppression of a group of genes that is linked to the quiescence program [6, 7]. Transcription factors and components in cell cycle control play a central role in the quiescence regulation. Recently, ubiquitination degradation pathway has also been added into the growing list of the quiescence-associated factors [8].

A common characteristic shared by most of these quiescence-associated molecules is their high abundance in the naïve T cell but the expression has rapidly vanished upon cell activation. Quiescence molecules are different from other negative regulators of T cells such as cytotoxic T lymphocyte antigen 4 (CTLA4) and program cell death protein 1 (PD-1). Although both impose inhibitory signals on T cell proliferation and effector activity, it is important to note that the expression of quiescence molecules is usually high in naïve T cells but reduce upon cell activation. In contrast, CTLA4 and PD1-1 are expressed only after T cell activation.

Deficiency or dysfunction of the quiescence molecules often results in loss of the quiescence control marked by the cell's semi-activation to hyperactivation with robust proliferation, accompanied by exert activities such as cytokines secretion and predisposition to apoptotic cell death. The direct physical consequence to loss of T cells quiescence is impaired immune tolerance and development of autoimmune diseases in an individual. In this chapter, we will discuss several quiescence factors along with the mechanisms utilized to promote lymphocyte quiescence and longevity.

2. KLF2

The Sp/Kruppel-like factor (KLF) family of zinc-finger transcription factors contains at least 20 identified members, which include numerous Kruppel-like factors that have different roles across the mammalian system [9]. Kruppel-like family 2 (KLF2, also known as lung Kruppel-like factor or LKLF) has been implicated in programming T cell quiescence [10]. KLF2 is highly expressed in mature $CD4^+$ and $CD8^+$ T cells. Similar to many other key players in quiescence control, its expression is rapidly switched off after T cell activation [11]. KLF2 can also be detected in thymocytes at single-positive (SP) stage but not during earlier double-negative (DN) or double-positive (DP) stages [11]. KLF2 controls mature T cell egress from thymus [12] and recirculation through secondary lymphoid tissues [13] by regulating transcription of sphingosine-1-phosphate receptor 1 (S1Pr1). KLF2-deficient thymocytes show impaired thymocyte emigration, whereas KLF2-transduced T cells are prone to homing in lymphoid organs following adoptive transfer [14].

The conventional KLF2-deficient mice died between embryonic days, from 12.5 to 14.5, due to severe intra-embryonic and intra-amniotic hemorrhage resulting from defects in the smooth muscle cells migration during blood vessel maturation [15, 16]. To study KLF2-deficient T cells, a $Rag\text{-}2^{-/-}KLF2^{-/-}$ chimeric mouse system was applied, in which $KLF2^{-/-}$ embryonic stem cells were injected into $RAG2^{-/-}$ blastocyst to populate the T cell pool [11]. This model provides strong evidence supporting the role of KLF2 in the quiescence control. First, a massive loss (up to 90%) of the peripheral T cell is observed. Intriguingly, these KLF2-deficient T cells displayed stigmata of activated phenotype, that is, an increased cell size and surface expression of activation markers ($CD69^{hi}$ $CD44^{hi}$ $CD62L^{lo}$); however, these cells are non-proliferative. A large number of KLF2-deficient T cells are apoptotic, attributable to high surface expression of Fas ligand (FasL) [11].

In a different experiment using an overexpression model, in vitro forced expression of KLF2 in Jurkat T cells using doxycycline inducible system programs the cells into a quiescent phenotype [17]. KLF2 overexpression dramatically inhibits proliferation of Jurkat T cells and prevents synthesis of surface molecules such as CD30 and CD71, by which this effect can be reversible when the KLF2 expression is removed. KLF2-mediated regulation of quiescent T cells is partially achieved through its suppression of c-Myc. Conversely, transient expression of MadMyc, a dominant negative form of c-Myc, recapitulates the phenotype produced by KLF2 overexpression [17]. On the other hand, expression of neurotransmitter dopamine D4 receptor on resting T cells promotes T cell quiescence by upregulating KLF2 expression and an administration of U101958; a D4 antagonist could diminish the effect [18]. KLF2-deficient B cells showed increased apoptosis and impaired proliferation after B-cell receptor cross-linking [19]. B cell distribution and trafficking are disturbed due to low surface expression of CD62L and β7-integrin expression. Percentages of B cell subsets is also disturbed as B1 cells are almost disminished accompanied by increased in the number of MZ and transitional B cells. [19, 20]. These suggest a potential role of KLF2 in control of B-cell quiescence.

Another KLF family member, KLF4, also known as gut-enriched Kruppel-like factor or GKLF, is also important in T cell biology by regulating thymocyte development and IL-17 expression during Th17 differentiation [21]. Both thymocytes and mature T cells express high level of KLF4. In KLF4 knock-out mice, the proliferation of thymocytes at double-negative stage was significantly reduced, attributed to loss of KLF4 control on Cdkn1b, a cell cycle molecule. KLF4 is also involved in Th17 differentiation and IL-17 expression by which its deficiency contributes to reduced IL-17 production and thus ameliorates the severity of in vivo experimental autoimmune encephalomyelitis [21]. KLF4 is able to exert a global inhibitory effect on macromolecular biosynthesis, including protein biosynthesis, transcription, and cholesterol biosynthesis [22]. The expression pattern of KLF4 in B cells highly resembles those in T cells, whereby the expression is abundant in mature resting cells but rapidly decreased upon cell activation. In KLF4-deficient mice, a modest decrease in the numbers of pre-B cells in the bone marrow and mature B cells in the spleen can be observed [23]. Fewer B cells enter S phase of the cell cycle and complete cell division in response to BCR and/or CD40L engagement, in vitro, in the absence of KLF4, suggesting its role in maintaining quiescence in B cells. This could be a result of decreased expression of cyclin D2 in B cells because KLF4 regulates cyclin B2 through a direct binding to its promoter [23]. Thus, we can also postulate a potential role of KLF4 in controlling T or B lymphocytes quiescence.

3. Foxo

Forkhead box (Foxo) family genes are the orthologs of DAF-16 gene identified in nematode worm *Caenorhabditis elegans,* which programs cells for resistance to oxidative stress and cell cycle control to maintain cells at a dauer (non-action) state [24]. In mammals, there are three members in Foxo family, Foxo1, Foxo3, and Foxo4. The Foxo family of transcription factors triggers the induction or suppression of multiple target genes dependent on context molecules [25] and hence plays multiple functions in cell quiescence control [3, 26–29], including maintenance of stem cells pluripotency [30], oxidative stress control [31], cell cycle, cancer progress [32], and others. In T cells, Foxo molecules have multiple roles by controlling cell-surface molecules, signaling proteins, and nuclear factors that control gene expression [33]. Foxo1 is also detected in thymocyte subsets, dominant negative inhibition of Foxo1 causes increased proliferation capacity of thymocytes, thus interferes with central tolerance control [34].

In the animal model, Foxo1 deletion causes spontaneous T cell activation that leads to development of colitis [35]. Higher percentages of activated/memory T phenotypes have been reported in T cell-specific Foxo1 knock-out mice model [35, 36]. Besides, inflammatory bowel disease is also observed in the wildtype mice after receiving Foxo1-deficient T cells. In a mouse model with CD4 promoter-driven T cell-specific deletion of Foxo1, mice develop exocrine pancreatitis, hind limb paralysis, and multiorgan lymphocyte infiltration. Anti-nuclear antibodies and formation of germinal centers are detected in mice, suggesting Foxo1 suppresses cells from differentiating into follicular helper (T_{FH}) subtypes [37]. Foxo1-deficient T cells demonstrate a highly defective ability for cell homing to lymph nodes, due to impaired L-selectin [38] and CCR7 expression [36]. Although some argue that Foxo is not a true quiescence factor stating the activated phenotype may be due to its functions like cell trafficking, these distinct roles of Foxo may directly or indirectly impose lymphocyte quiescence.

In contrast to Foxo1's specific expression in lymphocytes, Foxo3 is ubiquitously expressed in many tissues in the body. It mediates cell death in many cells including T and B lymphocytes. The role of Foxo3 in the regulation of cell quiescence remains controversial. An earlier report using Fox3TRAP mice (created by retroviral gene-trap technique) demonstrates typical autoimmune characteristics including spontaneous lymphoproliferation, hyperactivation, and lymphocyte infiltration into multiple organs [39]. However, another two mice generated, using gene-trap, show no such symptoms except for abnormal ovary development [40, 41]. Different mice generated with targeted recombinant techniques demonstrated only some decrease in the number of pre-B and circulating B cells [42, 43]. Foxo3 protects quiescent cells from oxidative stress through regulation of antioxidant manganese superoxide dismutase (MnSOD) [44] and growth arrest, and damage response gene (Gadd45a) is a direct target of Foxo3a [45].

In the last decade, increasing numbers of target genes regulated by Foxo transcription factor have been identified. These include KLF2 [36], GTPase of immunity-associated protein 5 (Gimap5) [46], IL-7Ra, homing molecules (L-selectin, CCR7, and Fam65b), CTLA4 [37], and shingosine-1 phosphate receptor [38], among others. A major target of Foxo is KLF2, an essential transcription factor for quiescence control. Introduction of Foxo1 into T cells causes induction of KLF2 transcription factor while T cell's specific deletion of Foxo1 showed lower expression of KLF2 [36]. Foxo1 binds directly to promoter of KLF2 gene to induce its expression [47].

4. Foxp1

A member in the subfamily P of the large Fox family, Forkhead box protein P1 (Foxp1), has an essential role in B lymphopoiesis to control the expression of recombination-activating genes 1 and 2 and transition from pro B to pre B cells [48]. Foxp1 has been implicated in the quiescence control of naïve T cells by inhibiting IL-7Ra expression and diminishing signaling by the kinase Erk [49, 50]. Acute deletion of Foxp1 induces naïve T cells to gain effector phenotype. Homeostatic proliferation of quiescence cells is regulated by IL7 signaling pathway, which can be negatively regulated by autocrine feedback control of IL7Ra expression [51]. Transcription factor Foxp1 helps maintain the quiescence of naïve T cells by binding to 3.5 kb upstream of IL7R transcription start site and inhibiting IL-7Ra expression [36]. Foxp1 is a negative regulator of Foxo1 as they compete with each other for the forkhead binding site at IL7R enhancer region [49].

5. Tob

A member of the Tob family shares a highly conserved NH_2 terminal sequence. Tob is expressed in resting T cells as well as in anergic T cells [52]. Its expression is diminished upon T cell activation by anti-CD3/anti-CD28 or mitogen PMA stimulation. Forced expression of exogenous Tob molecule inhibits T cell proliferation. Tob interacts with Smad2 and Smad4 molecules and enhances Smad4, signaling to suppress the transcription of multiple cytokines including IL-2. Overexpression of Tob also blocks cell cycle progression by promoting p27kip1, a negative regulator of cell cycle. In contrast, the positive regulator of cell cycle molecules including cyclin E, cyclin A, and Cdk2 was suppressed. Elimination of Tob protein synthesis using antisense oligonucleotide reduces the threshold of T cell activation.

6. Tsc1

Tuberous sclerosis 1 (Tsc1) functions as a GTPase-activating protein (GAP) that binds small GTPase RHEB and negatively regulates mTOR1 signaling. Tsc1 is important in T cell biology in memory cell differentiation, effector, and regulatory functions [53, 54]. Tsc1 is also implicated in anergy T cells, and its expression is higher in anergy as compared to activated T cells [55]. Tsc1$^{-/-}$ T cells in mice model loss quiescence as demonstrated by increased cell surface marker (CD44^{hi}CD122^{-}) and prominent upregulation of activation markers such as CD69, CD25 and CD71 [56]. Besides, Tsc1$^{-/-}$ T cells demonstrated increased cell size, proliferation, reactive oxygen species (ROS) generation, and susceptibility to apoptosis. Tsc1 deficiency also dampens anti-bacterial immune response in animal model as reduced OVA-reactive tetramer-positive T cells and interferon-producing CD8^{+} T cells. The effect of Tsc1 deficiency is attributed to its ability to inhibit mTORC1 as this effect can be reverted by rapamycin treatment.

7. Slfn2

The word "schlafen" means sleeping in German. Schlafen (Slfn) family of genes, so-called owing to their ability to promote cells into an inactive state, consists of six genes with RNA helicase-like motif in human. Schlafen proteins promote growth inhibitory responses and play roles in thymocytes development [57], effector, and regulatory T cells [58]. Slfn2 was added to the gaining list of quiescence factors coincidentally when scientists investigate the phenotype in elektra mouse, a G_3 mice homozygous for chemically induced random germline mutation [59]. The eureka mice carry a single mutation in Slfn2, which results in isoleucine-to-asparagine substitution of amino acid residue 135, which is induced after exposure to N-ethyl-N-nitrosourea. Eureka mice are defenseless and succumb to lymphocytic choriomeningitis virus and *Listeria monocytogenes* infection due to immunodeficient phenotype. This increased susceptibility to bacterial and viral infections can be reversed with bacteria artificial chromosome (BAC) transgenesis of Sfln2 gene, thus confirming the role of Sfln2. Interestingly, T cells from eureka mice exist in a semi-activated state [59]. The T cells are generally lesser in amount but express higher surface activation marker (CD44^{hi}) and proliferate strongly and are more prone to apoptosis in response to anti-CD3/anti-CD28 activation signal. A chronic ER stress under steady-state conditions observed in Eureka T cells could explain the loss of immune cell quiescence [60]. Slfn2 has been suggested as a promising target for treating human T-ALL malignancy [61]. In T-ALL mice model, impaired Slfn2 functions rescue the mice from disease progress as the proliferation potential and survival of leukemic T cells are affected. In addition, the symptoms of severe lymphoproliferative disease in Fas deficient mice can also be rescued by Sfln2 loss-of-function mutation.

8. Runx1

Runx family comprise three members: Runx1 and Runx3 play crucial roles in T cell development and differentiation [62], whereas Runx2 is a key player in osteoblast differentiation during bone formation [63]. Runx1 knock-out mice die of impaired fetal hematopoiesis at embryonic day E12.5 [64]. Conditional knock-out mice driven by CD4-Cre promoter lead to low number of CD4+ T cell population attributed to apoptotic cell death. When an anti-apoptotic Bcl-2 transgene is introduced to rescue the T cells, Runx1$^{-/-}$ T cells demonstrate spontaneous hyperactivation (CD44^{hi}CD62L^{lo}) phenotype. This mouse model displays a breakdown of immune tolerance as the signs and complications of systemic inflammatory response syndrome (SIRS) such as cytokine storm, monocytosis, blood coagulation, and muscle wasting syndrome can be observed. Infiltration of Runx1$^{-/-}$ cells into the lung causes autoimmune lung disease similar to human pulmonary alveolar proteinosis (PAP) [65]. In addition, increased surface activation markers, CD40L and CD69, were observed along with increased cytokine, chemokines, and other signaling molecules [66]. It is noteworthy that similar to other quiescence factors such as KLF2, Runx1 is abundantly expressed in naïve T cells, and TCR signaling results in rapid reduction of Runx1 expression [67]. One possible mechanism of Runx1 to exert quiescence is through silencing the expression of cytokines IL-2. Besides, Runx1 may control quiescence indirectly through transcriptional control of Foxp1, Foxo1, and KLF2 by binding to their promoter region [66].

9. Peli

Ubiquitination is a post-translational mechanism for protein degradation. During ubiquitination, small ubiquitin proteins attach to the lysine residues of substrate protein catalyzed by sequential action of E1, E2, and E3 ubiquitin-activating enzymes. Ubiquitination process has been shown to involve in immune regulation [8, 68, 69]. Peli family is composed of three members, Peli1, Peli2, and Peli3 [70], among which E3 ligase Peli1 has been implicated in T cell quiescence control. CD4^{+} and CD8^{+} T cells from Peli-deficient mice demonstrate hyperactivation and increased proliferation response upon TCR-CD28 signaling [8]. Most of the Peli1$^{-/-}$ T cells turn into memory cells. Peli$^{-/-}$ mice develop autoimmune diseases, as demonstrated by multiorgan inflammation, detection of antinuclear autoantibody, and prominent immune complex deposition in kidney, and more pathogenic potentials are induced in experimental autoimmune encephalitis model [8].

10. Gimap5

Gimap5 stands for GTPase of immunity-associated protein 5. A missense mutation in the Gimap5 results in abrogation of quiescence and reduced number and survival of lymphocytes [46]. Gimap5-deficient CD4^{+} T cells from the mice are Th1/Th17 polarized and thus promotes colitis and early mortality. Gimap5 also plays a role in regulatory T cells because in its absence, regulatory T cells become reduced in frequency in the peripheral tissues and their immunosuppressive capacity becomes impaired.

11. Summary

Mature T lymphocytes in our body can remain in a quiescence state for a prolonged duration in the absence of infectious or stimulatory factors. Loss of T cell quiescence control leads to breakdown of immune tolerance and is the main causative factor for various types of autoimmune diseases, lymphoma, and leukemia. The understanding of the interaction among the multiple factors that are involved in intrinsic control of quiescence status is hence crucial to control the balance between immune tolerance and activation.

Acknowledgements

This study is supported by Fundamental Research Grant Scheme (FP030-2014A) from Malaysia Ministry of Higher Education.

Abbreviations

VDJ	variable, diversity and joining
Sp	Specificity protein transcription factors
IL	interleukin
BCR	reakpoint cluster region protein
PMA	phorbol 12-myristate 13-acetate
OVA	ovalbumin
ER	endoplasmic reticulum
CD	cluster of differentiation
Th17	helper T 17
RHEB	Ras homolog enriched in brain
CDKH1b	Cyclin-dependent kinase inhibitor 1B
CCR7	C-C chemokine receptor type 7
Fam65b	Family With Sequence Similarity 65 Member B
T-ALL	T-cell acute lymphoblastic leukaemia
Runx	Runt-related transcription factor
Peli	Pellino E3 Ubiquitin Protein Ligase
BCL-2	B-cell lymphoma 2

Author details

Ahmed Fadhil Neama[1], Chung Yeng Looi[2] and Won Fen Wong[3]*

Address all correspondence to: wonfen@um.edu.my

1 Center of Biotechnology Researches, University of Al-Nahrain, Baghdad, Iraq

2 School of Biosciences, Taylor's University, Subang Jaya, Malaysia

3 Department of Medical Microbiology, Faculty of Medicine, University of Malaya, Kuala Lumpur, Malaysia

References

[1] Tzachanis D, Boussiotis VA. Tob, a member of the APRO family, regulates immunological quiescence and tumor suppression. Cell Cycle. 2009;**8**:1019-1025. DOI: 10.4161/cc.8.7.8033

[2] Horton MR, Powell JD. Quieting T cells with Slfn2. Nature Immunology. 2010;**11**:281-282. DOI: 10.1038/ni0410-281

[3] Yusuf I, Fruman DA. Regulation of quiescence in lymphocytes. Trends in Immunology. 2003;**24**:380-386. DOI: S1471490603001418 [pii].

[4] Tzachanis D, Lafuente EM, Li L, Boussiotis VA. Intrinsic and extrinsic regulation of T lymphocyte quiescence. Leukemia & Lymphoma. 2004;**45**:1959-1967. DOI: 10.1080/1042819042000219494

[5] Feske S, Giltnane J, Dolmetsch R, Staudt LM, Rao A. Gene regulation mediated by calcium signals in T lymphocytes. Nature Immunology. 2001;**2**:316-324. DOI: 10.1038/86318

[6] Glynne R, Ghandour G, Rayner J, Mack DH, Goodnow CC. B-lymphocyte quiescence, tolerance and activation as viewed by global gene expression profiling on microarrays. Immunological Reviews. 2000;**176**:216-246

[7] Teague TK, Hildeman D, Kedl RM, Mitchell T, Rees W, Schaefer BC, Bender J, Kappler J, Marrack P. Activation changes the spectrum but not the diversity of genes expressed by T cells. Proceedings of the National Academy of Sciences of the United States of America. 1999;**96**:12691-12696

[8] Chang M, Jin W, Chang JH, Xiao Y, Brittain GC, Yu J, Zhou X, Wang YH, Cheng X, Li P, et al. The ubiquitin ligase Peli1 negatively regulates T cell activation and prevents autoimmunity. Nature Immunology. 2011;**12**:1002-1009. DOI: 10.1038/ni.2090

[9] Black AR, Black JD, Azizkhan-Clifford J. Sp1 and kruppel-like factor family of transcription factors in cell growth regulation and cancer. Journal of Cellular Physiology. 2001;**188**:143-160. DOI: 10.1002/jcp.1111

[10] Di Santo JP. Lung Krupple-like factor: A quintessential player in T cell quiescence. Nature Immunology. 2001;**2**:667-668. DOI: 10.1038/90598

[11] Kuo CT, Veselits ML, Leiden JM. LKLF: A transcriptional regulator of single-positive T cell quiescence and survival. Science. 1997;**277**:1986-1990

[12] Carlson CM, Endrizzi BT, Wu J, Ding X, Weinreich MA, Walsh ER, Wani MA, Lingrel JB, Hogquist KA, Jameson SC. Kruppel-like factor 2 regulates thymocyte and T-cell migration. Nature. 2006;**442**:299-302. DOI: 10.1038/nature04882

[13] Yamada T, Park CS, Mamonkin M, Lacorazza HD. Transcription factor ELF4 controls the proliferation and homing of CD8+ T cells via the Kruppel-like factors KLF4 and KLF2. Nature Immunology. 2009;**10**:618-626. DOI: 10.1038/ni.1730

[14] Bai A, Hu H, Yeung M, Chen J. Kruppel-like factor 2 controls T cell trafficking by activating L-selectin (CD62L) and sphingosine-1-phosphate receptor 1 transcription. Journal of Immunology. 2007;**178**:7632-7639

[15] Kuo CT, Veselits ML, Barton KP, Lu MM, Clendenin C, Leiden JM. The LKLF transcription factor is required for normal tunica media formation and blood vessel stabilization during murine embryogenesis. Genes & Development. 1997;**11**:2996-3006

[16] Wu J, Bohanan CS, Neumann JC, Lingrel JB. KLF2 transcription factor modulates blood vessel maturation through smooth muscle cell migration. Journal of Biological Chemistry. 2008;**283**:3942-3950. DOI: 10.1074/jbc.M707882200

[17] Buckley AF, Kuo CT, Leiden JM. Transcription factor LKLF is sufficient to program T cell quiescence via a c-Myc-dependent pathway. Nature Immunology. 2001;**2**:698-704. DOI: 10.1038/90633

[18] Sarkar C, Das S, Chakroborty D, Chowdhury UR, Basu B, Dasgupta PS, Basu S. Cutting edge: Stimulation of dopamine D4 receptors induce T cell quiescence by up-regulating Kruppel-like factor-2 expression through inhibition of ERK1/ERK2 phosphorylation. Journal of Immunology. 2006;**177**:7525-7529

[19] Hart GT, Wang X, Hogquist KA, Jameson SC. Kruppel-like factor 2 (KLF2) regulates B-cell reactivity, subset differentiation, and trafficking molecule expression. Proceedings of the National Academy of Sciences of the United States of America. 2011;**108**:716-721. DOI: 10.1073/pnas.1013168108

[20] Winkelmann R, Sandrock L, Porstner M, Roth E, Mathews M, Hobeika E, Reth M, Kahn ML, Schuh W, Jack HM. B cell homeostasis and plasma cell homing controlled by Kruppel-like factor 2. Proceedings of the National Academy of Sciences of the United States of America. 2011;**108**:710-715. DOI: 10.1073/pnas.1012858108

[21] An J, Golech S, Klaewsongkram J, Zhang Y, Subedi K, Huston GE, Wood WH 3rd, Wersto RP, Becker KG, Swain SL, et al. Kruppel-like factor 4 (KLF4) directly regulates proliferation in thymocyte development and IL-17 expression during Th17 differentiation. FASEB Journal. 2011;**25**:3634-3645. DOI: 10.1096/fj.11-186924

[22] Whitney EM, Ghaleb AM, Chen X, Yang VW. Transcriptional profiling of the cell cycle checkpoint gene kruppel-like factor 4 reveals a global inhibitory function in macromolecular biosynthesis. Gene Expression. 2006;**13**:85-96

[23] Klaewsongkram J, Yang Y, Golech S, Katz J, Kaestner KH, Weng NP. Kruppel-like factor 4 regulates B cell number and activation-induced B cell proliferation. Journal of Immunology. 2007;**179**:4679-4684

[24] Burgering BM. A brief introduction to FOXOlogy. Oncogene. 2008;**27**:2258-2262. DOI: 10.1038/onc.2008.29

[25] van der Vos KE, Coffer PJ. FOXO-binding partners: It takes two to tango. Oncogene. 2008;**27**:2289-2299. DOI: 10.1038/onc.2008.22

[26] Coffer PJ. Transcriptional regulation of lymphocyte quiescence: As cunning as a FOX. Trends in Immunology. 2003;**24**:470-471; author reply 471

[27] Eijkelenboom A, Burgering BM. FOXOs: Signalling integrators for homeostasis maintenance. Nature Reviews Molecular Cell Biology. 2013;**14**:83-97. DOI: 10.1038/nrm3507

[28] Hedrick SM. The cunning little vixen: Foxo and the cycle of life and death. Nature Immunology. 2009;**10**:1057-1063. DOI: 10.1038/ni.1784

[29] Ouyang W, Li MO. Foxo: In command of T lymphocyte homeostasis and tolerance. Trends in Immunology. 2011;**32**:26-33. DOI: 10.1016/j.it.2010.10.005

[30] Zhang X, Yalcin S, Lee DF, Yeh TY, Lee SM, Su J, Mungamuri SK, Rimmele P, Kennedy M, Sellers R, et al. FOXO1 is an essential regulator of pluripotency in human embryonic stem cells. Nature Cell Biology. 2011;**13**:1092-1099. DOI: 10.1038/ncb2293

[31] Sandri M. FOXOphagy path to inducing stress resistance and cell survival. Nature Cell Biology. 2012;**14**:786-788. DOI: 10.1038/ncb2550

[32] Fu Z, Tindall DJ. FOXOs, cancer and regulation of apoptosis. Oncogene. 2008;**27**:2312-2319. DOI: 10.1038/onc.2008.24

[33] Hedrick SM, Hess Michelini R, Doedens AL, Goldrath AW, Stone EL. FOXO transcription factors throughout T cell biology. Nature Reviews Immunology. 2012;**12**:649-661. DOI: 10.1038/nri3278

[34] Leenders H, Whiffield S, Benoist C, Mathis D. Role of the forkhead transcription family member, FKHR, in thymocyte differentiation. European Journal of Immunology. 2000;**30**:2980-2990. DOI: 10.1002/1521-4141(200010)30:10<2980::AID-IMMU2980>3.0.CO;2-9

[35] Ouyang W, Beckett O, Flavell RA, Li MO. An essential role of the Forkhead-box transcription factor Foxo1 in control of T cell homeostasis and tolerance. Immunity. 2009;**30**:358-371. DOI: 10.1016/j.immuni.2009.02.003; S1074-7613(09)00107-1 [pii]

[36] Kerdiles YM, Beisner DR, Tinoco R, Dejean AS, Castrillon DH, DePinho RA, Hedrick SM. Foxo1 links homing and survival of naive T cells by regulating L-selectin, CCR7 and interleukin 7 receptor. Nature Immunology. 2009;**10**:176-184. DOI: 10.1038/ni.1689

[37] Kerdiles YM, Stone EL, Beisner DR, McGargill MA, Ch'en IL, Stockmann C, Katayama CD, Hedrick SM. Foxo transcription factors control regulatory T cell development and function. Immunity. 2010;**33**:890-904. DOI: 10.1016/j.immuni.2010.12.002; S1074-7613 (10)00460-7 [pii]

[38] Fabre S, Lang V, Harriague J, Jobart A, Unterman TG, Trautmann A, Bismuth G. Stable activation of phosphatidylinositol 3-kinase in the T cell immunological synapse stimulates Akt signaling to FoxO1 nuclear exclusion and cell growth control. Journal of Immunology. 2005;**174**:4161-4171. DOI: 174/7/4161 [pii].

[39] Lin L, Hron JD, Peng SL. Regulation of NF-kappaB, Th activation, and autoinflammation by the forkhead transcription factor Foxo3a. Immunity. 2004;**21**:203-213. DOI: 10.1016/j.immuni.2004.06.016; S1074761304002055 [pii].

[40] Castrillon DH, Miao L, Kollipara R, Horner JW, DePinho RA. Suppression of ovarian follicle activation in mice by the transcription factor Foxo3a. Science. 2003;**301**:215-218. DOI: 10.1126/science.1086336301/5630/215 [pii].

[41] Hosaka T, Biggs WH 3rd, Tieu D, Boyer AD, Varki NM, Cavenee WK, Arden KC. Disruption of forkhead transcription factor (FOXO) family members in mice reveals their functional diversification. Proceedings of the National Academy of Sciences of the United States of America. 2004;**101**:2975-2980. DOI: 10.1073/pnas.0400093101

[42] Dengler HS, Baracho GV, Omori SA, Bruckner S, Arden KC, Castrillon DH, DePinho RA, Rickert RC. Distinct functions for the transcription factor Foxo1 at various stages of B cell differentiation. Nature Immunology. 2008;**9**:1388-1398. DOI: 10.1038/ni.1667

[43] Hinman RM, Nichols WA, Diaz TM, Gallardo TD, Castrillon DH, Satterthwaite AB. Foxo3−/− mice demonstrate reduced numbers of pre-B and recirculating B cells but normal splenic B cell sub-population distribution. International Immunology. 2009;**21**:831-842. DOI: 10.1093/intimm/dxp049

[44] Kops GJ, Dansen TB, Polderman PE, Saarloos I, Wirtz KW, Coffer PJ, Huang TT, Bos JL, Medema RH, Burgering BM. Forkhead transcription factor FOXO3a protects quiescent cells from oxidative stress. Nature. 2002;**419**:316-321. DOI: 10.1038/nature01036

[45] Tran H, Brunet A, Grenier JM, Datta SR, Fornace AJ Jr, DiStefano PS, Chiang LW, Greenberg ME. DNA repair pathway stimulated by the forkhead transcription factor FOXO3a through the Gadd45 protein. Science. 2002;**296**:530-534. DOI: 10.1126/science.1068712

[46] Aksoylar HI, Lampe K, Barnes MJ, Plas DR, Hoebe K. Loss of immunological tolerance in Gimap5-deficient mice is associated with loss of Foxo in CD4+ T cells. Journal of Immunology. 2012;**188**:146-154. DOI: 10.4049/jimmunol.1101206

[47] Fabre S, Carrette F, Chen J, Lang V, Semichon M, Denoyelle C, Lazar V, Cagnard N, Dubart-Kupperschmitt A, Mangeney M, et al. FOXO1 regulates L-selectin and a network of human T cell homing molecules downstream of phosphatidylinositol 3-kinase. Journal of Immunology. 2008;**181**:2980-2989. DOI: 181/5/2980 [pii].

[48] Hu H, Wang B, Borde M, Nardone J, Maika S, Allred L, Tucker PW, Rao A. Foxp1 is an essential transcriptional regulator of B cell development. Nature Immunology. 2006;**7**:819-826. DOI: 10.1038/ni1358

[49] Feng X, Wang H, Takata H, Day TJ, Willen J, Hu H. Transcription factor Foxp1 exerts essential cell-intrinsic regulation of the quiescence of naive T cells. Nature Immunology. 2011;**12**:544-550. DOI: 10.1038/ni.2034

[50] Feng X, Ippolito GC, Tian L, Wiehagen K, Oh S, Sambandam A, Willen J, Bunte RM, Maika SD, Harriss JV, et al. Foxp1 is an essential transcriptional regulator for the generation of quiescent naive T cells during thymocyte development. Blood. 2010;**115**:510-518. DOI: 10.1182/blood-2009-07-232694

[51] Park JH, Yu Q, Erman B, Appelbaum JS, Montoya-Durango D, Grimes HL, Singer A. Suppression of IL7Ralpha transcription by IL-7 and other prosurvival cytokines: A novel mechanism for maximizing IL-7-dependent T cell survival. Immunity. 2004;**21**:289-302. DOI: 10.1016/j.immuni.2004.07.016; S1074761304002031 [pii].

[52] Tzachanis D, Freeman GJ, Hirano N, van Puijenbroek AA, Delfs MW, Berezovskaya A, Nadler LM, Boussiotis VA. Tob is a negative regulator of activation that is expressed in anergic and quiescent T cells. Nature Immunology. 2001;**2**:1174-1182. DOI: 10.1038/ni730

[53] Park Y, Jin HS, Lopez J, Elly C, Kim G, Murai M, Kronenberg M, Liu YC. TSC1 regulates the balance between effector and regulatory T cells. Journal of Clinical Investigation. 2013;**123**:5165-5178. DOI: 10.1172/JCI69751

[54] Shrestha S, Yang K, Wei J, Karmaus PW, Neale G, Chi H. Tsc1 promotes the differentiation of memory CD8+ T cells via orchestrating the transcriptional and metabolic programs. Proceedings of the National Academy of Sciences of the United States of America. 2014;**111**:14858-14863. DOI: 10.1073/pnas.1404264111

[55] Xie DL, Wu J, Lou YL, Zhong XP. Tumor suppressor TSC1 is critical for T-cell anergy. Proceedings of the National Academy of Sciences of the United States of America. 2012;**109**:14152-14157. DOI: 10.1073/pnas.1119744109

[56] Yang K, Neale G, Green DR, He W, Chi H. The tumor suppressor Tsc1 enforces quiescence of naive T cells to promote immune homeostasis and function. Nature Immunology. 2011;**12**:888-897. DOI: 10.1038/ni.2068

[57] Schwarz DA, Katayama CD, Hedrick SM. Schlafen, a new family of growth regulatory genes that affect thymocyte development. Immunity. 1998;**9**:657-668

[58] Condamine T, Le Luduec JB, Chiffoleau E, Beriou G, Louvet C, Heslan M, Tilly G, Cuturi MC. Characterization of Schlafen-3 expression in effector and regulatory T cells. Journal of Leukocyte Biology. 2010;**87**:451-456. DOI: 10.1189/jlb.0609410

[59] Berger M, Krebs P, Crozat K, Li X, Croker BA, Siggs OM, Popkin D, Du X, Lawson BR, Theofilopoulos AN, et al. An Slfn2 mutation causes lymphoid and myeloid immunodeficiency due to loss of immune cell quiescence. Nature Immunology. 2010;**11**:335-343. DOI: 10.1038/ni.1847

[60] Omar I, Lapenna A, Cohen-Daniel L, Tirosh B, Berger M. Schlafen2 mutation unravels a role for chronic ER stress in the loss of T cell quiescence. Oncotarget. 2016;**7**:39396-39407. DOI: 10.18632/oncotarget.9818

[61] Goldshtein A, Zerbib SM, Omar I, Cohen-Daniel L, Popkin D, Berger M. Loss of T-cell quiescence by targeting Slfn2 prevents the development and progression of T-ALL. Oncotarget. 2016;**7**:46835-46847. DOI: 10.18632/oncotarget.9390

[62] Wong WF, Kohu K, Chiba T, Sato T, Satake M. Interplay of transcription factors in T-cell differentiation and function: The role of Runx. Immunology. 2011;**132**:157-164. DOI: 10.1111/j.1365-2567.2010.03381.x

[63] Komori T. Regulation of osteoblast differentiation by Runx2. Advances in Experimental Medicine and Biology. 2010;**658**:43-49. DOI: 10.1007/978-1-4419-1050-9_5

[64] Okuda T, van Deursen J, Hiebert SW, Grosveld G, Downing JR. AML1, the target of multiple chromosomal translocations in human leukemia, is essential for normal fetal liver hematopoiesis. Cell. 1996;**84**:321-330

[65] Wong WF, Kohu K, Nakamura A, Ebina M, Kikuchi T, Tazawa R, Tanaka K, Kon S, Funaki T, Sugahara-Tobinai A, et al. Runx1 deficiency in CD4+ T cells causes fatal autoimmune inflammatory lung disease due to spontaneous hyperactivation of cells. Journal of Immunology. 2012;**188**:5408-5420. DOI: 10.4049/jimmunol.1102991

[66] Wong WF, Kohu K, Nagashima T, Funayama R, Matsumoto M, Movahed E, Tan GM, Yeow TC, Looi CY, Kurokawa M, et al. The artificial loss of Runx1 reduces the expression of quiescence-associated transcription factors in CD4(+) T lymphocytes. Molecular Immunology. 2015;**68**:223-233. DOI: 10.1016/j.molimm.2015.08.012

[67] Wong WF, Kurokawa M, Satake M, Kohu K. Down-regulation of Runx1 expression by TCR signal involves an autoregulatory mechanism and contributes to IL-2 production. Journal of Biological Chemistry. 2011;**286**:11110-11118. DOI: 10.1074/jbc.M110.166694

[68] Chang M, Jin W, Sun SC. Peli1 facilitates TRIF-dependent Toll-like receptor signaling and proinflammatory cytokine production. Nature Immunology. 2009;**10**:1089-1095. DOI: 10.1038/ni.1777

[69] Chen ZJ, Bhoj V, Seth RB. Ubiquitin, TAK1 and IKK: Is there a connection? Cell Death & Differentiation. 2006;**13**:687-692. DOI: 10.1038/sj.cdd.4401869

[70] Schauvliege R, Janssens S, Beyaert R. Pellino proteins: Novel players in TLR and IL-1R signalling. Journal of Cellular and Molecular Medicine. 2007;**11**:453-461. DOI: 10.1111/j.1582-4934.2007.00040.x

Chapter 6

Regulatory T Lymphocytes (Treg): Modulation and Clinical Application

Cadiele Oliana Reichert, Joel da Cunha,
Débora Levy, Luciana Morganti Ferreira Maselli,
Sérgio Paulo Bydlowski and Celso Spada

Additional information is available at the end of the chapter

http://dx.doi.org/10.5772/intechopen.69152

Abstract

Treg cells CD4+CD25+FOXP3+ have a specific function in the tolerance of autoantigens and regulation of the immune response. Modulation of differentiation pathways and the use of Treg cells in cell therapy have been reported in autoimmune diseases, systemic lupus erythromatosis, autoimmune hepatitis, type 1 diabetes mellitus, multiple sclerosis, rheumatoid arthritis, graft-versus-host disease, bone marrow transplantation and solid organs. The expansion of Treg cells *in vivo* occurs through low-dose IL-2 treatment. However, because of the heterogeneity and variability of Treg cells, the isolation of peripheral blood cells, through the technique of leucopheresis by GMP (good manuring practice), for *in vitro* expansion is difficult, necessitating a large combination of specific and reliable cellular markers. Currently, two specific markers, Helios and neuropilin-1, are being studied to facilitate the differentiation of thymus Treg cells and peripheral Treg cells. However, Treg cells induced in vitro are unstable. Modulation of the FOXP3 gene in the CNS1 and CNS2 region is an alternative to maintaining the stability of expanded Treg cells *in vitro*.

Keywords: autoimmune tolerance, cell therapy, heterogeneity treg, FOXP3+, regulatory T

1. Introduction

Regular T lymphocytes (Treg) were first described in the year 1970 in murine models [1]. They are subpopulations of T lymphocytes defined by the expression of CD4+ and CD25+ molecules, as well as by the transcription factor FOXP3 (*forkhead box P3*). Treg cells maintain self-tolerance and immune homeostasis through immune responses against self and non-self antigens and in fetal-maternal self-tolerance. Regulation of the immune response occurs through suppression of effector T cells, minimizing the production of cells of adaptive immunity and innate immunity [2, 3]. The suppressor function of Treg cells is directed by the transcription factor FOXP3, occurring in a non-random manner. However, a deregulation in the Treg cells can make them autoreactive with the recognition of autoantigens, developing autoimmune diseases [4]. The organism acts naturally against self-reactive T cells through the process of negative selection by inactivation or clonal deletion in the thymic tissue, and genetic mutations contribute to self-tolerance in the thymus [5].

FOXP3 expression is initiated through a combination of antigen recognition, microenvironmental influences, and epigenetic factors. FOXP3 is present in about 10–20% of the T cells. Peripheral induction of FOXP3 expression may occur in the colon and placenta [6, 7]. Treg cells exhibit high expression of the IL-2α receptor (CD25) and low expression of CD127 [8]. Changes or loss of FOXP3 is associated with the development of collagenases and vasculitis, rheumatoid arthritis, mixed connective tissue disease, Kawasaki disease, Wegener's granulomatosis, systemic lupus erythematosus and Sjögren's syndrome, enteropathies, type 1 diabetes, thyroiditis and eczema [9]. The various clinical alterations of which Treg cells are present, the use of Treg as cell therapy with *in vitro* and *ex vivo* expansion has been a research alternative for certain treatments with the development of tolerance and autoimmunity [10].

2. Treg cell heterogeneity

Treg cells account for 5–10% of peripheral CD4+ T cells in humans and rats. Treg cells that grow in the thymus are called natural (nTreg) or thymic (tTreg) Tregs, and Treg cells that develop at the periphery by specific stimuli of conventional CD4+ T cells are termed pTreg cells. When Treg cells are induced *in vitro* are called iTreg [11]. Treg cell generation in the thymus and peripheral tissues occurs in response to T cell receptor (TCR) and cytokine receptor signaling. Natural Treg cells are generated during the period of positive selection of CD4+ T cells by expression of the transcription factor of the FOXP3 gene in the thymus. FOXP3 expression is controlled by conserved noncoding sequences (CNS) in the promoter region of the gene and by intronic regulatory sequences [12]. TGF-β, IL-2, and TCR are required for FOXP3 gene expression during cell differentiation [13]. The promoter region of the FOXP3 gene is activated by the NF-kB pathway, NFAT (nuclear factor of activated T), the transcription factor SMAD-3, the retinoic acid produced by dendritic cells and epithelial cells, rapamycin and NR4As proteins [14–16].

However, there is a small portion of Treg that does not express FOXP3 is known as regulatory T type 1 (Tr1) with phenotype CD41+CD49b1+LAG-31+CD2261+FOXP3−. These cells are induced by the chronic activation of CD4+ by antigens in the presence of IL-10 and are responsible for peripheral immunotolerance. It is possible to distinguish the Tr1 from other CD4+ populations from the expression of the cytokines: IL-10++TGF-b+IFN-γ+IL-5+IL-4

IL-2–$^{low/neg}$ [10]. T cells expressing FOXP3 circulate through the secondary lymphoid tissues as "central" Tregs. Activation signals involving T cell receptors (TCR), co-stimulation of CD28 and/or interleukin-2 (IL-2) induce positive regulation of interferon regulating factor 4 (IRF4) expression, promoting the differentiation of Treg cells "central" in "effector" Treg cells. Unknown stimuli induce the polarization of Treg cells by upregulation of transcription factors that may act in conjunction with FOXP3 to induce the expression of chemokine receptors that mediate recruitment to tissues or sites of inflammation [17, 18]. During activation of TCR in a cytokine medium, T CD4+ cells can differentiate into various T cell lines, T helper (Th), including Th1, Th2, Th17, Th17, and iTreg, as defined by their production standard and function of cytokines [19].

Thymic Treg cells are generated in the medulla and/or the medullo-cortex junctions in the thymus and arise from a thimocyte CD4+CD8–. TCR plays an essential role in the differentiation of Treg cells, but it does not act alone. TCR signaling along with co-stimulation of nuclear factor activated T-cell (NF-AT), an activator of protein-1 (AP-1) and CARMA1/Bcl10/Malt1 NF-kB, acts on the FOXP3 gene to induce its expression. In addition, signaling via tumor growth factor β (TGF-β), interleukin-2 (IL-2) and transcription activator-5 (STAT5) induce signs of stimuli for expression of the Foxp3 gene, so that differentiation of naive T occurs Treg. Through stimuli by TGF-β tTreg can differentiate into pTreg [20–22]. The deficiency of TCR signaling mediators such as TAK1, Bcl10, CARMA1, PKCh, and IKKb reduces the number of Treg cells generated in the thymus without affecting the generation of conventional T cells. This decrease in Treg compromises immunotolerance and equilibration of the immune system [23].

2.1. Treg cell subtypes

Treg naive cells are recognized by the phenotype FOXP3loCD45RA+CD45RO–, and Treg cells are FOXP3hiCD45RA–CD45RO+ and express both the Fas receptor (CD95) and cytotoxic T-lymphocyte antigen (CTLA-4). A small part of Treg has a phenotype ICOS+IL-10+. Treg cells expressing FOXP3 exhibit their immunoregulatory activity by a variety of effector mechanisms such as CTLA-4 uptake, IL-2 uptake, IL-10, TGF-β, IL-35 and galactin-1 production. The environment in which Treg cells are found alters the mechanisms by which they exert suppressive activity. Identification of CD45RA or CD45RO molecules, when combined with CD25 and/or FOXP3, is useful for identifying naive reg T cells. Human CD45RO+CD25hiCD4+Treg cells are similar to rat Treg cells in CD25 expression. The Treg CD45RA+FOXP3+ and CD45RO+FOXP3+ cells are functionally different but are related to the development of immunosuppression. Expression of the transcription factor of the B lymphocyte-induced maturation protein (Blimp-1) is common to all Treg cells [15, 24–26].

Differentiation of naive Treg gives rise to subtypes of Treg CD4+CD25FOXP3+: tTreg, pTreg, and iTreg. With the use of Treg cells in the therapy of human diseases, it is important to distinguish between cell subtypes. Expression in the Helios molecule can be effective in differentiating between the subtypes of tTreg and iTreg/pTreg [21]. Helios is expressed in the thymus, so it may be a marker to identify tTreg from the other populations of Treg, and it acts as upregulation in FOXP3 protein [27–29]. However, the Helios molecule can be found in iTregs and pTregs depending on the type of antigen presenting cells and signals found. Cells that super-expression Helios have a superior effect of peripheral immunosuppression. This feature can be used in treatments for autoimmune diseases such as systemic lupus erythematosus (SLE) and rheumatoid arthritis (RA) [30]. Through *in vitro* induction of Helios in Treg cells, it was found that CD103 and GITR are expressed at high levels in a subset of cells Treg Helios+. These markers together can be used to differentiate Treg subtypes from each other [21, 31]. Another alternative, the Nrp1 protein (neuropilin-1) is expressed in tTreg cells as opposed to iTreg and pTreg cells [31].

The pTreg cells are present in the intestine and mucosa. Dendritic cells present in the mucosa, especially CD103+ induce FOXP3+ Tregs through the production of TGF-β and retinoic acid [32]. Retinoic acid binds to its receptor, RAR, generating induction signals in the CNS1 region of the FOXP3 gene. This signal induction leads to increased histone acetylation in the region of the CNS1, the SMAD3 binding sites, and increased phosphorylated SMAD3 binding, inducing expression of FOXP3, and originating pTreg cells in the gut. The microbiota also promotes cell differentiation of TCD4+ in Treg CD4+FOXP3+. Most of the Tregs in the intestine coexpress FOXP3 and RORgt, a Th17 regulator, as well as T-bet, GATA3 or IRF4, proteins that present suppression role in the Th1/Th2 response, maintaining the immunological tolerance and acting in the resistance to pathological infections originated microorganisms present in the mucosae [33].

2.2. FOXP3 and autoimmunity

FOXP3 is the main labeled Treg cell. The key role of FOXP3 in the immune response of Treg has been described in patients with immune dysregulation, polyendocrinopathy, enteropathy, X-linked (IPEX) and in rats scurfy [34, 35]. Patients and scurfy mice present monogenic mutations in the FOXP3 gene, which confers a phenotype with dysregulation of the immune system with the development of autoimmunity due to lack of Treg cells [36, 37]. Patients with IPEX present mutations in a Phe367 residue of the F367V protein, F367L, and F367C, which make up the FOXP3 protein [38]. Polymorphic changes in the promoter region of the FOXP3 gene contribute to loss of function and dysregulation of FOXP3, as well as the development of polygenic autoimmune diseases [39]. However, there is no dominant mechanism for the development of autoimmunity. Factors affecting FOXP3 function, effects of genetic alterations, altered signaling, and expression of FOXP3 messenger RNA (mRNA) or mature protein are related to the development of autoimmunity with an imbalance between conventional Treg cells and pathogenic Tregs [40].

IPEX is a rare genetic disease resulting from the lack of functional Treg cells due to the loss of functional mutations in FOXP3. It affects men exclusively because of its recessive pattern of heredity linked to the X chromosome and is often fatal in the first year of life unless it is rescued with bone marrow transplantation. Clinically, IPEX presents a triad of autoimmune enteropathy, autoimmune endocrinopathy, and eczematous dermatitis. The most common manifestation is enteropathy followed by endocrinopathy, especially type 1 insulin-dependent diabetes mellitus. Additional manifestations described include immune-mediated cytopenia, which may present as neutropenia, anemia and/or thrombocytopenia, and autoimmune nephropathy, hepatitis, and pulmonary disease. Food allergy with high serum IgE and eosinophilia. Patients with IPEX generally have a wide range of autoantibodies due to adaptive immune dysregulation. The only curative treatment available for this disease is the allogeneic hematopoietic stem cell transplantation with chemotherapy of reduced intensity. Prior to transplantation, patients require nutritional support and immunosuppressive therapy, which may include glucocorticoids and/or steroid-sparing agents, such as calcineurin inhibitors, rapamycin inhibitor (mTOR) [11].

Single nucleotide polymorphism (SNP) 7340C>T is related to the development of autoimmune diseases and allergies in children. This polymorphism alters the stability of FOXP3 mRNA by preventing translation. In addition to SNPs in FOXP3 itself, SNPs in three other loci indirectly affect FOXP3 expression and are associated with autoimmunity: CD25, PTPN2, and PTPN22. All three genes are involved in the response to IL-2. Tregs do not produce IL-2, but this interleukin is essential for its survival and function. The low expression of CD25 is associated as STAT5 after exposure to IL-2, with decreased Tregs throughout life in patients with type 1 diabetes and multiple sclerosis. The polymorphism rs3761549 G/A is related to the development of Graves' disease in children. These changes related to FoxP3 protein are commonly known as IPEX-type changes [40–43].

3. Treg-cell therapy

The use of Treg cells in clinical practice was made possible after isolation and enhancement of GMP (good manuring practice) CD4+CD25+ Treg cells with a yield of approximately 90% Treg, allowing the cryopreservation and expansion of these cells. Cell therapy with Treg has a purpose in the treatment of diseases, which result in a decompensated or undesired suppressed Treg activity in cancer, immunoglobulin deficiency, autoimmune or inflammatory diseases, and deleterious consequences of immunosuppression after organ transplantation. Therefore, the manipulation of Treg cells can control the progression of cancer through cell configurations, solid organ transplantation and hematopoietic cells, transplant rejection, and autoimmune diseases. The concept of cellular immunotherapy with Treg is to give the patient Treg cells to decrease the exaggerated immune response to autoimmune diseases, organ transplants and bone marrow [44–47]. The nTreg cells, *in vitro*, can be expanded by antigenic stimulation in the presence of a high concentration of IL-2. *In vivo*, low-dose IL-2 treatment increases Treg expansion and is used in the treatment of graft versus host disease (GVHD) and hepatitis C virus-induced cryoglobulinemic vasculitis and, together with rapamycin. Low dose IL-2 was chosen to preferentially expand Treg cells without also expanding activated effector T cells. Modulation of IL-2 homeostasis is an important mechanism by which Treg modulates effector differentiation of CD8+ under strongly immunogenic conditions [48, 49]. Some authors suggest the use of rapamycin for Treg expansion *in vivo* with an approximately 75–80% yield of pure cells and total depletion of CD8 and CD19 [50–52].

Three categories of GMP-grade clinical Treg can define: first generation (CD4+CD25+); second generation, bone fide Treg (CD4+CD25+CD127$^{low/-}$) and third generation naive Treg (CD4+CD25+CD127$^{low/-}$CD45Ra+). These three types of Treg can be isolated and expanded by Il-2 [46]. The main obstacle to Tregs expansion in the laboratory is iTregs instability. The use of the Nrp1 protein reduces the phosphorylation of the Akt protein, promoting cell stability. Demethylation of the CpG islands in the CNS2 region at the FOXP3 locus recruits transcription factors, including STAT5, NFAT, Runx1/Cbfb, CREB and FOXP3 itself, making the tTregs stable. However, demethylation in the CNS2 region of FOXP3 is known to render iTregs unstable. The control of the methylation/demethylation processes of the CNS1 and CNS2 regions of the FOXP3 gene of the iTregs is still not possible with 100% efficacy in the laboratory. In this way, it compromises clonal expansion *in vitro*, and several transcription factors are involved [47, 53].

3.1. Graft-versus-host disease (GVHD)

Allogeneic stem cell transplantation presents a series of problems, among which we can highlight GVHD, with high mortality rates of 15–30% in transplanted patients and 50% of morbidity. Treg cells are a novel approach based on cellular immunotherapy to reduce the risk of severe acute lesions of graft versus host disease (aGVHD). These lesions may occur within 100 days after transplantation. Chronic GVHD takes about 2–5 years for the signs and symptoms of the diseases to appear in the transplanted patient due to the presence of effector T cells in the marrow receptor tissue. To combat this reaction, aggressive immunosuppressive therapies are started, often unsuccessful. Despite the advances in GVHD treatment, the high rates of death are still high [54–56]. The development of acute and chronic forms of GVHD is different with signs and symptoms because it involves cells cytotoxic TCD8+ and helper TCD4+, and these cells activate different pathways in the autoimmune response. The pathway involving donor TCD8+ cells is activated when binding of TCR to major class I histocompatibility complex (MHC-I) peptides occurs, and interaction the patient antigen-presenting cells (APCs), with the release of granzins, perforins, and production of inflammatory cytokines. Although activation of donor TCD4+ cells results in the activation of a Th1 inflammatory response with high production of INF-Y, IL-12, and IL-2, or a Th2-mediated inflammatory response with extensive production of IL-4, IL-5, IL-6 and IL-10 [54, 57].

After the haematopoietic stem cell transplantation (HSCT), reconstituted Treg cells express markers of recent thymic emigrants. These markers increase the number of native Treg cells in the population of graft-derived Treg cells after HSCT. Second, Treg Helios+ cells from patients receiving HSCT express higher levels of naive markers (such as CD45RA and CD31) than those from patients with active systemic lupus erythromatosus. This increase in Treg controls the immune responses of Th1 and Th2. Infusion of Treg cells into HSCT has been explored in murine and human models. Infusion of Treg cells during allogenic HSCT reduces acute and chronic graft-versus-host disease [58]. Patients with HSCT demonstrated that the use of IL-2 at the dose of 1×10^6 IU per square meter decreases the chances of developing GVHD, in which the number of Treg increased due to activation of the FOXP3+ gene by IL-2, and the amount of Tcon decreased [51]. The immunological reaction of cGVHD exhibits phosphorylation of the transcription factor STAT5, increase of IL-17, IL-15 and deficiency or decrease of IL-2, The IL-2 therapy increased cell proliferation in the thymic and decrease apoptosis by activates phosphorylation of STAT5 [59]. Another alternative for Treg expansion is CD28 stimulation of pTregs, which results in a polyclonal expansion and preservation of a Treg phenotype and function as indicated by the high level FOXP3/Helios expression, reduced prokaryotic cytokine expression, inflammatory and powerful suppressive function [60]. Tr1 cells express CD49b and Lag3, producing IL-10. Tr1 cells play a role in tolerance but are distinct from FOXP3+ Tregs. Studies to examine these cells in organ transplantation are being initiated. The association between immunosuppressive drugs that increase the serum concentration of IL-2 to induce Treg has also been gaining strength in the treatment of GVHD [61–65].

3.2. Type 1 diabetes

Type 1 diabetes mellitus (T1DM) is a chronic disease that results from the autoimmune destruction of insulin-producing pancreatic beta cells. May be associated with the development of IPEX [66]. The death of β cells occurs due to exposure of their antigens to MHC class II complex APC cells and presentation to TCD4+ lymphocytes in the lymphatic modules of the pancreas. After presentation, TCD4+ cells differentiate into self-reactive effector TCD4+ (Teffs). The fractions of the complement system C3a and C5a facilitate the expansion and the function of Teff. In pancreatic islets, activated Teffs release cytokines including IFN-γ and IL-2, resulting in the recruitment of cytotoxic T lymphocytes and TCD8+ lymphocytes. Cytotoxic inflammatory cells eventually infiltrate and destroy the islet cells in a process called "insulite", with the release of perforins and granzins AND release of IFN-γ, TNF α, IL-1β by macrophages. Chemokines released by the injured β-cells promote recruitment of additional mononuclear cells and the release of additional autoantigens allows the expansion and propagation of the self-reactive Teff response [67–71]. In the pathogenesis of T1DM, the immune response is exaggerated against its own antigens. There is an imbalance between Tregs and effector T cells. Isolation and expansion ex vivo of Tregs CD25+CD127$^{low/-}$CD25+ showed improved function and retained their diversity of T cell receptors, then these cells were used in T1DM patients. The infusions were well tolerated and with good safety. The use of pharmacotherapy including anti-CD3 therapy, glutamic acid decarboxylase (GAD) injection, hematopoietic stem cell transplantation (HSCT), autologous umbilical cord blood transfusion and stem cell educator therapy has demonstrated efficacy with increased levels of C-peptides and decrease in the daily dose of insulin [72, 73].

The subpopulations of Tregs in T1DM are different when compared to healthy individuals. The proportion of cells CD25$^{low/-}$ between cells Treg CD4+FOXP3+In T1DM patients was higher than in healthy patients. Low or no CD25 expression implies a decrease in Treg cell differentiation with decreased peripheral suppressor activity and increased Teff cell growth [74, 75]. The difficulty in using expanded Tregs ex vivo in patients with T1DM is found in the cells themselves since these cells express CD45RO+ memory phenotype. Another issue is the expression of Helios by lymphocytes in peripheral blood. Expanded lymphocytes in vitro have a lower expression of the molecule on their surface when compared to their own lymphocytes. However, the activity of suppressing autologous or allogeneic TCD8+ effector cells is maintained. Thus, it becomes a good alternative in the treatment of T1DM in the long term. Some studies have conflicting results on the use of Treg cells in the treatment of T1DM since several mechanisms are involved in the T1DM pathology; however, they are in line with lack, dysregulation or deficiency of local and peripheral Treg [76]. Studies with the use of IL-2 in the treatment of T1DM have demonstrated effective results in the expansion of Treg [77].

3.3. Autoimmune hepatitis and systemic lupus erythematosus

The inflammatory response of autoimmune hepatitis (AIH) involves the B-lymphocytes, T cells, Th1, Th17 and cytotoxic T cells. Studies have shown that the function of the mature FOXP3 protein shows inactivity in T CD4+ cells. Cell therapy, such as the infusion of autologous, antigen-specific and hepatic regulatory T cells to restore hepatic immune tolerance, may soon be a potential future treatment for patients with AIH [78, 79]. Hepatic tolerance is involved in the pathogenesis of autoimmune hepatitis, with an imbalance of immune responses. There are controversies in scientific research regarding the number of Treg present in AHI. Though the modulating function of the cell appears to be compromised [80, 81]. However, in treated patients with IL-2, the Treg number is higher than untreated patients. This fact supports the hypothesis of treating patients with autologous Tregs expanded *ex vivo* and may lead to tolerance to hepatic antigens during the development of chronic disease, with remission of the clinical signs and symptoms of AIH. The use of IL-2 for Treg expansion *in vivo* is an option for treatment in patients with reduced Treg numbers [82–84].

SLE is a chronic autoimmune disease characterized by the production of antinuclear autoantibodies of the IgG type. Symptoms of the disease include light hypersensitivity, impaired joints, thyroid dysfunction, changes in the central nervous system and renal filtration [85]. There is growing evidence that Th1, Th2, Th9, and Th17 cells are associated with the pathogenesis of SLE. Disorders related to the amount, function of Treg show a worse evolution in the disease and decrease the production of IL-2. But studies that demonstrate this commitment are not homogeneous [86]. The use of IL-2 in the treatment of SLE demonstrated decreased exaggerated inflammatory response and increased proliferation of Tregs *in vivo* [87–90]. Treg cells expressing Helios are used with functional suppressive capacity and migratory potential in inflamed tissues is expanded in active SLE, presumably by γ-chain signaling cytokines and TCR stimulation, to compensate for autoreactive effector responses [91]. Treatment with melatonin increases the frequency of CD3+CD4+FOXP3+ cells and the mean fluorescence intensity of FOXP3 in patients with SLE [92].

3.4. Rheumatoid arthritis and multiple sclerosis

Rheumatoid arthritis is characterized by chronic inflammation of the joints, with severe pain and in the long term, loss of movement of the affected joint. In the development of rheumatoid arthritis, Treg cells are unable to suppress inflammatory responses, with an imbalance between Treg effector cells and TCD4+ cells. Low doses of IL-2 increase Treg stimulation in rheumatoid arthritis [93, 94]. In rats, depletion of Treg cells results in the onset of a variety of autoimmune diseases, including arthritis. Treg's cellular replacement relieves the symptoms of the disease. The importance of Treg cells in rheumatoid arthritis is supported by the efficacy of CTLA4-Ig therapy, an increased ratio of Treg cells/effector

http://dx.doi.org/10.5772/intechopen.69152

T cells after treatment with anti-IL-6R or anti-TNF-α and the identification of CTLA-4 associated with rheumatoid arthritis. FOXP3+ T cells are able to convert into pathogenic Th17 cells. Th17 cells are increased in rheumatoid arthritis, being responsive for the production of inflammatory cytokines and the activation of inflammation in severe cases. The modulation between Treg/Th17 is an alternative for the immunocellular treatment of rheumatoid arthritis [95–97]. Tregs play a key role in protecting individuals against autoimmunity. Many studies suggest that the amount of Treg may be a protective factor against the development of multiple sclerosis. The use of TGF-β may be an alternative aid in the treatment of multiple sclerosis, since Treg and effector T cells are defective. The causes of multiple sclerosis are still unknown, but the immune system plays a central role in the development of the disease [98, 99].

4. Conclusion

The success of Treg cell therapy depends initially on the isolation and characterization of cells. New studies are emerging, with the discovery of new cell markers for the identification of Treg. However, current research does not use a universally applicable standard for Treg identification. This gap in identification leads to conflicting and doubtful research results. The cellular variability of Treg is wide. It is important to characterize the phenotype and suppressor function of each subtype of Treg present in the periphery or in the thymus. The deregulation of these cells leads to the development of autoimmune diseases or the worsening of the clinical picture of these diseases. The FOXP3 protein is responsive to Treg cell suppressor activity, together with other molecules. Understanding the modulation pathway to activate the FOXP3 gene is important for the expansion of stable Tregs in vitro and that in the future we will have effective cellular therapy without damage to the organism.

Conflict of interests

The authors declare that there is no conflict of interest

Author details

Cadiele Oliana Reichert[1]*, Joel da Cunha[1,2], Débora Levy[2], Luciana Morganti Ferreira Maselli[2], Sérgio Paulo Bydlowski[2] and Celso Spada[1]

*Address all correspondence to: kadielli@hotmail.com

1 Clinical Analysis Department, Health Sciences Center, Federal University of Santa Catarina (FUSC), Florianópolis, Brazil

2 Laboratory of Genetics and Molecular Hematology, LIM31, University of São Paulo School of Medicine (USPSM), São Paulo, Brazil

References

[1] Gershon RK, Kondo K. Cell interactions in the induction of tolerance: The role of thymic lymphocytes. Immunology. 1970;**18**(5):723-737

[2] Sakaguchi S, Yamaguchi T, Nomura T. and Ono M. Regulatory T cells and imune tolerance. Cell. 2008;**133**:775-787

[3] Ghaebi M, Nouri M, Ghasemzadeh A, Farzadi L, Jadidi-Niaragh F, Ahmadi M, Yousefi M. Immune regulatory network in successful pregnancy and reproductive failures. Biomedicine & Pharmacotherapy. 2017;**88**:61-73. DOI: 10.1016/j.biopha.2017.01.016

[4] Rosenblum MD, Way SS, Abbas AK. Regulatory T cell memory. Nature Reviews Immunology. 2016;**16**(2):90-101. DOI: 10.1038/nri.2015.1

[5] Paiva RS, Lino AC, Bergman M-L, et al. Recent thymic emigrants are the preferential precursors of regulatory T cells differentiated in the periphery. Proceedings of the National Academy of Sciences of the United States of America. 2013;**110**(16):6494-6499. DOI: 10.1073/pnas.1221955110

[6] Schumacher A, Zenclussen AC. Regulatory T cells: regulators of life. American Journal of Reproductive Immunology. 2014;**72**(2):158-170. DOI: 10.1111/aji.12238

[7] Churchman SM, El-Jawhari JJ, Burska AN, et al. Modulation of peripheral T-cell function by interleukin-7 in rheumatoid arthritis. Arthritis Research & Therapy. 2014;**16**(6):511. DOI: 10.1186/s13075-014-0511-3

[8] Li X, Zheng Y. Regulatory T cell identity: Formation and maintenance. Trends in immunology. 2015;**36**(6):344-353. DOI: 10.1016/j.it.2015.04.006

[9] Gomez-Tourino I, Arif S, Eichmann M, Peakman M. T cells in type 1 diabetes: Instructors, regulators and effectors: A comprehensive review. Journal of Autoimmunity. 2016;**66**:7-16. DOI: 10.1016/j.jaut.2015.08.012

[10] Zeng H, Zhang R, Jin B, Chen L. Type 1 regulatory T cells: A new mechanism of peripheral immune tolerance. Cellular & Molecular Immunology. 2015;**12**(5):566-571. DOI: 10.1038/cmi.2015.44

[11] Alroqi FJ, Chatila TA. T Regulatory cell biology in health and disease. Current Allergy and Asthma Reports. 2016;**16**(4):27. DOI: 10.1007/s11882-016-0606-9

[12] Wing JB, Sakaguchi S. Foxp3$^+$ T(reg) cells in humoral immunity. International Immunology. 2014;**26**(2):61-69. DOI: 10.1093/intimm/dxt060

[13] Kim CH. FOXP3 and its role in the immune system. Advances in Experimental Medicine and Biology. 2009;**665**:17-29

[14] Won HY, Hwang ES. Transcriptional modulation of regulatory T cell development by novel regulators NR4As. Archives of Pharmacal Research. 2016;**39**(11):1530-1536

[15] Sakaguchi S, Miyara M, Costantino CM, Hafler DA. FOXP3+ regulatory T cells in the human immune system. Nature Reviews Immunology. 2010;**10**(7):490-500. DOI: 10.1038/nri2785

[16] Sekiya T, Kashiwagi I, Inoue N, Morita R, Hori S, Waldmann H, et al. The nuclear orphan receptor Nr4a2 induces Foxp3 and regulates differentiation of CD4+ T cells. Nature Communications. 2011;**2**:269. DOI: 10.1038/ncomms1272

[17] Lu L, Zhou X, Wang J, Zheng SG, Horwitz DA. Characterization of protective human CD4CD25 FOXP3 regulatory T cells generated with IL-2, TGF-β and retinoicacid. PLoS One. 2010;**5**(12):e15150. DOI: 10.1371/journal.pone.0015150

[18] Miyara M, Yoshioka Y, Kitoh A, Shima T, Wing K, Niwa A, et al. Functional delineation and differentiation dynamics of human CD4 + T cells expressing the FoxP3 transcription factor. Immunity. 2009;**30**(6):899-911. DOI: 10.1016/j.immuni.2009.03.019

[19] Zhu J, Yamane H, Paul WE. Differentiation of effector CD4 T cell populations (*). Annual Review of Immunology. 2010;**28**:445-489. DOI: 10.1146/annurev-immunol-030409-101212

[20] Chen W, Konkel JE. The development of thymic Foxp3+ regulatory T cells: TGF-β matters. European Journal of Immunology. 2015;**45**(4):958-965. DOI: 10.1002/eji.201444999

[21] Yuan X, Cheng G, Malek TR. The importance of regulatory T-cell heterogeneity in maintaining self-tolerance. Immunological Reviews. 2014;**259**(1):103-114. DOI: 10.1111/imr.12163

[22] Hall BM, Tran GT, Robinson CM, Hodgkinson SJ. Induction of antigen specific CD4(+) CD25(+)Foxp3(+)T regulatory cells from naïve natural thymic derived T regulatory cells. International Immunopharmacology. 2015;**28**(2):875-886. DOI: 10.1016/j.intimp.2015.03.049

[23] Oh H, Ghosh S. NF-κB: Roles and regulation in different CD4(+) T-cell subsets. Immunological Reviews. 2013;**252**(1):41-51. DOI: 10.1111/imr.12033

[24] Cretney E, Kallies A, Nutt SL. Differentiation and function of Foxp3(+) effector regulatory T cells. Trends in Immunology. 2013;**34**(2):74-80. DOI: 10.1016/j.it.2012.11.002

[25] Ohkura N, Sakaguchi S. Regulatory T cells: Roles of T cell receptor for their development and function. Seminars in Immunopathology. 2010;**32**(2):95-106. DOI: 10.1007/s00281-010-0200-5

[26] Beyer M, Schultze JL. Plasticity of T(reg) cells: Is reprogramming of T(reg) cells possible in the presence of FOXP3? International Immunopharmacology. 2011;**11**(5):555-560. DOI: 10.1016/j.intimp.2010.11.024

[27] John LB, Ward AC. The Ikaros gene family: Transcriptional regulators of hematopoiesis and immunity. Molecular Immunology. 2011;**48**(9-10):1272-1278. DOI: 10.1016/j.molimm.2011.03.006

[28] Shevach EM, Thornton AM. tTregs, pTregs, and iTregs: Similarities and differences. Immunological reviews. 2014;**259**(1):88-102. DOI: 10.1111/imr.12160

[29] Grzanka J, Leveson-Gower D, Golab K, Wang XJ, Marek-Trzonkowska N, Krzystyniak A, et al. FoxP3, Helios, and SATB1: Roles and relationships in regulatory T cells. International Immunopharmacology. 2013;**16**(3):343-347. DOI: 10.1016/j.intimp.2013.02.004

[30] Müller M, Herrath J, Malmström V. IL-1R1 is expressed on both Helios(+) and Helios(−) FoxP3(+) CD4(+) T cells in the rheumatic joint. Clinical & Experimental Immunology. 2015;**182**(1):90-100. DOI: 10.1111/cei.12668

[31] Zabransky DJ, Nirschl CJ, Durham NM, Park BV, Ceccato CM, Bruno TC, et al. Phenotypic and functional properties of Helios+ regulatory T cells. PLoS One. 2012;**7**(3):e34547. DOI: 10.1371/journal.pone.0034547

[32] Hadaschik EN, Enk AH. TGF-β1-induced regulatory T cells. Human Immunology. 2015;**76**(8):561-564. DOI: 10.1016/j.humimm.2015.06.015

[33] Kanamori M, Nakatsukasa H, Okada M, Lu Q, Yoshimura A. Induced regulatory T cells: Their development, stability, and applications. Trends in Immunology. Nov 2016;**37**(11):803-811. DOI: 10.1016/j.it.2016.08.012

[34] Bacchetta R, Barzaghi F, Roncarolo MG. From IPEX syndrome to FOXP3 mutation: A lesson on immune dysregulation. Annals of the New York Academy of Sciences. 2016. 1-18. DOI: 10.1111/nyas.13011

[35] Gambineri E, Torgerson TR, Ochs HD. Immune dysregulation, polyendocrinopathy, enteropathy, and X-linked inheritance (IPEX), a syndrome of systemic autoimmunity caused by mutations of FOXP3, a critical regulator of T-cell homeostasis. Current Opinion in Rheumatology. 2003;**15**(4):430-435

[36] Zhan H, Sinclair J, Adams S, Cale CM, Murch S, Perroni L, et al. Immune reconstitution and recovery of FOXP3 (forkhead box P3)-expressing T cells after transplantation for IPEX (immune dysregulation, polyendocrinopathy, enteropathy, X-linked) syndrome. Pediatrics. 2008;**121**(4):e998-e1002. DOI: 10.1542/peds.2007-1863

[37] Blanco Quirós A, Arranz Sanz E, Bernardo Ordiz D, Garrote Adrados JA. Fromautoimmune enteropathy to the IPEX (immune dysfunction, polyendocrinopathy, enteropathy, X-linked) syndrome. Allergologia et Immunopathologia. 2009;**37**(4):208-215. DOI: 10.1016/j.aller.2009.04.002

[38] Colobran R, Álvarez de la Campa E, Soler-Palacín P, Martín-Nalda A, Pujol-Borrell R, de la Cruz X, et al. Clinical and structural impact of mutations affecting the residue Phe367 of FOXP3 in patients with IPEX syndrome. Clinical Immunology. 2016;**163**:60-65. DOI: 10.1016/j.clim.2015.12.014

[39] Jmaa MB, Abida O, Bahloul E, Toumi A, Khlif S, Fakhfakh R, Elloumi N, Sellami K, Masmoudi A, Turki H, Masmoudi H. Role of FOXP3 gene polymorphism in the susceptibility to Tunisian endemic Pemphigus Foliaceus. Immunology Letters. 2017;**184**:105-111. DOI:10.1016/j.imlet.2017.02.005

[40] Pesenacker AM, Cook L, Levings MK. The role of FOXP3 in autoimmunity. Current Opinion in Immunology. 2016;**43**:16-23. DOI: 10.1016/j.coi.2016.07.004

[41] Parackova Z, Kayserova J, Danova K, Sismova K, Dudkova E, Sumnik Z, et al. T regulatory lymphocytes in type 1 diabetes: Impaired CD25 expression and IL-2 induced STAT5 phosphorylation in pediatric patients. Autoimmunity. 2016;**49**(8):523-531

[42] Cerosaletti K, Schneider A, Schwedhelm K, Frank I, Tatum M, Wei S, et al. Multiple autoimmune-associated variants confer decreased IL-2R signaling in CD4+ CD25(hi) T cells of type 1 diabetic and multiple sclerosis patients. PLoS One. 2013;**8**(12):e83811. DOI: 10.1371/journal.pone.0083811

[43] Bossowski A, Borysewicz-Sańczyk H, Wawrusiewicz-Kurylonek N, Zasim A, Szalecki M, Wikiera B, et al. Analysis of chosen polymorphisms in FoxP3 gene in children and adolescents with autoimmune thyroid diseases. Autoimmunity. 2014;**47**(6):395-400. DOI: 10.3109/08916934.2014.910767

[44] Peters JH, Preijers FW, Woestenenk R, Hilbrands LB, Koenen HJ, Joosten I. Clinical grade Treg: GMP isolation, improvement of purity by CD127 Depletion, Treg expansion, and Treg cryopreservation. PLoS One. 2008;**3**(9):e3161. DOI: 10.1371/journal.pone.0003161

[45] Hoffmann P, Boeld TJ, Eder R, Albrecht J, Doser K, Piseshka B, Dada A, Niemand C, Assenmacher M, Orsó E, Andreesen R, Holler E, Edinger M. Isolation of CD4+CD25+ regulatory T cells for clinical trials. Biology of Blood and Marrow Transplantation. 2006;**12**(3):267-274

[46] Jeffery HC, Braitch MK, Brown S, Oo YH. Clinical potential of regulatory T cell therapy in liver diseases: An overview and current perspectives. Frontiers in Immunology. 2016;**7**:334. DOI: 10.3389/fimmu.2016.00334

[47] Li Z, Li D, Tsun A, Li B. FOXP3+ regulatory T cells and their functional regulation. Cellular and Molecular Immunology. 2015;**12**(5):558-565. DOI: 10.1038/cmi.2015.10

[48] Horch M, Nguyen VH. Regulatory T-cell immunotherapy for allogeneic hematopoietic stem-cell transplantation. Therapeutic Advances in Hematology. 2012;**3**(1):29-44. DOI: 10.1177/2040620711422266

[49] Miyara M, Ito Y, Sakaguchi S. TREG-cell therapies for autoimmune rheumatic diseases. Nature Reviews Rheumatology. 2014;**10**(9):543-551. DOI: 10.1038/nrrheum.2014.105

[50] Velaga S, Alter C, Dringenberg U, Thiesler CT, Kuhs S, Olek S, et al. Clinical-grade regulatory T cells: Comparative analysis of large-scale expansion conditions. Experimental Hematology. 2017;**45**:27-35.e1. DOI: 10.1016/j.exphem.2016.09.008

[51] Koreth J, Matsuoka K, Kim HT, McDonough SM, Bindra B, Alyea EP 3rd, et al. Interleukin-2 and regulatory T cells in graft-versus-host disease. The New England Journal of Medicine. 2011;**365**(22):2055-2066. DOI: 10.1056/NEJMoa1108188

[52] Brunstein CG, Miller JS, Cao Q, McKenna DH, Hippen KL, Curtsinger J, et al. Infusion of ex vivo expanded T regulatory cells in adults transplanted with umbilical cord blood: Safety profile and detection kinetics. Blood. 2011;**117**(3):1061-1070. DOI: 10.1182/blood-2010-07-293795

[53] Mackay LK, Kallies A. Transcriptional regulation of Tissue-Resident lymphocytes. Trends in Immunology. 2017;**38**(2):94-103. DOI: 10.1016/j.it.2016.11.004

[54] Schroeder MA, DiPersio JF. Mouse models of graft-versus-host disease: advances and limitations. Disease Models & Mechanisms. 2011;**4**(3):318-333. DOI: 10.1242/dmm.006668

[55] Wingard JR, Majhail NS, Brazauskas R, Wang Z, Sobocinski KA, Jacobsohn D, et al. Long-term survival and late deaths after allogeneic hematopoietic cell transplantation. Journal of Clinical Oncology. 2011;**29**(16):2230-2239. DOI: 10.1200/JCO.2010.33.7212

[56] Battiwalla M, Hashmi S, Majhail N, Pavletic S, Savani BN, Shelburne N. National institutes of health hematopoietic cell transplantation late effects initiative: Developing recommendations to improve survivorship and long-term outcomes. Biology of Blood and Marrow Transplantation. 2017;**23**(1):6-9. DOI: 10.1016/j.bbmt.2016.10.020

[57] Hülsdünker J, Zeiser R. Insights into the pathogenesis of GvHD: What mice can teach us about man. Tissue Antigens. 2015;**85**(1):2-9. DOI: 10.1111/tan.12497

[58] Swart JF, Delemarre EM, van Wijk F, Boelens JJ, Kuball J, van Laar JM, Wulffraat NM. Haematopoietic stem cell transplantation for autoimmune diseases. Nature Reviews Rheumatology. 2017. DOI: 10.1038/nrrheum.2017.7

[59] Matsuoka K, Koreth J, Kim HT, Bascug G, McDonough S, Kawano Y, et al. Low-dose interleukin-2 therapy restores regulatory T cell homeostasis in patients with chronic graft-versus-host disease. Science Translational Medicine. 2013;**5**(179):179ra43. DOI: 10.1126/scitranslmed.3005265

[60] He X, Smeets RL, van Rijssen E, Boots AM, Joosten I, Koenen HJ. Single CD28 stimulation induces stable and polyclonal expansion of human regulatory T cells. Scientific Reports. 2017;**7**:1-11. DOI: 10.1038/srep43003

[61] Bacchetta R, Lucarelli B, Sartirana C, Gregori S, Lupo Stanghellini MT, Miqueu P, et al. Immunological outcome in Haploidentical-HSC transplanted patients treated with IL-10-Anergized donor T cells. Frontiers in Immunology. 2014;**5**:16. DOI: 10.3389/fimmu.2014.00016

[62] Andolfi G, Fousteri G, Rossetti M, Magnani CF, Jofra T, Locafaro G, et al. Enforced IL-10 expression confers type 1 regulatory T cell (Tr1) phenotype and function to human CD4(+) T cells. Molecular Therapy. 2012;**20**(9):1778-1790. DOI: 10.1038/mt.2012.71

[63] Hippen KL, Riley JL, June CH, Blazar BR. Clinical perspectives for regulatory T cells in transplantation tolerance. Seminars in Immunology. 2011;**23**(6):462-468. DOI: 10.1016/j.smim.2011.07.008

[64] McDonald-Hyman C, Turka LA, Blazar BR. Advances and challenges in immunotherapy for solid organ and bone marrow transplantation. Science Translational Medicine. 2015;**7**(280):280rv2. DOI: 10.1126/scitranslmed.aaa6853

[65] Blazar BR, Murphy WJ, Abedi M. Advances in graft-versus-host disease biology and therapy. Nature Reviews Immunology. 2012;**12**(6):443-58. DOI: 10.1038/nri3212

[66] Charbonnier LM, Janssen E, Chou J, Ohsumi TK, Keles S, Hsu JT, et al. Regulatory T-cell deficiency and immune dysregulation, polyendocrinopathy, enteropathy, X-linked-like disorder caused by loss-of-function mutations in LRBA. Journal of Allergy and Clinical Immunology. 2015;**135**(1):217-227. DOI: 10.1016/j.jaci.2014.10.019

[67] Cabrera SM, Rigby MR, Mirmira RG. Targeting regulatory T cells in the treatment of type 1 diabetes mellitus. Current Molecular Medicine. 2012;**12**(10):1261-1272

[68] Barcala Tabarrozzi AE, Castro CN, Dewey RA, Sogayar MC, Labriola L, Perone MJ. Cell-based interventions to halt autoimmunity in type 1 diabetes mellitus. Clinical & Experimental Immunology. 2013;**171**(2):135-146. DOI: 10.1111/cei.12019

[69] Bordignon C, Canu A, Dyczko A, Leone S, Monti P. T-cell Metabolism as a Target to control autoreactive T cells in β-cell autoimmunity. Current Diabetes Reports. 2017;**17**(5):24. DOI: 10.1007/s11892-017-0848-5

[70] Frumento D, Nasr MB, Essawy BE, D'Addio F, Zuccotti GV, Fiorina P. Immunotherapy for type 1 diabetes. Journal of Endocrinological Investigation. 2017. DOI: 10.1007/s40618-017-0641-y

[71] Papadopoulou-Marketou N, Chrousos GP, Kanaka-Gantenbein C. Diabetic nephropathy in type 1 diabetes: A review of early natural history, pathogenesis, and diagnosis. Diabetes/Metabolism Research and Reviews. 2017;**33**(2). DOI: 10.1002/dmrr.2841

[72] Gitelman SE, Bluestone JA. Regulatory T cell therapy for type 1 diabetes: May the force be with you. Journal of Autoimmunity. 2016;**71**:78-87. DOI: 10.1016/j.jaut.2016.03.011

[73] Tan T, Xiang Y, Chang C, Zhou Z. Alteration of regulatory T cells in type 1 diabetes mellitus: a comprehensive review. Clinical Reviews in Allergy & Immunology. 2014;**47**(2):234-243. DOI: 10.1007/s12016-014-8440-0

[74] Zóka A, Barna G, Somogyi A, Műzes G, Oláh Á, Al-Aissa Z, et al. Extension of the $CD4^{+}Foxp3^{+}CD25(-/low)$ regulatory T-cell subpopulation in type 1 diabetes mellitus. Autoimmunity. 2015;**48**(5):289-297. DOI: 10.3109/08916934.2014.992518

[75] Putnam AL, Brusko TM, Lee MR, Liu W, Szot GL, Ghosh T, et al. Expansion of human regulatory T-cells from patients with type 1 diabetes. Diabetes. 2009;**58**(3):652-662. DOI: 10.2337/db08-1168

[76] Du W, Shen YW, Lee WH, Wang D, Paz S, Kandeel F, et al. Foxp3+ Treg expanded from patients with established diabetes reduce Helios expression while retaining normal function compared to healthy individuals. PLoS One. 2013;**8**(2):e56209. DOI: 10.1371/journal.pone.0056209

[77] Todd JA, Evangelou M, Cutler AJ, Pekalski ML, Walker NM, Stevens, et al. Regulatory T cell responses in participants with type 1 diabetes after a single dose of Interleukin-2: A non-randomised, open label, adaptive dose-finding trial. PLoS Medicine. 2016;**13**(10):e1002139. DOI: 10.1371/journal.pmed.1002139

[78] Than NN, Jeffery HC, Oo YH. Autoimmune hepatitis: Progress from global immunosuppression to personalised regulatory T cell therapy. Canadian Journal of Gastroenterology and Hepatology. 2016;2016:7181685. DOI: 10.1155/2016/7181685

[79] Manns MP, Lohse AW, Vergani D. Autoimmune hepatitis—Update 2015. Journal of Hepatology. 2015;**62**:S100-S111. DOI: 10.1016/j.jhep.2015.03.005

[80] Sebode M, Lohse AW. Future perspective: Immunomodulatory therapy for autoimmune hepatitis. Digestive Diseases and Sciences. 2014;**32**(5):502-506. DOI: 10.1159/000360493

[81] Peiseler M, Sebode M, Franke B, Wortmann F, Schwinge D, Quaas A, et al. FOXP3+ regulatory T cells in autoimmune hepatitis are fully functional and not reduced in frequency. Journal of Hepatology. 2012;**57**(1):125-132. DOI: 10.1016/j.jhep.2012.02.029

[82] Taubert R, Hardtke-Wolenski M, Noyan F, Wilms A, Baumann AK, Schlue J, et al. Intrahepatic regulatory T cells in autoimune hepatitis are associated with treatment response and depleted with current therapies. Journal of Hepatology. 2014;**61**(5):1106-1114. DOI: 10.1016/j.jhep.2014.05.034

[83] Christen U, Hintermann E. Immunopathogenic mechanisms of autoimmune hepatitis: How much do we know from animal models? Haybaeck J, editor. International Journal of Molecular Sciences. 2016;**17**(12):2007. DOI: 10.3390/ijms17122007

[84] Cassim S, Bilodeau M, Vincent C, Lapierre P. Novel immunotherapies for autoimmune hepatitis. Frontiers in Pediatrics. 2017;**5**:8. DOI: 10.3389/fped.2017.00008

[85] Edens C, Robinson AB. Systemic lupus erythematosus, bone health, and osteoporosis. Current Opinion in Endocrinology, Diabetes and Obesity. 2015;**22**(6):422-431. DOI: 10.1097/MED.0000000000000197

[86] Shu Y, Hu Q, Long H, Chang C, Lu Q, Xiao R. Epigenetic variability of CD4+CD25+ tregs contributes to the pathogenesis of autoimmune diseases. Clinical Reviews in Allergy & Immunology. Apr 2017;**52**(2):260-272. DOI: 10.1007/s12016-016-8590-3

[87] Mizui M, Tsokos GC. Low-Dose IL-2 in the treatment of lupus. Current Rheumatology Reports. 2016;**18**(11):68

[88] Von Spee-Mayer C, Siegert E, Abdirama D, Rose A, Klaus A, Alexander T, et al. Low-dose interleukin-2 selectively corrects regulatory T cell defects in patients with systemic lupus erythematosus. Annals of the Rheumatic Diseases. 2016;**75**(7):1407-1415. DOI: 10.1136/annrheumdis-2015-207776

[89] Jiang SH, Shen N, Vinuesa CG. Posttranscriptional T cell gene regulation to limit Tfh cells and autoimmunity. Current Opinion in Immunology. 2015;**37**:21-27. DOI: 10.1016/j.coi.2015.09.003

[90] Ohl K, Tenbrock K. Regulatory T cells in systemic lupus erythematosus. European Journal of Immunology. 2015;**45**(2):344-355. DOI: 10.1002/eji.201344280

[91] Alexander T, Sattler A, Templin L, Kohler S, Groß C, Meisel A, et al. Foxp3+ Helios+ regulatory T cells are expanded in active systemic lupus erythematosus. Annals of the Rheumatic Diseases. 2013;**72**(9):1549-1558. DOI: 10.1136/annrheumdis-2012-202216

[92] Ren W, Liu G, Chen S, Yin J, Wang J, et al. Melatonin signaling in T cells: Functions and applications. Journal of Pineal Research. 2017;**62**(3):1-15. DOI: 10.1111/jpi.12394

[93] Byng-Maddick R, Ehrenstein MR. The impact of biological therapy on regulatory T cells in rheumatoid arthritis. Rheumatology (Oxford). 2015;**54**(5):768-775. DOI: 10.1093/rheumatology/keu487

[94] Kosmaczewska A, Ciszak L, Swierkot J, Szteblich A, Kosciow K, Frydecka I. Exogenous IL-2 controls the balance in Th1, Th17, and Treg cell distribution in patients with progressive rheumatoid arthritis treated with TNF-alpha inhibitors. Inflammation. 2015;**38**(2):765-774. DOI: 10.1007/s10753-014-9987-x

[95] Komatsu N, Takayanagi H. Regulatory T cells in Arthritis. Progress in Molecular Biology and Translational Science. 2015;**136**:207-215. DOI: 10.1016/bs.pmbts.2015.07.021

[96] Wang T, Sun X, Zhao J, Zhang J, Zhu H, Li C, et al. Regulatory T cells in rheumatoid arthritis showed increased plasticity toward Th17 but retained suppressive function in peripheral blood. Annals of the Rheumatic Diseases. 2015;**74**(6):1293-1301. DOI: 10.1136/annrheumdis-2013-204228

[97] Asnagli H, Martire D, Belmonte N, et al. Type 1 regulatory T cells specific for collagen type II as an efficient cell-based therapy in arthritis. Arthritis Research & Therapy. 2014;**16**(3):R115. DOI: 10.1186/ar4567

[98] Noori-Zadeh A, Mesbah-Namin SA, Bistoon-Beigloo S, Bakhtiyari S, Abbaszadeh HA, Darabi S, et al. Regulatory T cell number in multiple sclerosis patients: A meta-analysis. Multiple Sclerosis and Related Disorders. 2016;**5**:73-76. DOI: 10.1016/j.msard.2015.11.004

[99] Lee PW, Severin ME, Lovett-Racke AE. TGF-β regulation of encephalitogenic and regulatory T cells in multiple sclerosis. European Journal of Immunology. 2017;**47**(3):446-453. DOI: 10.1002/eji.20164

Chapter 7

Innate Lymphoid Cells (Non-NK ILCs)

Ahmet Eken and Hamiyet Donmez-Altuntas

Additional information is available at the end of the chapter

http://dx.doi.org/10.5772/intechopen.68893

Abstract

Until a decade ago, natural killer (NK) cells constituted the major—if not the sole—player of innate lymphoid cell populations. The discovery of the presence and execution of curial functions by lymphoid tissue inducer-like cells (LTi) in adults is followed by the discovery of Th2-like innate cells and later Th1-like helper group 1 ILCs. With these findings, the innate lymphocyte family has expanded and a new paradigm has emerged. Apparently, innate versions of helper subsets of CD4+ T cells existed in humans and mice. These cells, unlike their adaptive counterparts, lack CD3, T and B cell receptors, do not rearrange their antigen receptors and get activated by microbial products or cytokines. Furthermore, these cells rely on similar transcription factors that helper CD4+ T cells use for their development and functions (such as T-bet, Gata3 and Rorγt); they produce similar effector cytokines (such as IFN-γ; IL-5, IL-13, IL-4; IL-17A, IL-22, GMCSF, respectively). Moreover, these cells assume crucial functions as an immediate, first line source of cytokines/chemokines against pathogens during protective immune responses. Lastly, very much like their adaptive counterparts, they are present and contribute to pathogenesis in various chronic inflammatory diseases of mice and humans in several tissues.

Keywords: ILC1, ILC2, ILC3, innate lymphoid cell, LTi cell

1. Introduction

In this review, recently described ILC subsets (group 1, 2 and 3 innate lymphoid cells,) which are phenotypically and functionally distinct from NK cells, are introduced (**Figure 1**). The origin of these cells, their development, the genes that are necessary for their generations as well as functions are described. The signature cytokines produced by ILC subsets and the parallels between their adaptive counterparts, namely T helper lineages (Th1, Th2, Th17) are discussed. For each ILC type, their phenotypic diversity and subsets, unique and discriminating surface markers are explained. For each cell type, their role in protective immunity, as well as their

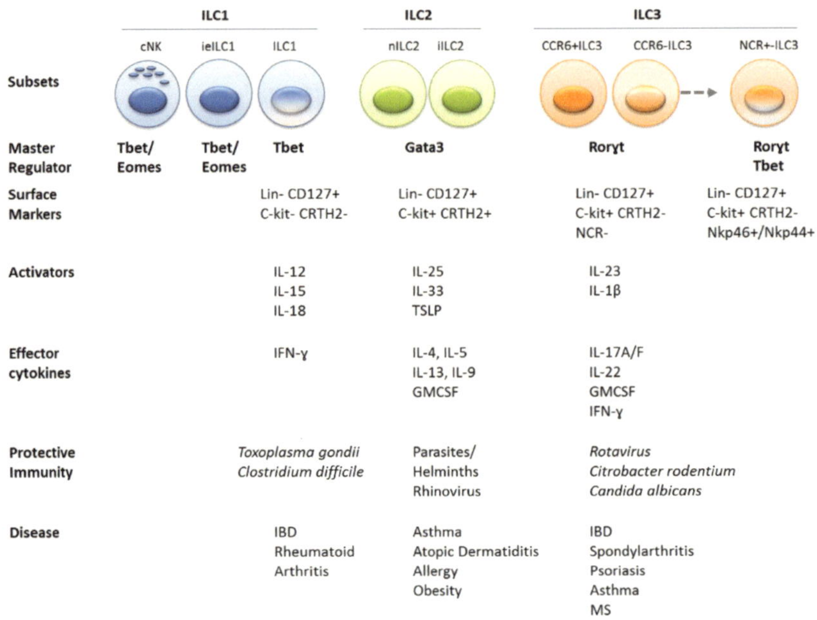

Figure 1. Human innate lymphoid cell classification, signature cytokines and immune processes they are involved in.

involvement in the pathogenesis of various inflammatory diseases, is discussed based on the various data from animal models and human patients. Finally, the plasticity of these cells and the experimental evidence indicating a transition between each lineage are laid out.

2. Group 1 innate lymphoid cells (ILC1)

Group 1 ILCs include Natural killer cells and non-NK ILC1s [1]. We will not be describing NK cells, but concentrate non-NK ILC1s in this review. The distinction between NK cells and non-NK ILC1s is a difficult one to make due to shared use of many markers across tissues [2, 3]. Furthermore, a criterion valid for discrimination of NK cells from non-NK ILC1s in one tissue does not appear to hold for other tissues. Having said that, conventional NK (cNK) cells differ from ILC1 in some regards. ILC1s are found in liver, intestines, uterine tissue, lung, tonsils, peritoneum, spleen and blood [2, 3]. Unlike circulating NK cells, non-NK ILC1s are considered to be mostly tissue resident [4, 5]. ILC1s, like other ILC subsets, express CD127 (IL-7R) whereas mature NK cells do not. T-bet deficiency does not impact cNK cells ontogeny (although it is important in mature NK cells). In contrast, ILC1s are missing in T-bet-deficient mice. Moreover, cNK cells need eomesodermin (Eomes) in addition to T-bet for their function; ILC1s, however, do not express Eomes, though this may change with the tissue of interest. Eomes could also be expressed in low quantity by some NK cells, thus it may not always be a unique NK cell definer.

In humans and mice, both CD127+ and CD127- ILC1s have been described; however, the difference of the latter subset from the cNK cells have been still debated [2, 3, 6]. CD127+ ILC1s were described as Lineage-ckit-CD161+ NKp44+ cells which lacked NK cell markers CD56, CD94, granzyme B and perforin and responsive to IL-12 to produce IFN-γ [7]. CD127+ ILC1s described in the intestinal lamina propria, tonsils and blood as well. These cells are Eomes- and T-bet+, which enforced the idea that they are different than cNK cells. In mice, similar T-bet+ NKp46+ ILC1 were identified by Vonarbourg et al. [8].

CD127- ILC1s, however, are phenotypically closer to cNK cell. They were described in the human intestinal intraepithelial region (named as ieILC1) and tonsils; they express CD56, also CD103 allowing them to interact with epithelial cell [9]. ieILC1s express CD160 in mice. ieILC1s express Eomes and T-bet-like cNK cells but develop from distinct progenitors [10, 11]. In the liver of humans and mice, ILC1s have been reported. $CD3\varepsilon^{-}NK1.1^{+} DX5^{-}$ CD49a+ cells are considered to be liver non-NK ILC1s and lack Eomes; in humans, a small fraction of CD49+ Eomes- ILC1 is presently likely to be the human equivalent of mouse liver ILC1s [3].

In salivary glands, ILC1s are described; however, they express DX5 and Eomes like cNK cells and produce low levels of IFN-γ, and thus, it is unclear if they are truly different than NK cells or ILC1s [3, 12, 13].

2.1. ILC1 development and activation

Hematopoietic common lymphoid progenitors (CLP) differentiate into, first, early innate lymphoid progenitor (EILP) that later give rise to more specialized progenitor positive for TCF-1 [14]. EILP can make both NK cells and ILCs [15]. EILP further differentiates into an ID2+ common helper innate lymphoid progenitor (CHILP) which has lost potential to make NK cells and can generate all helper ILC subsets. CHILP further differentiates into transcription factor promyelocytic leukemia zinc finger (PLZF)+ precursors, which can make, again all ILC subsets with the exception of true LTi cells [16, 17]. PLZF is not expressed in ILC1s; however, ILC1s come from progenitors who expressed PLZF for a period of time during their development [16]. Similar to other ILC subsets, ID2 and Tox are needed for ILC1 development [18, 19]. Nfil3 requirement for ILC1 is controversial [20–23]. Nfil3-independent ILC1s have been reported in breast and prostate tumor tissues, salivary glands, skin, uterus and kidney [3, 12, 13, 24]. Runx3 was also shown to regulate ILC1 as well as ILC3 development [25, 26]. Lastly, at least some of the ILC1s arise as a result of the conversion of ILC3s or ILC2s to ILC1. Ex-ILC3 ILC1s develop from CCR6- ILC3s through upregulation of NKp46 and gradual loss of Rorγt upon IL-12 and IL-15 stimulation [6, 8]. ILC2s can also give rise to ILC1 upon IL-12 and Il-1β exposure, thus a fraction of ILC1 would be ex-ILC2s [27–29].

IFN-γ is the signature cytokine of ILC1s. And ILC1s are activated by IL-12, IL-18 or IL-15 to produce those cytokines.

2.2. ILC1s in protective immunity

ILC1s are thought to be important in immunity against viruses, intracellular bacteria or protozoans owing to their production of IFN-γ [30]. Several infectious agents have been used to assess the role of ILC1s in protective immunity.

A study from Diefenbach's laboratory showed that during *Toxoplasma gondii* infection ILC1s contribute to IFN-γ and TNF-α production and thus, to protective immunity; in T-bet-deficient mice, in which ILC1s are missing, the infection progresses more severely [31]. Though T-bet also functions in NK cells, this study suggests that ILC1s might be important in immunity to *Toxoplasma gondii.* Another study by the same group showed that ILC1s substantially contribute to IFN-γ production during *Salmonella enterica* infection, and the bacteria-induced colitis is alleviated if these cells were depleted [6].

ILC1-based protective immunity to another pathogen was tested by Eric Pamer's group. They showed that due to the absence of ILC1 (but not ILC3), Rag2-/-Il2Rγc-/- mice are more susceptible to *Clostridium difficile* infection. Accordingly, those mice are protected after adoptive transfer of ILC1s, suggesting that ILC1s may play a crucial role in protective immunity to *C. difficile* infections [32].

2.3. ILC1s during inflammatory diseases

Synovial fluids of psoriatic arthritis have been reported to be enriched in ILC1 content [33]. Although a similar increase in NCR+ ILCs in rheumatoid arthritis patients' synovial fluid has been reported, it is unclear whether these cells were conventional NK cells or not.

ILC1 enrichment, particularly in the intestines, has been reported in inflammatory bowel diseases (IBD) patients as well as in various murine models of IBD than found in any other disease [7, 8, 34, 35]. These ILC1s appear to be ex-ILC3s who lost Rorγt expression over time and became a major source of IFN-γ.

3. Group 2 innate lymphoid cells (ILC2)

ILC2s are found in mucosal surfaces, such as lungs and intestines, and the mesentery, fat-associated lymphoid clusters (FALC) as well as blood. They are identified by various groups at about the same time under different names as nuocytes, natural helper cells, innate type 2 helper (Ih2) cells, or multipotent progenitor type 2 (MPP^{type2}) cells [36–38]. Although these innate cells have been previously reported by McKenzie's group and others as a source of Th2 cytokines, naming and a through characterization of them came after these initial reports [39, 40].

Currently, ILC2 s in mice can be categorized into two subsets. Natural ILC2s (nILC2) and inflammatory ILC2s (iLC2). nILC2 was shown to be regulated by IL-33 and rely more on IL-33R (IL-1βLR), whereas iILC2 reportedly express IL-25R and is regulated by IL-25 [41]. nILC2s produce Th2 cytokines IL-5 and IL-13. iILC2, however, can produce IL-13 and IL-17 together.

Human ILC2s that can produce both IL-13 and IL-22 with low Rorγt expression has been defined [42].

Although T-bet is a Th1-specific transcription factor important in driving IFN-γ expression (in NK cells and ILC1), its deletion in ILC2s revealed that it also assumes important functions particularly suppressing IL-9 production by ILC2s. In IL-33-induced airway inflammation mouse models, Tbx21 deficiency lead to exacerbated eosinophilic inflammation mediated by unleashed IL-9 production [43].

3.1. ILC2 development and activation

All the ILC subsets differentiate from a common lymphoid progenitor (CLP) that can also give rise to adaptive lymphoid cells. Further specialization of this progenitor proceeds to a branching point after which inhibitory DNA binding protein 2 (Id2) is derepressed in newly formed progenitors. This branching by upregulating Id2 is believed to commit the precursor to a helper ILC lineage. This $Id2^+$ precursor is named as common helper innate lymphoid progenitor (CHILP), and so far, lacks potential to make cNK cells. Although Id2 is also reported to be required for cNK cells development, its upregulation occurs after $Id2^-$NK cell precursor branches off to an NK cell fate before the CHILP stage. In other words, current literature suggest that NK lineage branches off from CLP before CHILP does. Phenotypically, CHILP is defined to be $Lin^-Id2^+Flt3^-IL\text{-}7R\alpha^+$ CD25- or more recently $Lin^-Flt3^-IL\text{-}7R\alpha^+\alpha_4\beta_7^+$ PD-1^{high} and have Tox2, Tcf-1, Gata3 expression and differentiate into all ILC subsets after adoptive transfer [44].

Deletion of Gata3 in hematopoietic cells blocks development of all helper ILC subsets, but spares cNK cells [45]. However, spatiotemporal deletion driven by stage-specific promoters revealed that Gata3 deletion after Id2 is turned on, only blocks ILC2 generation, whereas its deletion after the initiation of Ncr-1 expression impacts ILC1 [46].

Notch signaling has also been shown to be required for the development of all three ILC subsets to varying degrees both *in vitro* and *in vivo* [47].

Bcl11b is particularly required for specialization into ILC2, its absence blocks ILC2 generation [48].

Rorα is also crucial in ILC2 development. As such Rorα-/- mice lacks ILC2, whereas Th2 cells appear to develop normally. Furthermore, Rorα-/- mice fail to mount protease-induced asthma consistent with the role of ILC2s in this process [49, 50].

T-cell factor 1 (TCF1) is another transcription factor required for ILC2 development. TCF-1 is produced by its gene *Tcf7*. TCF-1 is crucial in early thymic T cell development and is also expressed by ILC2s [51, 52]. Studies show that its deletion impairs ILC2 development and that TCF-1 works downstream of Notch signaling during ILC2 development. Thus, papain-induced inflammation or protective immunity is diminished in Tcf7-/- mice [15].

Nuclear factor IL-3 (*Nfil3*), also known as *E4BP4,* is a transcription factor previously reported to be required for generation of some of the hematopoietic cells, including CD8+ DCs and, although controversial, NK cells. Nfil3-/- mice have been shown to lack Peyer's patches, both ILC3 and ILC2 cells have been shown to be greatly reduced in the Nfil3-/- mice. Consistent with these results, Nfil3-/- mice mounts a weak immune response to *Citrobacter rodentium* infection and a reduced airway inflammation to papain-induced allergy [53].

Gfi1 (growth factor independent 1) is also another gene reported to regulate ILC2 development ad function. Its genetic deletion results in reduced number and function of ILCs, and render mice more susceptible to worm infection and more resistant to papain-induced lung inflammation [54].

ILC2 cells interact with Th2 cells, via costimulatory molecules OX40/OX40L, MHCII as well as cytokines such as IL-4; by doing so, they allow generation of a robust immunity [55].

IL-25, IL-33, TSLP, leukotriene D4 and IL-4 are the most notable activators of ILC2s.

Activation of Th2 cells through TCR leads to activation and translocation of NFAT to the nucleus, in addition to mobilization of AP1 and NF-κB, all of which lead to the expression of Th2 cytokines. The latter two were described for ILC2s, how NFAT gets activated was not known. More recently, leukotriene receptors have been shown to activate NFAT in ILC2s [56].

Another protein important for Th2 activation is PKC-θ. PKC-θ was also expressed by ILC2 and its absence results in reduced ILC2 numbers, in addition to Th2 cell reduction. Moreover, IL-5, IL-13 as well as IRF4 production by ILC2s are regulated by PKC-θ, thus its deletion or inhibition blocks their production in HDM allergen-induced airway hypersensitivity model [57].

IL-33 in the lung is produced by epithelial cells (mostly pneumocytes) and antigen presenting cells (DCs and macrophages) [58].

ILC2s also express IL-4R and expand in response to IL-4 (produced by basophils) during atopic dermatitis [59].

3.2. ILC2s in protective immunity

ILC2s are important in defense against helminths/worms and rhinoviruses. *Nippostrongylus brasiliensis* or *Strongyloides venezuelensis* infection models are widely used in ILC2 studies, the infection of mice with these pathogens results in accumulation and activation of ILC2 s in the lungs [60, 61]. Using IL-33KO mice, it was shown that ILC2 expansion and IL-13 production by ILC2s are important in immunity against hookworm *N. brasiliensis* in mice [62].

ILC2s has also been shown to expand during rhinovirus infection in mice in an IL-25-dependent fashion [63].

ILC2s also support the generation of a robust Th2 response. ILC2s function as a IL-4 source and by providing IL-4 they support Th2 differentiation or maintenance. Thus, during *H. polygyrus* infection in mice ILC2 specific deletion of the IL-4 result in diminished Th2 response [64].

3.3. ILC2s during inflammatory diseases

ILC2s are implicated in various chronic inflammatory conditions, including asthma, atopic dermatitis (AD) and chronic rhinosinusitis.

AD patient skins have increased ILC2 (as well as other ILC subsets) [65]. Studies with mouse models of AD also showed that ILC2 cells can induce AD symptoms in the absence of T cells in Rag-/- mice. IL-5, IL-13 and/or IL-2 may be important in driving pathology in these contexts [66–68].

Chemoattractant receptor-homologous molecule expressed on Th2 cells (CRTH2) is expressed by Th2, ILC2, eosinophils and basophils. A humanized antibody targeting CRTH2 can deplete these cells along with ILC2 and have been shown to effectively ameliorate airway inflammation developed by various means in a humanized mouse model [69].

The contribution of ILC2 to the development of asthma in various mice models have been shown. Even in the presence of Th2 cells, ILC2s make a substantial contribution to pathogenesis through the production of IL-4, IL-5 and IL-13 during IL-25/IL-33 induced as well as house dust mite-induced asthma models [70]. The contribution of ILC2s to allergic inflammation was assessed most notably in Rag-/- mice which lack adaptive immune cells. House dust mite (HDM), as well as papain protease-induced models of asthma/airway inflammation, was ameliorated in Rag1-/- animals when ILC2s were deleted, and disease was restored when ILC2s were adoptively transferred in to Rag2-/-IL2rgc-/- animals which lack ILC2s [49].

Furthermore, virally induced airway inflammation via H3N1 (within 5 days of infection) has also been shown to be dependent on ILC2 [71] and manifested itself in either the WT or Rag1-/- mice. As expected, the inflammation was dependent on IL-33 and the downstream IL-13.

Tuft cells in the intestine constitutively produce IL-25 and regulate ILC2 homeostasis. After helminth infection, ILC2 activation relies on tuft cell-derived IL-25 which also further stimulates ILC2 for IL-13 production leading eventually to epithelial regeneration [72].

In a mouse model of cutaneous injury, ILC2 was suggested to promote wound healing through their activation by IL-33 [73]. ILC2s were found enriched in the nasal polyps of chronic rhinosinusitis patients as well [74].

For the eosinophilia associated with asthma or other allergen induced asthma models, ILC2-derived IL-13 was shown to be necessary. Additionally, ILC2s were proposed to cause the eosinophilia observed in some patients with autoimmune disease who are receiving experimental IL-2 therapy. This is shown to be mediated via IL-5 rather than IL-13 [75].

ILC2s were reported to be involved in obesity in various reports. ILC2s are present in the adipose tissue both in humans and mice and were shown to regulate adipocyte differentiation directly via ILC2-derived methionine-enkephalin peptides that act on adipocytes or indirectly by mobilizing eosinophils which eventually leads to adipocyte beiging. Thus, modulating ILCs or activatory cytokines IL-25 or IL-33 presents themselves as potential therapeutic approaches [76–79].

4. Group 3 innate lymphoid cells (ILC3)

Various subsets of RORgt+ group 3 ILCs have been reported both in humans and mice [80–82]. ILC3s are characterized as lineage—(CD3-Tcrab-Tcrγδ-CD11b-Cd19-) CD45+ CD127+ Ckit+ Rorγt+ IL-23R+ in both mice and humans. Currently, the ILC3 community categorizes them into two major groups (LTi cells/NCR-ILC3s/CCR6+ ILC3s and NCR+ ILC3s); however, these two major groups do not represent final states, likely vary in their expression of various cell surface markers upon exposure to different microenvironment-specific stimuli.

LTi cells (CCR6+ ILC3s or NCR-ILC3s): Lymphoid tissue inducer (LTi) cells are the prototype of group 3 ILCs. They were found initially in the fetal liver of mice and were reported to be required for the generation of peripheral secondary lymphoid organs such as lymph nodes and Peyer's patches via their interactions with stromal cells. In the absence or dysfunction of LTi cells (shown through genetic deletion of the genes including Rorγt, IL-2Rγc, IL-7R (CD127) and LTα, or LTβR), these organs fail to develop. LTi cells are also important for the development of cryptopatches and isolated lymphoid follicles in the intestine whose formation take place early after birth [83, 82]. Fetal LTi cells are characterized by the expression of CD127 (IL-7Ra), CCR6, Rorγt, IL-23R and lymphotoxin $\alpha 1\beta 2$ [84]. LTi cells do not express natural cytotoxicity receptor (NKp46 or NKp44). Adult human and mice also harbor such LTi-like cells (adult LTi cells) with potential to induce lymphoid organogenesis and with similar surface markers [44, 85].

LTi cells also have subsets. Neuropilin+ subset is identified which mainly reside in tissues and nearby high endothelial venules [86]. LTi cell can also be categorized based on a CD4 expression.

NCR+ ILC3s (CCR6-ILC3s): The second major ILC3 subset express natural cytotoxicity receptors NKp44 or NKp46 in humans and mice, respectively [81, 87, 44]. It was debated whether these cells develop through a separate lineage than that of LTi cells. The most current evidence indicates that a branching occurs in the developmental pathway allowing progress of two different lineage pathways one leading to the precursors of NKp46+ ILC3, which do not give rise to true LTi cells. The other branch, on the other hand, leads to LTi development. NKp46+ ILC3, unlike LTi cells, express low levels of CCR6 and interestingly co-express the Th1 master regulator T-bet and Rorγt. NCR+ ILC3s, in mice, have been shown to derive from CCR6-NCR- ILC3s, which expand shortly after birth in the intestines upon exposure to various dietary ligands. CCR6-NCR- ILC3s then can give rise to NCR+T-bet+ILC3s; further conditioning of these cells with IL-12 pushes them to ILC1 phenotype. Upregulation of NKp46 in CCR6-NCR- ILC3 requires T-bet and Notch signaling, thus in Tbx21-/- mice, although CCR6+ and CCR6- ILC3 are present, upregulation of NKp46+ and transition from NCR-CCR6- state to NKp46+ ILC3 does not occur due to a block [6, 8, 88].

4.1. ILC3 development and activation

RORγt transcription factor is a common requirement for all ILC3 subset's development. As such, its genetic deletion results in complete absence of all ILC3 subsets and lack of lymph nodes and Peyer's patches as well as crypto patches and isolated lymphoid follicles in mice [89–91]. Like all other ILCs, Id2, tox2 and IL-7 are crucial for the development of ILC3s. Indeed, genetic deletion of any of these genes in mice results in a reduction in the ILC3 population [92]. Tox 2 is transcription factor is necessary for upregulation of Id2. Also, TCF-1, NFIL3, Gata3 were also shown to regulate ILC3 development [44]. AhR is another transcription factor required for the generation of CCR6- ILC3 subset. Genetic deletion of AhR in mice or removal of AhR ligands from the diet result in a reduction in CCR6-ILC3 subsets [6, 44]. These studies also showed that CCR6- ILC3 subsets are involved in crypto patches and isolated lymphoid follicle formation in the small intestine. Our studies revealed that cytoskeleton protein dedicator of cytokinesis 8 (Dock8) is required for the generation/maintenance and function of adult ILC3s [93]. In the Dock8-/- mice ILC3 cells are missing in the adult mice despite the fact that Dock8-/- mice have normal lymph nodes and Peyer's patches suggesting that fetal LTi cells are spared. Lastly, as alluded above, T-bet is necessary for the development of NCR+ ILC3s; thus, in Tbx21-/- mice these cells are missing [6].

All ILC3 subsets express the IL-23 receptor (IL-23R) and are activated by IL-23 produced by antigen presenting cells upon activation with various PAMPs [94]. IL-23 also regulates the expansion of ILC3s [95–97]. IL-23R signaling activates STAT3, which subsequently translocates to the nucleus, and turns on several ILC3 signature cytokine genes (IL-22, IL-17A/F etc.). In addition, IL-1β was also shown to activate and expand ILC3s [97].

4.2. ILC3s in protective immunity

In the steady state, ILC3s assume critical functions in the mucosal surfaces for the containment of the commensals at an arms distance of epithelial cells [98, 99]. This is mainly achieved via ILC3-derived IL-22, which act on epithelial cells, in turn resulting in the production of various anti-microbial molecules, including Reg3γ, Reg3β, S100A8, S100A9 and mucins. Indeed, in the absence of ILC3s, microbial translocation across intestinal epithelium and detection of microbes in the distant organs/tissues has been reported [100].

Viral, bacterial, as well as fungal infection models have been used to dissect the role ILC3s during these infections. Rotavirus infection is cleared much more efficiently with the help of IL-22 coming from the innate sources (mainly ILC3). IL-22 was shown to synergize with IFN-γ to boost the production IFN-γ-mediated expression of antiviral genes [101, 102].

ILC3s also fight some enteric bacteria. The most notable example is attaching-effacing *Citrobacter rodentium*, which is widely used by the ILC3 community in murine models. ILC3s and innate IL-22 are necessary for protection from infection in mice lacking adaptive cells [93, 103, 104]. In the lymphoreplete mice, it was controversial whether ILC3s are absolutely required owing to the presence of Th17 cells, and data indicate in the immunocompetent mice that the redundant mechanisms may eventually save the mice [104].

To dissect the role of ILC3s in fungal immunity *Candida albicans* has been used in murine models. *Rag1-/-* mice became susceptible when ILC3s are depleted, or when *Rorc* is deleted [105, 106]. Given that absence of Th17 axis leads to susceptibility to *Candida* infections, ILC3s are likely important, however, how essential they are, whether Th17 and ILC3 redundantly control the immunity is unknown.

4.3. ILC3s during inflammatory diseases

ILC3 are implicated in several chronic inflammatory diseases based on data obtained from murine models and human patients. Accumulation of ILC3-like cells (defined as NK-22 in the paper with ability to produce IL-22 and TNF-a) or LTi cells in the synovial fluid of rheumatoid arthritis patients have reported [107, 108].

IL-23 pathway and IL-17 has been shown to drive the pathogenesis of spondylarthritis. Antibodies against IL-17 are being tested in trials. In the synovial fluid of psoriatic arthritis patients, increased IL-17+ NKp44+ ILC3s were reported; augmented amounts of CCL20 in the synovial fluid imply that CCR6+ ILC3s may be attracted through this ligand [30, 33, 109].

NKp44+ ILC3s enrichment in the tissues (ileum, synovial fluid, blood bone marrow) of ankylosing spondylitis have been reported. Some of the studies found IL-17 production by these ILC3s, others reported them as an IL-22 source [30].

NKp44+ ILC3 are also implicated in systemic sclerosis and systemic lupus erythematosus [30, 110].

In various mouse models of IBD, ILC3s were shown to play critical roles [111]. In infection-induced colitis (by *Citrobacter rodentium* or *Helicobacter pylori*), these cells mediate pathology via IL-17 and IFN-γ [95]. ILC3s, via IL-22, have also been shown to drive pathology in some IBD models [96, 104], whereas in other murine models ILC3-derived IL-22 was shown to be protective [112]. In human Crohn's disease patients' intestines, ILC3s were enriched. CD56+ ILC3s were shown to produce IL-22, whereas CD56- ILC3s produced IL-17 and F [113]. Others, however, reported enrichment of IFN-γ+ ILC1s, rather a reduction in NCR+ IL-22 ILC3s [7, 114]. IFN-γ+ ILC1s presence in the intestine appear to be a common theme in both human IBD and murine IBD models, in fact, by fate map experiments, IFN-γ+ ILC1s have been shown to derive from ILC3s via gradual loss of Rorγt [6, 8, 35].

ILC3s have also been shown to be crucial for the induction of peripheral tolerance to commensal antigens via MHCII molecules they express along with low levels of costimulatory molecules. Deletion of MHCII in ILC3s break this tolerance and results in IBD-like disease in mice models [115, 116].

Increased ILC3 number and/or activity have been reported in other autoimmune diseases [30]. In psoriasis patients, both in the skin and blood, elevated frequency of ILC3s either producing IL-22 or IL-17A has been described [117, 118]. Similarly, in the mouse model of multiple sclerosis, EAE, ILC3 presence in the brain was reported. More importantly, ILC3 number or activity is also described in MS patients blood and CSF [119–122]. In both of these autoimmune conditions, how actually ILC3s impact the disease progression is yet to be defined.

5. Plasticity of ILCs

Most recent research indicates that ILCs could modify their transcriptional program and convert to another type in the presence of environmental cues that favor the effector functions of one over the other. This was proposed to occur between ILC3 and ILC1, via modulating the availability of IL-23 or IL-12. Similar plasticity has been reported between ILC2 and ILC1. A summary and discussion of the current information regarding the plasticity between ILC subsets are presented below.

5.1. ILC2 to ILC1 or ILC2 to ILC3 plasticity

A few intracellular molecules that maintain ILC2 identity have been defined. Bcl11b and Gfi1 maintain the expression of ILC2 genes associated with ILC2 identity, the deletion of either gene in mice blocks ILC2 master regulator Gata3 expression and, subsequently, IL-5 and IL-13 production [54, 123]. Bcl11b or Gif1 KO ILC2 can also produce IL-17. Lysine methyltransferase G9a gene was shown to also suppress ILC3-related genes' expression in ILC2. Additionally, Zhang et al. showed that Notch signaling can promote Rorc and IL-17 production by iILC2 cells that are primarily responsive to IL-25 [124].

External stimuli that drive phenotypic switch from ILC2 to other innate lineages have been demonstrated recently in murine models [27, 29, 125]. IL-12 and/or IL-18 have been shown to push ILC2 to an ILC1-like phenotype (with increased production of IFN-γ and reduced Gata-3 expression). This conversion appears to be driven by viruses (influenza, RSV) and bacteria (*S. aureus*). Observations in human patients of chronic obstructive pulmonary disease (COPD) or chronic rhinosinusitis with nasal polyps (CRSwNP) have been shown to harbor elevated levels of ILC1 and ILC2 cells, and their signature cytokines imply that this phenotypic conversion may occur in humans as well. A detailed examination of ILC2 fate in human hematopoietic cells-engrafted IL2rγ-/-Nod/scid mice suggested that these cells indeed can assume an ILC1 phenotype with IL-12 exposure [27]. IL-1β was shown to prime ILC2s at high concentrations and potentiate the IL-12 driven phenotypic switch to Gata3+ T-bet+ ILC1 fate [125].

5.2. ILC3 to ILC1 plasticity

The plasticity of ILC3 lineage was first described by Vonarbourg et al. in a study which employed Rorγt fate map mice [8]. In this work the authors demonstrated that Rorγt+ ILC3s downregulated this transcription factor, gradually upregulated T-bet and NKp46, this eventually led to a cell population termed as "ex- ILC3". This transition requires T-bet, notch signaling. IL-12 and IL-15 were shown to promote this transition. Conversion of ILC3s to ILC1s has been observed by many other investigators in mice. More importantly, ILC3-to ILC1 conversion has been shown to operate for human ILC3s in a reversible fashion, dictated by the presence of IL-12 in ILC3 to ILC1 direction and by IL-23 in the other direction [7, 35, 114].

6. Conclusions

The discovery of ILCs brought a paradigm shift in our understanding of both innate and adaptive immunology. From a developmental standpoint, understating the lineage specification in ILCs, their similarities to and differences from helper T cells need to be worked out in better detail moving forward. Ambiguities regarding ILC1-NK cell classifications require more studies. Various gene expression studies have been done to identify such unique and distinctive molecules, and hopefully, more functional studies will remove the confusion. More importantly, the extent and nature of the involvement of these cells in the inflammatory diseases and tissue homeostasis will be further evaluated beyond diseases described for the past 7 years. Also, the discovery of more specific surface markers and inhibitors that will target exclusively ILCs are needed for both understanding the possible redundancy between ILCs and helper T cells and for potential use as therapeutics.

Author details

Ahmet Eken and Hamiyet Donmez-Altuntas*

*Address all correspondence to: donmezh@erciyes.edu.tr

Department of Medical Biology, Medical Faculty, Erciyes University, Kayseri, Turkey

References

[1] Cortez VS, Colonna M. Diversity and function of group 1 innate lymphoid cells. Immunology Letters. 2016; **179**:19-24

[2] Spits H, Bernink JH, Lanier L. NK cells and type 1 innate lymphoid cells: Partners in host defense. Nature Immunology. 2016;**17**:758-764

[3] Fuchs A. ILC1s in Tissue Inflammation and Infection. Frontiers in Immunology. 2016 **7**:104

[4] Gasteiger G, Fan X, Dikiy S, et al. Tissue residency of innate lymphoid cells in lymphoid and nonlymphoid organs. Science. (80-); 2015;**350**:981-985

[5] Peng H, Jiang X, Chen Y, et al. Liver-resident NK cells confer adaptive immunity in skin-contact inflammation. Journal of Clinical Investigation. 2013;**123**:1444-1456

[6] Klose CSN, Kiss EA, Schwierzeck V, et al. A T-bet gradient controls the fate and function of CCR6-RORγt+ innate lymphoid cells. Nature. 2013;**494**:261-265

[7] Bernink JH, Peters CP, Munneke M, et al. Human type 1 innate lymphoid cells accumulate in inflamed mucosal tissues. Nature Immunology. 2013;**14**:221-229

[8] Vonarbourg C, Mortha A, Bui VL, et al. Regulated expression of nuclear receptor RORγt confers distinct functional fates to NK cell receptor-expressing RORγt(+) innate lymphocytes. Immunity. 2010;**33**:736-751

[9] Chen Y, Chou K, Fuchs E, et al. Protection of the intestinal mucosa by intraepithelial gamma delta T cells. Proceedings of the National Academy of Sciences of United States of America. 2002;**99**:14338-14343

[10] Daussy C, Faure F, Mayol K, et al. T-bet and Eomes instruct the development of two distinct natural killer cell lineages in the liver and in the bone marrow. The Journal of Experimental Medicine. 2014;**211**:563-577

[11] Peng H, Tian Z. Re-examining the origin and function of liver-resident NK cells. Trends in Immunology. 2015;**36**:293-299

[12] Tessmer MS, Reilly EC, Brossay L. Salivary gland NK cells are phenotypically and functionally unique. PLOS Pathogens; 2011;**7**: e1001254

[13] Cortez VS, Fuchs A, Cella M, et al. Cutting edge: Salivary gland NK cells develop independently of Nfil3 in steady-state. The Journal of Immunology. 2014;**192**:4487-4491

[14] Zook EC, Kee BL. Development of innate lymphoid cells. Nature Immunology. 2016; **17**:775-782

[15] Yang Q, Li F, Harly C, et al. TCF-1 upregulation identifies early innate lymphoid progenitors in the bone marrow. Nature Immunology. 2015;**16**:1044-1050

[16] Constantinides MG, McDonald BD, Verhoef PA, et al. A committed precursor to innate lymphoid cells. 2014 Nature. **508**:397-401

[17] Constantinides MG, Gudjonson H, McDonald BD, et al. PLZF expression maps the early stages of ILC1 lineage development. Proceedings of the National Academy of Sciences. 2015;**112**:5123-5128

[18] Seehus CR, Aliahmad P, de la Torre B, et al. The development of innate lymphoid cells requires TOX-dependent generation of a common innate lymphoid cell progenitor. Nature Immunology. 2015;**16**:599-608

[19] Yokota Y, Mansouri A, Mori S, et al. Development of peripheral lymphoid organs and natural killer cells depends on the helix-loop-helix inhibitor Id2. Nature. 1999;**397**:702-706

[20] Xu AT, Li Y, Zhao D, et al. High suppressor of cytokine signaling-3 expression impairs STAT3-dependent protective effects of interleukin-22 in ulcerative colitis in remission. Inflammatory Bowel Diseases. 2015;**21**:241-250

[21] DiSanto JP, Müller W, Guy-Grand D, et al. Lymphoid development in mice with a targeted deletion of the interleukin 2 receptor gamma chain. Proceedings of the National Academy of Sciences of the United States of America. 1995;**92**:377-381

[22] Xu W, Domingues RG, Fonseca-Pereira D, et al. NFIL3 Orchestrates the emergence of common helper innate lymphoid cell precursors. 2015 Cell Reports. **10**:2043-2054

[23] Yu X, Wang Y, Deng M, et al. The basic leucine zipper transcription factor NFIL3 directs the development of a common innate lymphoid cell precursor. Elife;**3**. Epub ahead of print 13 October 2014. DOI: 10.7554/eLife.04406

[24] Dadi S, Chhangawala S, Whitlock BM, et al. Cancer Immunosurveillance by tissue-resident innate lymphoid cells and innate-like T cells. Cell. 2016;**164**:365-377

[25] Ebihara T, Song C, Ryu SH, et al. Runx3 specifies lineage commitment of innate lymphoid cells. Nature Immunology. 2015;**16**:1124-1133

[26] Levanon D, Negreanu V, Lotem J, et al. Transcription factor Runx3 regulates interleukin-15-dependent natural killer cell activation. Molecular and Cellular Biology. 2014;**34**:1158-1169

[27] Bal SM, Bernink JH, Nagasawa M, et al. IL-1β, IL-4 and IL-12 control the fate of group 2 innate lymphoid cells in human airway inflammation in the lungs. Nature Immunology. 2016;**17**:636-645

[28] Lim AI, Menegatti S, Bustamante J, et al. IL-12 drives functional plasticity of human group 2 innate lymphoid cells. The Journal of Experimental Medicine. 2016;**213**:569-583

[29] Silver JS, Kearley J, Copenhaver AM, et al. Inflammatory triggers associated with exacerbations of COPD orchestrate plasticity of group 2 innate lymphoid cells in the lungs. Nature Immunology. 2016;**17**:626-635

[30] Shikhagaie MM, Germar K, Bal SM, et al. Innate lymphoid cells in autoimmunity: emerging regulators in rheumatic diseases. Nature Reviews Rheumatology. 2017;**13**:164-173

[31] Klose CSN, Flach M, Möhle L, et al. Differentiation of Type 1 ILCs from a common progenitor to all helper-like innate lymphoid cell lineages. 2014 Cell. **157**:340-356

[32] Abt MC, Lewis BB, Caballero S, et al. Innate immune defenses mediated by two ILC subsets are critical for protection against acute clostridium difficile Infection. Cell Host & Microbe. 2015;;**18**:27-37

[33] Leijten EFA, van Kempen TS, Boes M, et al. Brief Report: Enrichment of activated group 3 innate lymphoid cells in psoriatic arthritis synovial fluid. Arthritis & Rheumatology. 2015;**67**:2673-2678

[34] Fuchs A, Vermi W, Lee JS, et al. Intraepithelial type 1 innate lymphoid cells are a unique subset of IL-12- and IL-15-responsive IFN-γ-producing cells. Immunity. 2013;**38**:769-781

[35] Qiu J, Guo X, Chen Z-ME, et al. Group 3 innate lymphoid cells inhibit T-cell-mediated intestinal inflammation through aryl hydrocarbon receptor signaling and regulation of microflora. Immunity. 2013;**39**:386-399

[36] Moro K, Yamada T, Tanabe M, et al. Innate production of TH2 cytokines by adipose tissue-associated c-Kit+Sca-1+ lymphoid cells. Nature. 2010;**463**:540-544

[37] Neill DR, Wong SH, Bellosi A, et al. Nuocytes represent a new innate effector leukocyte that mediates type-2 immunity. Nature. 2010;**464**:1367-1370

[38] Price AE, Liang H-E, Sullivan BM, et al. Systemically dispersed innate IL-13-expressing cells in type 2 immunity. Proceedings of the National Academy of Sciences. 2010;**107**:11489-11494

[39] Fallon PG, Ballantyne SJ, Mangan NE, et al. Identification of an interleukin (IL)-25–dependent cell population that provides IL-4, IL-5, and IL-13 at the onset of helminth expulsion. The Journal of Experimental Medicine. 2006;**203**:1105-1116

[40] Terashima A, Watarai H, Inoue S, et al. A novel subset of mouse NKT cells bearing the IL-17 receptor B responds to IL-25 and contributes to airway hyperreactivity. The Journal of Experimental Medicine. 2008;**205**:2727-2733

[41] Huang Y, Guo L, Qiu J, et al. IL-25-responsive, lineage-negative KLRG1hi cells are multipotential 'inflammatory' type 2 innate lymphoid cells. Nature Immunology. 2014;**16**:161-169

[42] Mjösberg JM, Trifari S, Crellin NK, et al. Human IL-25–and IL-33-responsive type 2 innate lymphoid cells are defined by expression of CRTH2 and CD161. Nature Immunology. 2011;**12**:1055-1062

[43] Matsuki A, Takatori H, Makita S, et al. T-bet inhibits innate lymphoid cell-mediated eosinophilic airway inflammation by suppressing IL-9 production. Journal of Allergy and Clinical Immunology. Epub ahead of print 23 September 2016. DOI: 10.1016/j.jaci.2016.08.022

[44] Diefenbach A, Colonna M, Koyasu S. Development, differentiation, and diversity of innate lymphoid cells. Immunity. 2014;**41**:354-365

[45] Yagi R, Zhong C, Northrup DL, et al. The transcription factor GATA3 is critical for the development of all IL-7Rα-expressing innate lymphoid cells. Immunity. 2014;**40**:378-388

[46] Hoyler T, Klose CSN, Souabni A, et al. The transcription factor GATA-3 controls cell fate and maintenance of type 2 innate lymphoid cells. Immunity. 2012;**37**:634-648

[47] Mielke LA, Groom JR, Rankin LC, et al. TCF-1 controls ILC2 and NKp46+ROR t+ innate lymphocyte differentiation and protection in intestinal inflammation. The Journal of Immunology. 2013;**191**:4383-4391

[48] Yu Y, Tsang JCH, Wang C, et al. Single-cell RNA-seq identifies a PD-1(hi) ILC progenitor and defines its development pathway. Nature. 2016;**539**:102-106

[49] Halim TYF, MacLaren A, Romanish MT, et al. Retinoic-Acid-Receptor-related orphan nuclear receptor alpha is required for natural helper cell development and allergic inflammation. Immunity. 2012;**37**:463-474

[50] Wong SH, Walker JA, Jolin HE, et al. Transcription factor RORα is critical for nuocyte development. Nature Immunology. 2012;**13**:229-236

[51] Germar K, Dose M, Konstantinou T, et al. T-cell factor 1 is a gatekeeper for T-cell specification in response to Notch signaling. Proceedings of the National Academy of Sciences of the United States of America. 2011;**108**:20060-20065

[52] Weber BN, Chi AW-S, Chavez A, et al. A critical role for TCF-1 in T-lineage specification and differentiation. 2011 Nature. **476**:63-68

[53] Seillet C, Huntington ND, Gangatirkar P, et al. Differential Requirement for Nfil3 during NK Cell Development. The Journal of Immunology. 2014;**192**:2667-2676

[54] Spooner CJ, Lesch J, Yan D, et al. Specification of type 2 innate lymphocytes by the transcriptional determinant Gfi1. Nature Immunology. 2013;**14**:1229-1236

[55] Drake LY, Iijima K, Kita H. Group 2 innate lymphoid cells and CD4+ T cells cooperate to mediate type 2 immune response in mice. Allergy. 2014;**69**:1300-1307

[56] von Moltke J, O'Leary CE, Barrett NA, et al. Leukotrienes provide an NFAT-dependent signal that synergizes with IL-33 to activate ILC2s. The Journal of Experimental Medicine. 2017;**214**:27-37

[57] Madouri F, Chenuet P, Beuraud C, et al. Protein kinase Cθ controls type 2 innate lymphoid cell and TH2 responses to house dust mite allergen. Journal of Allergy and Clinical Immunology. Epub ahead of print October 2016. DOI: 10.1016/j.jaci.2016.08.044

[58] Hardman CS, Panova V, McKenzie ANJ. IL-33 citrine reporter mice reveal the temporal and spatial expression of IL-33 during allergic lung inflammation. European Journal of Immunology. 2013;**43**:488-498

[59] Kim BS, Wang K, Siracusa MC, et al. Basophils Promote Innate lymphoid cell responses in inflamed skin. The Journal of Immunology. 2014;**193**:3717-3725

[60] Yasuda K, Muto T, Kawagoe T, et al. Contribution of IL-33-activated type II innate lymphoid cells to pulmonary eosinophilia in intestinal nematode-infected mice. Proceedings of the National Academy of Sciences. 2012;**109**:3451-3456

[61] Liang H-E, Reinhardt RL, Bando JK, et al. Divergent expression patterns of IL-4 and IL-13 define unique functions in allergic immunity. Nature Immunology. 2011;**13**:58-66

[62] Hung L-Y, Lewkowich IP, Dawson LA, et al. IL-33 drives biphasic IL-13 production for noncanonical Type 2 immunity against hookworms. Proceedings of the National Academy of Sciences of the United States of America. 2013;**110**:282-287

[63] Hong JY, Bentley JK, Chung Y, et al. Neonatal rhinovirus induces mucous metaplasia and airways hyperresponsiveness through IL-25 and type 2 innate lymphoid cells. Journal of Allergy and Clinical Immunology. 2014;**134**:429-439.e8

[64] Pelly VS, Kannan Y, Coomes SM, et al. IL-4-producing ILC2s are required for the differentiation of TH2 cells following heligmosomoides polygyrus infection. Mucosal Immunology. 2016;**9**:1407-1417

[65] Mjösberg J, Eidsmo L. Update on innate lymphoid cells in atopic and non-atopic inflammation in the airways and skin. Clinical & Experimental Allergy. 2014;**44**:1033-1043

[66] Imai Y, Yasuda K, Sakaguchi Y, et al. Skin-specific expression of IL-33 activates group 2 innate lymphoid cells and elicits atopic dermatitis-like inflammation in mice. Proceedings of the National Academy of Sciences of the United States of America. 2013;**110**:13921-13926

[67] Kim BS, Siracusa MC, Saenz SA, et al. TSLP elicits IL-33-independent innate lymphoid cell responses to promote skin inflammation. Science Translational Medicine. 2013;**5**:170ra16-170ra16

[68] Salimi M, Barlow JL, Saunders SP, et al. A role for IL-25 and IL-33–driven type-2 innate lymphoid cells in atopic dermatitis. The Journal of Experimental Medicine. 2013;**210**:2939-2950

[69] Huang T, Hazen M, Shang Y, et al. Depletion of major pathogenic cells in asthma by targeting CRTh2. JCI Insight; 2016 **1**

[70] Klein Wolterink RGJ, Serafini N, van Nimwegen M, et al. Essential, dose-dependent role for the transcription factor Gata3 in the development of IL-5+ and IL-13+ type 2 innate

lymphoid cells. Proceedings of the National Academy of Sciences of the United States of America. 2013;**110**:10240-10245

[71] Chang Y-J, Kim HY, Albacker LA, et al. Innate lymphoid cells mediate influenza-induced airway hyper-reactivity independently of adaptive immunity. Nature Immunology. 2011;**12**:631-638

[72] von Moltke J, Ji M, Liang H-E, et al. Tuft-cell-derived IL-25 regulates an intestinal ILC2–epithelial response circuit. Nature. 2015;**529**:221-225

[73] Rak GD, Osborne LC, Siracusa MC, et al. IL-33-Dependent Group 2 Innate Lymphoid Cells Promote Cutaneous Wound Healing. Journal of Investigative Dermatology. 2016;**136**:487-496

[74] van Drunen CM, Mjösberg JM, Segboer CL, et al. Role of innate immunity in the pathogenesis of chronic rhinosinusitis: Progress and new avenues. Current Allergy and Asthma Reports. 2012;**12**:120-126

[75] Van Gool F, Molofsky AB, Morar MM, et al. Interleukin-5-producing group 2 innate lymphoid cells control eosinophilia induced by interleukin-2 therapy. Blood. 2014;**124**:3572-3576

[76] Hams E, Locksley RM, McKenzie ANJ, et al. Cutting edge: IL-25 elicits innate lymphoid type 2 and type II NKT cells that regulate obesity in mice. The Journal of Immunology. 2013;**191**:5349-5353

[77] Flach M, Diefenbach A. Adipose tissue: ILC2 crank up the heat. Cell Metabolism. 2015; **21**:152-153

[78] Brestoff JR, Kim BS, Saenz SA, et al. Group 2 innate lymphoid cells promote beiging of white adipose tissue and limit obesity. 2014 Nature. 2014;**519**:242-246

[79] Lee M-W, Odegaard JI, Mukundan L, et al. Activated type 2 innate lymphoid cells regulate beige fat biogenesis. Cell. 2015;**160**:74-87

[80] Spits H, Artis D, Colonna M, et al. Innate lymphoid cells—A proposal for uniform nomenclature. Nature Reviews Immunology. 2013;**13**:145-149

[81] Klose CSN, Artis D. Innate lymphoid cells as regulators of immunity, inflammation and tissue homeostasis. Nature Immunology. 2016;**17**:765-774

[82] Cording S, Medvedovic J, Cherrier M, et al. Development and regulation of RORγt+ innate lymphoid cells. FEBS Letters. 2014;**588**:4176-4181

[83] Sawa S, Lochner M, Satoh-Takayama N, et al. RORγt+ innate lymphoid cells regulate intestinal homeostasis by integrating negative signals from the symbiotic microbiota. Nature Immunology. 2011;**12**:320-326

[84] Mebius RE, Rennert P, Weissman IL. Developing lymph nodes collect CD4+CD3-LT-beta+ cells that can differentiate to APC, NK cells, and follicular cells but not T or B cells. Immunity. 1997;**7**:493-504

[85] Hazenberg MD, Spits H. Human innate lymphoid cells. Blood. 2014;**124**:700-709

[86] Shikhagaie MM, Björklund ÅK, Mjösberg J, et al. Neuropilin-1 Is expressed on lymphoid tissue residing LTi-like group 3 innate lymphoid cells and associated with ectopic lymphoid aggregates. Cell Reports. 2017;**18**:1761-1773

[87] Melo-Gonzalez F, Hepworth MR. Functional and phenotypic heterogeneity of group 3 innate lymphoid cells. Immunology. 2017;**150**:265-275

[88] Juelke K, Romagnani C. Differentiation of human innate lymphoid cells (ILCs). Current Opinion in Immunology. 2016;**38**:75-85

[89] Eberl G, Marmon S, Sunshine M-J, et al. An essential function for the nuclear receptor RORgamma(t) in the generation of fetal lymphoid tissue inducer cells. Nature Immunology. 2004;**5**:64-73

[90] Kurebayashi S, Ueda E, Sakaue M, et al. Retinoid-related orphan receptor gamma (RORgamma) is essential for lymphoid organogenesis and controls apoptosis during thymopoiesis. Proceedings of the National Academy of Sciences of the United States of America. 2000;**97**:10132-10137

[91] Sun Z, Unutmaz D, Zou YR, et al. Requirement for RORgamma in thymocyte survival and lymphoid organ development. Science. 2000;**288**:2369-2673

[92] Aliahmad P, de la Torre B, Kaye J. Shared dependence on the DNA-binding factor TOX for the development of lymphoid tissue-inducer cell and NK cell lineages. Nature Immunology. 2010;**11**:945-952

[93] Singh AK, Eken A, Fry M, et al. DOCK8 regulates protective immunity by controlling the function and survival of RORγt+ ILCs. Nature Communications. 2014;**5**:4603

[94] Eken A, Singh AK, Oukka M. Interleukin 23 in Crohn's disease. Inflammatory Bowel Diseases. 2014;**20**:587-595

[95] Buonocore S, Ahern PP, Uhlig HH, et al. Innate lymphoid cells drive interleukin-23-dependent innate intestinal pathology. Nature. 2010;**464**:1371-1375

[96] Eken A, Singh AK, Treuting PM, et al. IL-23R+ innate lymphoid cells induce colitis via interleukin-22-dependent mechanism. Mucosal Immunology. 2014;7:143-154

[97] Coccia M, Harrison OJ, Schiering C, et al. IL-1β mediates chronic intestinal inflammation by promoting the accumulation of IL-17A secreting innate lymphoid cells and CD4(+) Th17 cells. The Journal of Experimental Medicine. 2012;**209**:1595-1609

[98] Cash HL, Whitham C V, Behrendt CL, et al. Symbiotic bacteria direct expression of an intestinal bactericidal lectin. Science. 2006 **313**:1126-1130

[99] Sonnenberg GF, Fouser LA, Artis D. Border patrol: Regulation of immunity, inflammation and tissue homeostasis at barrier surfaces by IL-22. 2011 Nature Immunology. **12**:383-390

[100] Sonnenberg GF, Monticelli LA, Alenghat T, et al. Innate lymphoid cells promote anatomical containment of lymphoid-resident commensal bacteria. Science (80-). 2012; **336**:1321-1325

[101] Hernández PP, Mahlakõiv T, Yang I, et al. Interferon-λ and interleukin 22 act synergistically for the induction of interferon-stimulated genes and control of rotavirus infection. Nature Immunology. 2015;**16**:698-707

[102] Zhang B, Chassaing B, Shi Z, et al. Viral infection. Prevention and cure of rotavirus infection via TLR5/NLRC4-mediated production of IL-22 and IL-18. Science. 2014;**346**:861-865

[103] Sonnenberg GF, Monticelli LA, Elloso MM, et al. CD4(+) lymphoid tissue-inducer cells promote innate immunity in the gut. Immunity. 2011;**34**:122-134

[104] Song C, Lee JS, Gilfillan S, et al. Unique and redundant functions of NKp46+ ILC3s in models of intestinal inflammation. The Journal of Experimental Medicine. 2015;**212**:1869-1882

[105] Gladiator A, LeibundGut-Landmann S. Innate lymphoid cells: New players in IL-17-mediated antifungal immunity. PLoS Pathogens. 2013;**9**:e1003763

[106] Gladiator A, Wangler N, Trautwein-Weidner K, et al. Cutting edge: IL-17-secreting innate lymphoid cells are essential for host defense against fungal infection. The Journal of Immunology. 2013;**190**:521-525

[107] REN J, FENG Z, LV Z, et al. Natural killer-22 cells in the synovial fluid of patients with rheumatoid arthritis are an innate source of interleukin 22 and tumor necrosis factor-α. The Journal of Rheumatology. 2011;**38**:2112-2118

[108] Koo J, Kim S, Jung WJ, et al. Increased lymphocyte infiltration in rheumatoid arthritis is correlated with an increase in LTi-like cells in synovial fluid. Immune Network. 2013;**13**:240

[109] Yeremenko N, Noordenbos T, Blijdorp I, et al. AB0049 human type 1 innate lymphoid cells accumulate in the inflamed synovium in spondyloarthritis. Annals of the Rheumatic Diseases. 2015;**74**:906.2-906

[110] Roan F, Stoklasek TA, Whalen E, et al. CD4+ Group 1 Innate lymphoid cells (ILC) form a functionally distinct ILC subset that is increased in systemic sclerosis. The Journal of Immunology. 2016;**196**:2051-2062

[111] Forkel M, Mjösberg J. Dysregulation of group 3 innate lymphoid cells in the pathogenesis of inflammatory bowel disease. Current Allergy and Asthma Reports. 2016;**16**:73

[112] Cox JH, Kljavin NM, Ota N, et al. Opposing consequences of IL-23 signaling mediated by innate and adaptive cells in chemically induced colitis in mice. Mucosal Immunology. 2012;**5**:99-109

[113] Geremia A, Arancibia-Cárcamo CV, Fleming MPP, et al. IL-23-responsive innate lymphoid cells are increased in inflammatory bowel disease. The Journal of Experimental Medicine. 2011;**208**:1127-1133

[114] Bernink JH, Krabbendam L, Germar K, et al. Interleukin-12 and -23 control plasticity of CD127(+) group 1 and group 3 innate lymphoid cells in the intestinal lamina propria. Immunity. 2015;**43**:146-160

[115] Hepworth MR, Fung TC, Masur SH, et al. Group 3 innate lymphoid cells mediate intestinal selection of commensal bacteria-specific CD4+ T cells. Science (80-). 2015;**348**:1031-1035

[116] Hepworth MR, Monticelli LA, Fung TC, et al. Innate lymphoid cells regulate CD4+ T-cell responses to intestinal commensal bacteria. Nature. 2013;**498**:113-117

[117] Villanova F, Flutter B, Tosi I, et al. Characterization of Innate lymphoid cells in human skin and blood demonstrates increase of NKp44+ ILC3 in psoriasis. Journal of Investigative Dermatology. 2014;**134**:984-991

[118] Teunissen MBM, Munneke JM, Bernink JH, et al. Composition of innate lymphoid cell subsets in the human skin: Enrichment of NCR+ ILC3 in lesional skin and blood of psoriasis patients. Journal of Investigative Dermatology. 2014;**134**:2351-2360

[119] Safavi F, Li H, Gonnella P, et al. c-kit plays a critical role in induction of intravenous tolerance in experimental autoimmune encephalomyelitis. Immunologic Research. 2015;**61**:294-302

[120] Hatfield JK, Brown MA. Group 3 innate lymphoid cells accumulate and exhibit disease-induced activation in the meninges in EAE. Cellular Immunology. 2015;**297**:69-79

[121] Perry JSA, Han S, Xu Q, et al. Inhibition of LTi cell development by CD25 blockade is associated with decreased intrathecal inflammation in multiple sclerosis. Science Translational Medicine. 2012;**4**:145ra106-145ra106

[122] Russi AE, Walker-Caulfield ME, Ebel ME, et al. Cutting edge: C-Kit signaling differentially regulates type 2 innate lymphoid cell accumulation and susceptibility to central nervous system demyelination in male and female SJL mice. The Journal of Immunology. 2015;**194**:5609-5613

[123] Califano D, Cho JJ, Uddin MN, et al. Transcription factor Bcl11b controls identity and function of mature type 2 innate lymphoid cells. Immunity. 2015;**43**:354-368

[124] Zhang K, Xu X, Pasha MA, et al. Cutting edge: Notch signaling promotes the plasticity of group-2 innate lymphoid cells. The Journal of Immunology. 2017;**198**:1798-1803

[125] Ohne Y, Silver JS, Thompson-Snipes L, et al. IL-1 is a critical regulator of group 2 innate lymphoid cell function and plasticity. Nature Immunology. 2016;**17**:646-655

Chapter 8

B Lymphocyte as a Target of Bacterial Infections

Jorge Ismael Castañeda-Sánchez,
Ana Rosa Muñoz Duarte,
María Lilia Domínguez-López,
Juan José de la Cruz-López and Julieta Luna-Herrera

Additional information is available at the end of the chapter

http://dx.doi.org/10.5772/intechopen.69346

Abstract

B lymphocytes are central players in the immune response; canonically, they have been recognized as precursors of antibody-producing cells: plasma cells. Recent findings have shown that the role of B lymphocytes goes far beyond the production of antibodies. There are different subtypes of B lymphocytes with different participations in innate and adaptive responses that include the recognition of the antigen, its processing, and its presentation to T lymphocytes, as well as the production of cytokines that impact and modulate the response toward the pathogen. Traditionally, it has been considered that B lymphocytes do not have phagocytic abilities that allow them to internalize, to process, or even to be infected by bacterial pathogens. The new information has shown that B lymphocytes can be readily infected by bacterial pathogens like *Salmonella, Francisella, Moraxella,* and *Mycobacterium,* among others, and respond to those infections. Some of the recent advances on these topics will be presented in this chapter.

Keywords: B lymphocyte, B1 lymphocytes, bacterial infection, *Brucella, Salmonella, Mycobacterium, Francisella,* endocytosis, macropinocytosis, innate response

1. Introduction

1.1. A brief history on the B-cell discovery

The immune response comprises cellular and humoral elements; among the cellular elements, macrophages were the first cells to be described by Metchnikoff in the year 1889 [1]. Almost simultaneously with Metchnikoff findings, began the recognition of one of the primordial elements of the specific humoral response: the antibodies. Von Bering and Kitasato in 1880 present their first work on serotherapy, showing that in the serum of animals immunized with diphtheria or tetanus toxins, there were specific elements of recognition for these toxins and that their use in patients conferred protection [2]. Later, Phlizalix and Calmette groups independently produce antisera against snake venoms [3], confirming the relevance of specific serum elements for the protective response. In those days, histological studies on organs of experimental animals subjected to immunization processes suggested that lymphoid organs were sites likely responsible for the synthesis of the serum elements responsible for protection against toxins and poisons [4]. Tisselius and Kabat in the 1930s demonstrated by electrophoretic techniques that humoral elements responsible for the serological protective response against toxins and poisons belong to the serum gamma globulin fraction [5]. Some years later, in the 1940s, ex vivo culture of plasma cells from the spleen of hyperimmune animals was achieved, and it was observed that, even in culture, the plasma cells were still producing the specific antibodies [6]. Later, the development and application of fluorescence techniques allowed the identification of antibodies in situ, locating them closely with the plasma cells present in secondary lymphoid organs [4]. Nossal's experiments demonstrated that antibodies produced by plasma cells isolated from immunized animals retained biological activity in vitro against the bacteria used in the immunization [7]. Human immunodeficiency studies, like Bruton's immunodeficiency, which is characterized by the absence of gamma globulin production and the absence of plasma cells in lymphoid organs [8, 9], demonstrated now in humans that antibodies were produced by plasma cells. The Landstainer and Chase experiments excluded antibodies as mediators of cell-mediated hypersensitivity responses [10], and it is in the 1960s when observations on the development of the immune response in thymectomized and reconstituted animals allowed to recognize the thymus as a fundamental organ of the immune response responsible for grafts rejection but also contributed to antibody production [11, 12]. The bird model for study of elements of the immune response initiated the identification of the organ responsible for B-lymphocyte production [13], and in 1965, in birds, it was demonstrated that in the thymus and in the bursa, the two cellular lineages fundamental for the immune response are generated [14]. Almost simultaneously, and thanks to the use of radioactive labels, it was demonstrated that circulating lymphocytes stimulated with antigen were the precursors of antibody-producing cells [15, 16], and by the year 1969, the two populations of lymphocytes were identified as T lymphocytes for those thymic-dependent, and those thymic-independent (bursa-equivalent) were referred as B lymphocytes [17]. Afterward, it was established in non-avian experimental models that a cooperative response of both lymphocyte species (T and B) was necessary for specific antibody production [18]; these observations prompted a large number of studies that recognized the complexity of T-B cooperation, resulting in specific responses to the antigen, including the production of specific high-affinity antibodies [19].

1.2. B lymphocytes: a bridge between innate and adaptive immune responses

It is now known that there are several types of B lymphocytes [20] and that B2 lymphocytes produce specific antibodies during the adaptive response [21]. On the other side, there are also natural antibodies of IgM class mainly [22]; unlike the adaptive antibodies, the natural antibodies are produced by B1 lymphocytes [23]. B1 lymphocytes are subdivided into B1-a and B1-b—subtype B1-a is responsible for natural antibody production—respond to T-independent antigenic challenges, are located mainly in the peritoneal and pleural cavity, and represent the first line of defense against microbial challenges [24]. In addition, B1-a lymphocytes may internalize and eliminate bacterial pathogens and have CD11b marker [25], resembling a macrophage phenotype. Some authors have suggested that the B1-a subset of lymphocytes and macrophages share lineage relationships, so these B/macrophage bi-phenotypic cells may represent an ancient B-lymphocyte lineage capable of adapting to bacterial challenges and innate responses [26]. The mammalian B1-a subset of lymphocytes could be evolutionary related to B cells from fishes, particularly teleost fishes like rainbow trout, catfish, etc.; circulating B cells in teleost fishes are morphologically similar to mammalian B lymphocytes; they also secrete and express immunoglobulin molecules at the membrane level with IgM, IgD, or IgT/Z isotypes and also possess phagocytic abilities [26]; this evolutionary theory of B cell supports the idea of an innate role of B1-a lymphocytes. In this context, B1-a lymphocytes and natural antibodies represent a bridge between innate and adaptive immunity [27].

2. B-cell subtypes

An important role of B lymphocytes in defense against pathogens is that B cells are part of a long-lived lymphocyte group that participates in the immune response by capturing and concentrating antigens for the presentation and production of antibodies. From the time that a B lineage cell becomes a mature B cell expressing the B-cell receptor (BCR) on its membrane, several transition steps have to occur [20]. During these steps, B cells are directed for negative and probably positive selection involved in generating a mature B-cell repertoire [28]. B lymphocytes have been divided into two subtypes, according to the origin of their development into B1 and B2 cells. B1 lymphocytes are the first cells produced in the ontogeny; in mice, B1 cells are produced in the fetus and are derived from distinct precursors. B1 cells are different from B2 lymphocytes by their capacity of spontaneous antibody production, self-renewal, impossibility for clonal expansion, and low somatic hypermutation [29].

B2 cell precursors in the bone marrow give origin to B-cell populations of the marginal zone and the follicular zone; these B cells are the main populations that respond to antigen contact then forming the germinal centers and therefore are long-term responders. These cell populations are the majority B lymphocytes in the host and are predominant in all lymphoid tissues. Marginal zone (MZ) B lymphocytes in the mouse are restricted to the splenic marginal zone, while their human counterparts appear to be also in blood circulation. In the mouse B1 cells are divided in two subsets, B1-a and B1-b, based on their expression of CD5; B1a cells (CD5+) and B1-b cells (CD5−) appear to share developmental precursors. Apart from the differential expression of CD5, they are phenotypically similar, with few functional differences like the ability for internalizing bacterial pathogens [24, 30].

The main function of B1 lymphocytes is the production of large amounts of natural antibodies of the IgM isotype that responds to encapsulated bacterial infections (among others bacterial challenges) and the production of IgA associated with mucosal defense against parasites. However, these cells are also able to produce IgG2 and IgG3 isotypes spontaneously, and under certain conditions, they may produce IgE. The production of antibodies by B1 lymphocytes is characterized by being spontaneous although it can be induced by T-cell-independent antigens and certain cytokines [31]. B1 lymphocytes predominate in fetal life but decrease with increasing age and have been reported to increase again in advanced age in mice as in humans. However, in the elderly, despite the increase, these cells are not fully functional, making older guests susceptible to acquire frequent lung infections associated with pneumonia. The natural antibodies have low specificity, so they are able to recognize self-antigens; for this, B1 cells have been identified as potential participants in the development of autoimmune diseases. A high number of B1-a cells have been associated with autoimmunity in human and mouse models. In addition, a greater number of B1 cells have been reported in patients with systemic lupus erythematosus, Sjögren's syndrome, and rheumatoid arthritis [32, 33].

B1 cells are the main population of B lymphocytes that are located in cavities such as the pleura and peritoneum (35–70%); these cells are mobilized between both cavities through the omentum, a process that requires the expression of the chemokine ligand CXCL13. In response to the pathogens, B1 cells are mobilized from their primary location within the peritoneum or pleura to secondary lymphoid organs such as the spleen and lymph nodes and at these sites begin to secrete IgM antibodies, so B1 lymphocytes represent a quick innate response toward bacterial challenges. B1 cells have been reported to be found in the spleen (1–2%), lymphoid nodes (0.1–0.3%), bone marrow (0.1–0.2%), lung parenchyma (0.4–0.6%), intestinal lamina propria (up to 50% are IgA + B cells), and blood (0.3–0.5%). In the peritoneal cavity, a subtype of B1 lymphocytes tend to lose expression of the CD43 molecule, but most of these cells in other tissues retain this marker; however, when B1 cells are activated, they overexpress CD43. In the peritoneal and pleura cavity, most of the B1-a and B1-b lymphocytes express the integrin CD11b but when these cells migrate to other organs such as the spleen downregulate its expression. In terms of functionality, B1 lymphocytes and marginal zone B cells are very similar; for this reason, the subgroup of marginal zone B cells (MZ) has been included in the group of "innate" type B cells, conformed then by B1-a cells, B1-b cells, and B cells of the marginal zone. B-cell MZ is also considered as B regulatory cell since after activation, it produces high levels of IL-10 (**Figure 1**) [34].

B1 lymphocytes in addition to producing the natural antibodies also actively contribute to the bacteria-induced immune response; several groups have explored B1 cell responses to pathogens like *Streptococcus pneumoniae*, *Salmonella* spp., *Francisella* spp., *Borrelia hermsii*, and influenza virus, among others. The antibody response analyzed for each case showed an increase of IgM produced by B1 cells in the spleen, regional lymph nodes, or serum. Some studies support the idea of a heterogeneity of B1 cells, but the causes of this heterogeneity are largely unknown and poorly explored. However, Baumgarth has considered three factors that can modulate the functions of B1 cells: (1) the multiple origin of B1 cells, (2) tissue-specific signals, and (3) differences in exposure and responsiveness of B1 cells toward self and foreign antigens. It has been suggested that it is important to determine the impact of these signals on the functionality of B1 cells, which could clarify much of the biology of this cell population and one of its most important products, the natural IgM [35].

http://dx.doi.org/10.5772/intechopen.69346

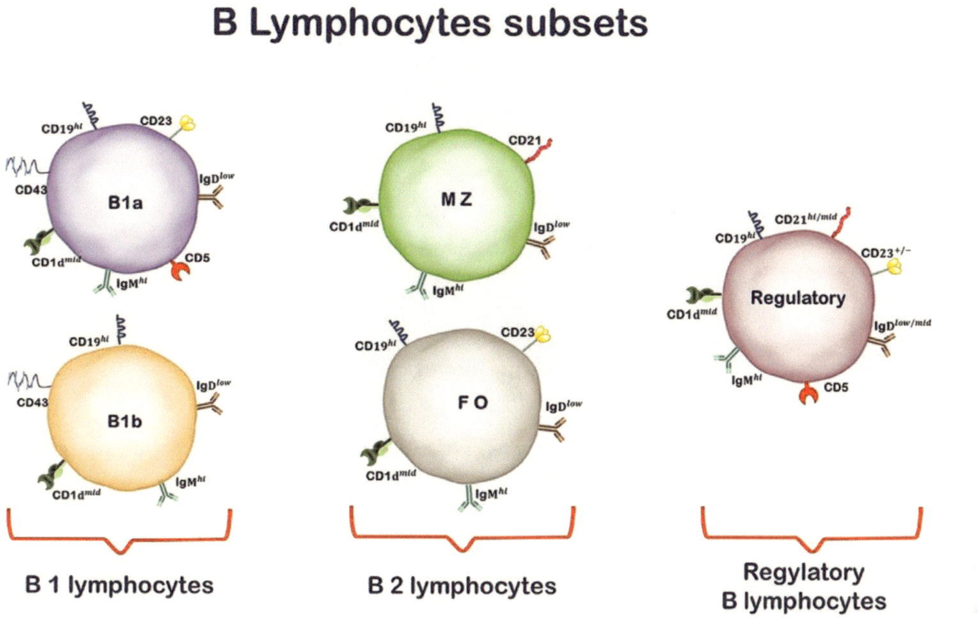

Figure 1. Immunophenotype of mature B-cell subpopulations. The B2-cell population constitutes the majority of spleen B cells formed by follicular cells (FZ) and marginal zone B cells (MZ). B1-a and B1-b cells are smaller populations in terms of frequency in the spleen; they can be distinguished based on CD5 expression: B1-a (CD5+) cells and B1-b (CD5−) cells. It appears that regulatory B cells have phenotypic markers of B1 and B2 cells.

3. B-cell receptors involved in bacterial recognition and uptake

As referred earlier B lymphocytes are not only plasma cell precursors but a heterogenic subset of cells with the capability to act as antigen-presenting cells (PCA) and produce pro- and anti-inflammatory cytokines. Some B-lymphocyte subsets are able, at different rates, to engulf several pathogens predominantly virus and bacteria; this event is mainly mediated by BCR, Toll-like receptors (TLR), and complement receptors (**Figure 2**). In some cases, after bacterial uptake, B lymphocytes are activated and settle a protective or suppressive immune response; also, they may act as pathogen niches or reservoirs that allow bacteria dissemination in the organism. The endocytic pathways developed by B lymphocytes that allow bacterial uptake depend on the receptors engaged during bacterial recognition. In other cases, bacterial components itself trigger in the host cell, mechanisms that allow their entrance into the B cells (**Figure 3**).We will describe some of these elements.

3.1. B-cell receptors

The B-cell receptor (BCR) for antigen is a complex of membrane immunoglobulin (mIg) of isotype IgM^{hi} and IGD^{low} in B1 and B2 lymphocytes and IgM^{hi} and $IgD^{low/mid}$ in B regulatory cells; this complex is responsible for extracellular antigen attachment and is linked to at least two other proteins, Ig α and Ig β forming a heterodimer. The mIg itself does not contain any

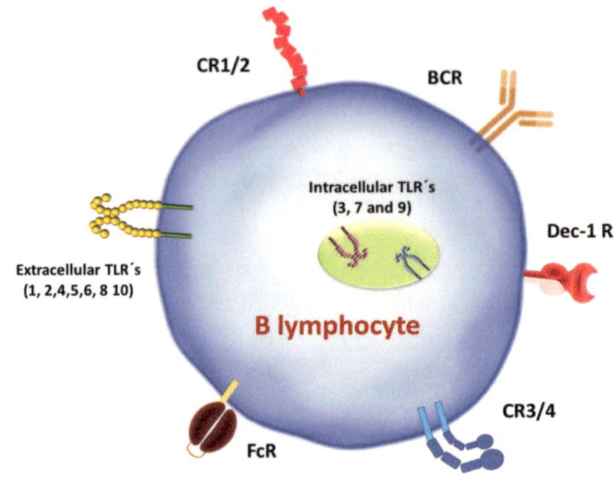

Figure 2. B-lymphocyte receptors involved in pathogens uptake. B lymphocytes displayed a wide number of receptors capable to recognize and engulf pathogens; they include intra- and extracellular innate receptors like TLRs, Dec-1, complement receptors, and the adaptive BCR receptor.

signaling motifs, but instead the Igα/β heterodimer contains immunoreceptor tyrosine-based activation motifs (ITAMs) responsible for initiating the signaling after antigen binding [36]. Membrane Ig (mIg) differs from circulatory antibody in the C-terminus of the heavy chain [37]. B-cell activation is triggered by BCR-antigen interaction and leads to multiple cellular events as BCR-antigen complex internalization, the signalosome assembly, regulation of gene

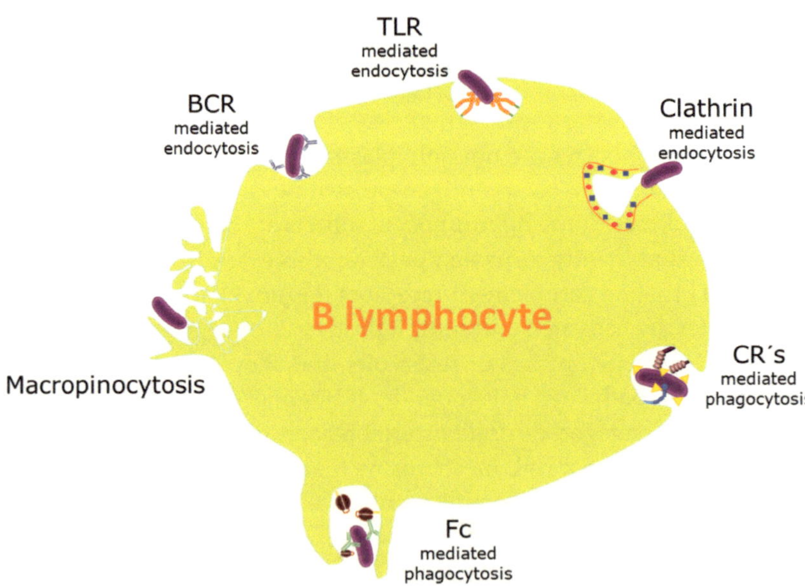

Figure 3. Endocytic pathways in B lymphocytes responsible for bacterial uptake. B lymphocytes are not only precursors of plasma cells but also a multitask cells. Several endocytic pathways may take place on the B cells to internalize bacterial pathogens; the cartoon depicts some of the pathways already described: clathrin-mediated endocytosis, Fc-mediated phagocytosis, CR (complement receptor)-mediated endocytosis, BCR-mediated endocytosis, TLR-mediated endocytosis, and macropinocytosis.

expression, cytoskeleton reorganization, and plasma and long-live B memory cell generation. Antigens internalized through BCR are processed and presented on the major histocompatibility complex II (MHC II). The idea that dimeric BCR complex binding the antigen was enough to activate B cells was accepted for years; nevertheless, it is known that B cells can form microclusters required for B-cell activation [38, 39], which involved around 10–100 BCR molecules; even in this microcluster, BCR complexes can interact in an oligomeric pattern [40]. Most of the studies related to antigen recognition by BCR have been related to soluble antigens [41]; however, more evidences have demonstrated that BCR also recognizes complete pathogens, like *Moraxella catarrhalis* [42] and more recently *Salmonella typhimurium* [43].

3.2. Toll-like receptors (TLRs)

Toll-like receptors (TLRs) are a family of transmembrane and cytoplasmic receptors that are phylogenetically ancient that share homology with the IL-1 receptor; TLRs are part of the group of molecules responsible of pathogen´s recognition that collectively receive the name of pathogen recognition receptors (PRRs) and are expressed in dendritic cells, macrophages, and NK cells (innate immune cells); B and T lymphocytes (cells of the adaptive immunity); and epithelial cells, endothelial cells, and fibroblasts (nonimmune cells). TLRs are responsible for activating the innate immune response [44]. The ligands of the TLRs, known as pathogen-associated molecular patterns (PAMPs), are highly conserved microbial molecules or harmful endogenous factors [damage-associated molecular patterns (DAMPs)]. When B cells-TLRs bound to their ligands, several activation pathways are engaged; two of the most studied are TLR4 and TLR9 activation pathways; TLR4 is expressed on the B-cell membrane along with MD-2 molecule, and this heterodimer participates in lipopolysaccharide (LPS) recognition to initiate several intracellular signaling pathways; one of the most important is the TIRAP-MyD88 pathway that regulates NF-κB activation and inflammatory cytokine production like IL-8, transforming growth factor alpha (TNF-α), etc. TLR9 is another important B cell-TLR, which is expressed in the endoplasmic reticulum and is recruited to endosomal/lysosomal compartments after stimulation with CpG DNAs, activating the MyD88 pathway without TIRAP, culminating in NF-κB activation, and resulting in the production of proinflammatory cytokines [45]. TLRs are classified based on their localization as cell surface TLRs (TLR1, TLR2, TLR4, TLR5, TLR6, and TLR10) or intracellular TLRs (TLR3, TLR7, TLR8, TLR9, TLR11, TLR12, and TLR13); on humans 10 members of the TLR family have been described, while murine cells express 13 TLRs [44]. B lymphocytes express ten types of TLR (TLR1-10) [46–48]; their expression depends on B-cell tissue localization and the stage of B-cell activation. TLRs 3, 4, and 5 and 8 are absent in naive and memory B cells but are present in plasma cells; TLRs 6–9 are highly expressed in naïve B cells, but when they are activated, the intracellular TLR9 is the most highly expressed [45, 49]. Recently, some authors have demonstrated that TLR ligands have a modulatory effect on the B-lymphocyte response, for instance, lipopolysaccharide (LPS) and CpG-containing DNAs promote proliferation, class switching, and plasma differentiation and are directly related with Th1 responses and autoimmune diseases [50–53]. Deficiencies in the downstream signaling pathways in B lymphocytes after TLRs activation favored pathogen infections specially the ones caused by *S. pneumoniae*, *S. aureus*, and *P. aeruginosa* [54]. TLR activation could be also detrimental for the B cells; for instance, B-lymphocyte TLR-2 interacting with *Shigella flexneri* promotes apoptosis of the host cell [55].

3.3. Dectin-1

Dectin-1 (Dec-1) is a transmembrane C-type lectin-like receptor (CTLR) that binds β-glucans; it is expressed mainly in myeloid cells; when Dec-1 recognizes its ligand, the interaction induces B-cell activation with the participation of SYK, the MAPK ERK and JNK, and the transcription factors AP-1 and NF-κB, leading to the production of proinflammatory cytokine production (like IL-8) and arachidonic metabolites synthesis [56, 57]. Dec-1 binds to numerous pathogens through their specific ligands β-1,3 glucans, most frequent in fungi pathogens like *Aspergillus, Candida, Coccidioides,* and *Pneumocystis* and in nonpathogenic *Penicillium* and *Saccharomyces;* beside Dec-1 can recognize mycobacteria [58]. Dec-1 was first described in dendritic cells; however, now it is known that Dec-1 is expressed in monocytes and lymphocytes. In B lymphocytes, Dec-1 activation leads to IL-8 production and neutrophil chemotaxis which shows that B lymphocytes can directly recognized pathogens via PRRs and have an important role in antifungal response [59].

3.4. Complement receptors

The complement system involves numerous plasma proteins that react with one another, in a cascade-like process that results in molecules that opsonize pathogens and promote inflammatory responses that help to fight infection. Complement proteins execute their biological functions by binding their corresponding receptors (CR1, CR3, and CR4) present in several cell types like macrophages, neutrophils, etc. B lymphocytes also express complement receptors, like CD35 (CR1) and CD21 (CR2) [60]. CR1 binds C3b and C4b, while CR2 binds C3d. It is known that CR2 interacts with CD19; this complex acts as a co-receptor for BCR [61].

Complement receptors CR1 and CR2 are expressed differentially during B-human-lymphocyte development. CR1 is more expressed in memory cells than in naïve cells, while CR2 is low expressed in memory cells. Changes in CR expression on B lymphocytes are related with breaking of B-cell tolerance and increased susceptibility to bacterial infections [62]. CR participates in bacteria internalization; *Francisella tularensis* is engulfed by B lymphocytes through complement receptors [63].

3.5. Fc receptors

Fc receptors (FcRs) belong to the immunoglobulin superfamily; they are expressed in many immune cells as monocytes, mastocytes, NK cells, and B lymphocytes and recognize the cristalizable fragment of the immunoglobulins (Fc) [64]. FcR activation results in many relevant responses like cytotoxicity, phagocytosis, mast cell activation, and pathogen clearance. FcRs are classified according to the antibody isotype; they recognized FcRγ (IgG), FcRε (IgE), and FcRα (IgA) [65].

FcR activation regulates many B lymphocyte activities, like activation and proliferation, class switching, and maturation of naive cells into plasma cells [65, 66]. Alterations in FcR functionality have been related to autoimmune diseases [67]. Some pathogens require immunoglobulin opsonization to be uptaken by B lymphocytes, coxsackievirus—opsonized with non-neutralizing antibodies infects and then replicates into B cells [68]. Bacterial pathogens like *Brucella abortus* require IgM opsonization to be internalized into B lymphocytes [69].

3.6. Mechanisms of bacterial uptake exerted by B lymphocytes

3.6.1. Phagocytosis

Phagocytosis was first described by Mechnikoff in 1884 and as a whole is one of the most important defense mechanisms against pathogens [1]. B lymphocytes have been considered as non-phagocytic cells or with much less internalization capabilities than macrophages [70, 71]. Still, it is a controversy upon the endocytic mechanism that the B lymphocyte exerts to internalize bacteria; it is not yet defined if internalization is by phagocytosis or by macropinocytosis (which is also known also as phagocytosis-like) or other mechanisms [72–74]. Recent evidence has shown that the B1-a lymphocyte subset can internalize pathogens [69, 75]; even some authors readily consider that B1-a lymphocytes are phagocytic [76]. However, still, it is not clear if bacterial recognition by B-lymphocyte receptors like BCR, FcR, CR, dectin-1, etc. activates the B cell to internalize the bacteria or if bacterial uptake is an active process triggered by bacterial components, as is the case of products from the pathogenicity islands of *Salmonella* [77].

In phagocytic cells (macrophages, neutrophils, monocytes), phagocytosis can be divided into type I and type II phagocytosis [78]. Type I phagocytosis is mediated by Fc receptors which recognize targets opsonized by immunoglobulins, being the most important the receptors FcRγ that recognizes different subclasses of IgG bound to the pathogen. Interaction between FcγR and IgG triggers phosphorylation of specific tyrosine residues in the ITAM-type motifs present in the intracellular domain of FcγR [79]. Later, the recruitment and activation of signaling proteins belonging to the Rho GTPases family, like Cdc42, resulting in actin polymerization, membrane protrusion formation, and bacterial internalization occur [80].

In the phagocytosis type II, particles opsonized by several complement fractions (like C3b and iC3b) are recognized by cells that have complement receptors CR1 and CR3 (CD11b), like macrophages or neutrophils. Complement-opsonized particles "sink" into the phagocyte; membrane disturbance is minimal without long membrane protrusion formation; particle internalization does not usually lead to an inflammatory response or oxidative burst. In this case, the small GTPase molecule activated is the GTPase RhoA, and they do not necessarily involve Cdc42 and Rac; after GTPase activation, the remodeling of the membrane driven by filamentous actin, phagosome closure, and pathogen internalization occurs [78, 79, 81].

Up today there are few studies on B-cell capabilities for bacterial internalization; there are descriptions of B-cell internalization of opsonized bacteria with immunoglobulin and with complement [63, 69, 74], but also there are descriptions that B cells can uptake non-opsonized bacteria [72]; so far there are no studies that clarified the role of small GTPases involved in bacterial internalization by B cells that could help to clarify if bacterial uptake by B cells is a phagocytic type I or type II process or if it is a unique endocytic mechanism for B cells.

3.6.2. Clathrin-mediated endocytosis (CME)

Clathrin-mediated endocytosis is a well-known endocytic mechanism performed by many cells, is involved in the intake of extracellular molecules recognized by cell membrane receptors, and is a major route of traffic from plasma membrane to endosomes [81, 82]. B cells recognize antigens by adaptive and innate mechanisms; the adaptive recognition is the most studied, also in the case for recognition of soluble antigens [83, 84]. Antigen adaptive recognition of B cells involves the antigen-specific B-cell receptor (BCR) expressed by B lymphocytes; BCR has two distinct tasks: the first one is to trigger cell activation after interaction with the specific antigen, and the second one is to internalize the antigen for subsequent processing and presentation on MHC class II molecules [85]. Clathrin is the scaffold of conserved cellular structures (pits) that are formed to capture membranal fractions where various cellular receptors are concentrated; once the ligand is bound to the membrane receptor, clathrin polymerization occurs resulting in a covered pit that detaches from the membrane as a coated vesicle that initiates an endosomal trafficking process [81, 82]. In B lymphocytes, clathrin-mediated endocytosis is a fundamental mechanism to translocate BCR-antigen complex to endosomal compartments; lipid rafts, microfilaments, and dynamin are required for this process [86, 87].

B lymphocytes can recognize bacterial antigens by their BCR, that is the case for *Salmonella* and *Francisella* pathogens. BCR-mediated internalization of *Salmonella Typhimurium* allowed bacterial internalization, antigen presentation into MHC class II molecules, and antibody production against *Salmonella* [88]. For the case of *Francisella,* evidence has demonstrated that *Francisella* is recognized by the B1-a cell by their BCRs alone; meanwhile, in the B1-b- and B2-cell subsets, bacterial recognition required simultaneous participation of BCR and complement receptors CR1 and CR2. *F. tularensis* was internalized by B cells at low rate, and internalized bacteria survive intracellularly [63]. In both studies the internalization process resembled more a cell membrane protrusion formation mechanism (like phagocytosis or macropinocytosis) rather than a clathrin-coated endocytosis mechanism. The size of the clathrin-coated pits is around 120 nm, being too small for a bacteria to fit in; however, recent studies have demonstrated that other larger structures coated with clathrin (clathrin plates) [82] are also formed into the cells; it will be interesting to find if bacteria could be uptaken by this mechanism.

3.6.3. *Macropinocytosis*

Macropinocytosis is a type of pinocytosis described for Warren Lewis in 1931 [89]. Eukaryotic cells have the capacity to internalize fluid (pinocytosis) and particles (phagocytosis) from the extracellular environment, using a variety of different processes [81]. Micropinocytosis is a common process in all cells; this mechanism results in the formation of small vesicles coated with clathrin, caveolin, or other proteins; also clathrin- and caveolin-independent mechanisms exist [81, 90]. Internalization of larger volume of fluids is mediated by a process called macropinocytosis; many signals trigger macropinocytosis, such as macrophage colony-stimulating factor-1 (CSF-1), epidermal growth factor (EGF), and phorbol myristate acetate [91]. Depending on the cell type, macropinocytosis can be a constitutive or an induced process. Macrophages and dendritic cells often utilize macropinocytosis to screen the extracellular environment for pathogenic or harmful materials [92]. Macropinocytosis is the main route for extracellular fluid uptake by the cells; it depends on energy and actin cytoskeleton rearrangements leading to the formation of filamentous and branched actin, supporting membrane modifications and lamellipodia formation; actin polymerization is initiated by the activation of the small Rho GTPase family (Rho, Cdc42, and Rac) working in parallel with phosphoinositides, to activate the WASp/Scar proteins, and the Arp2/3 complex, allowing actin branching, that force out plasma membrane and form membrane ruffles [93]. Macropinosomes are formed when these ruffles collapse with the plasma membrane enclosing a large volume of extracellular fluid phase; macropinosomes are spacious vesicles within the cytoplasm that can reach a size >0.2 μm [81]. Some pathogens take advantage of the macropinocytosis mechanism to enter into the non-phagocytic cells; *Shigella*, *Salmonella*, and *Mycobacterium* are bacteria known to use this mechanism [94–97]. The internalization process is characterized by the formation of actin-rich membrane protrusions known also as ruffles; for that, *Salmonella* produces the type III secretion system (T3SS) that translocate effectors from the *Salmonella* pathogenicity island I (SPI) into the host cytosol; these virulence factors target host mediators involved in cytoskeleton rearrangements like Rac, Cdc42, phosphoinositides, Arp2/3 complex, etc., resulting in actin cytoskeleton rearrangements and membrane ruffling [94, 98]. In the process of ruffling formation, the pathogen is captured among the ruffles that finally enclose the bacteria into a spacious macropinosome [93]. B lymphocytes can also be infected by bacterial pathogens that enter the B cell through a mechanism of macropinocytosis; *Salmonella*, *Francisella*, and *Mycobacterium* are some of these pathogens [28, 72, 99]; so far there is not a detailed description of the characteristics of this process in B lymphocytes.

4. Bacterial infections of B lymphocytes

B lymphocytes are central cells of the immune response being responsible of antibody production, but they are also cells that may modulate the immune response by the production of proinflammatory as well as anti-inflammatory cytokines [100, 101]. B lymphocytes can be the target of infection by various pathogens; the most recognized B infections are viral infections, especially infection caused by the Epstein-Barr virus (EBV). The susceptibility of B lymphocytes to this virus is primarily due to the expression of the CD21 molecule that is related to the gp350 viral protein [102]. In B lymphocytes EBV presents the lytic phase [103], while the latent phase of the virus is expressed in memory B lymphocytes [104]. B lymphocytes are also susceptible to viral infections caused by cytomegalovirus [105, 106] and smallpox virus [107, 108], among others. Viral infections in B lymphocytes modify the lymphocyte response to allow viral multiplication or persistence, alter apoptosis processes, interfere with antigenic presentation, etc., all to promote viral survival [55].

Although virus was among the earliest recognized pathogens with infective capabilities toward lymphocytes, perhaps the classic concept that B lymphocytes lacked phagocytic capabilities did not allow the recognition of bacterial infections in these cells [88, 109]. However, at present it is known that lymphocytes can internalize bacterial pathogens (mainly intracellular) and that these infections trigger different B-cell responses. Among the bacterial pathogens recognized with capacity to infect B lymphocytes are the genera: *Salmonella*, *Brucella*, *Francisella*, *Moraxella*, *Mycobacterium*, etc. Some characteristics of such infections will be described.

4.1. *Moraxella* B-cell infection

Moraxella catarrhalis is a Gram-negative bacterium that causes respiratory infections in children and causes chronic lung disease in adults; in children, it is highly associated with ear infections [110, 111]. *M. catarrhalis* produces the superantigen Moraxella IgD (MID)-binding protein, which binds to B-lymphocyte IgD, inducing lymphocyte proliferation, but cell proliferation requires also engagement of the innate TLR receptors [112]. In the particular case of *M. catarrhalis*, TLR-9 is required for B-lymphocyte proliferation; TLR-9 recognizes CpG motifs, distinctive of DNA of bacterial or viral origin [113]. The tonsil B lymphocytes are able to internalize *M. catarrhalis* by receptor-mediated endocytosis and after some time eliminate the internalized bacteria [112]. However, it has been described that *M. catarrhalis* is able to persist in pharyngeal lymphoid tissue including the adenoids and the tonsils, residing in macrophages and B lymphocytes [114].

4.2. *Brucella* B-cell infection

Among facultative intracellular microorganisms, *Brucella* spp. is one of the most representatives; this bacterium causes infections that become persistent in both humans and animals, representing a global zoonosis [115]. *Brucella* persists and replicates primarily in tissues and cells of the mononuclear phagocytic system, such as the spleen, bone marrow, lymph nodes, spleen, macrophages, and dendritic cells, and may also reside in cells of male and female reproductive systems including the uterus, placenta, and ovaries [116]; however, it has recently been recognized that B lymphocytes are not only infected but function as a reservoir of these bacteria [69]. *Brucella* also invades non-phagocytic cells such as epithelial cells, and the mechanism of internalization has been reported as zipper-like, promoting cytoskeleton rearrangement through the activation of Cdc42 by the pathogenic strains of *B. abortus* [117]. *Brucella* internalization into B cells depends on microfilaments and once internalized is allocated into late endosomal/lysosomal compartment allowing bacterial persistence and residency, infected B lymphocyte, thus producing anti-inflammatory cytokines such as TGF-β; interestingly mice lacking of B cell are more resistant to *Brucella* infection, pointing an important role of B cells as immunomodulators toward brucellosis [69].

4.3. *Francisella* B-cell infection

Francisella (especially *F. tularensis*) is another bacterium able to internalize and invade B lymphocytes; this bacterium is a facultative intracellular pathogen and has been reported that it infects phagocytic cells like macrophages, neutrophils [118, 119], and pulmonary and hepatic non-phagocytic cells [120, 121], among others. The main host cells of *F. tularensis* are the macrophages, where once the bacterium is internalized, it inhibits phagolysosomal fusion and leaves the cytoplasm, where it resides and actively replicates [122–124]. *Francisella*-infected macrophages promote a systemic anti-inflammatory reaction with high levels of TGF-β [125], with fatal consequences for the infected individual [126]. The first studies that highlighted the involvement of B lymphocytes in *F. tularensis* infection date back to the late 1990s, where it was found that B cells rather than antibodies were critical for protection against this bacterium [127].

The infective abilities of *F. tularensis* toward B lymphocytes were described in 2008, and it was found that the bacterium could be readily internalized by primary B lymphocytes and by B lymphocyte cell lines like Ramos or A20; lymphocytes allowed a moderate intracellular multiplication by 24 h after infection; however, from this time infected lymphocytes began to undergo apoptosis, which was accentuated at 48 h postinfection [128].

Among the B-lymphocyte (CD19+) subtypes, B1-a lymphocytes, classified as innate lymphocytes, are the best infected by *F. tularensis*, requiring only the BCR engagement for bacterial internalization, whereas B1-b and B2 lymphocytes are also susceptible to infection, although to a lesser extent; they require the joint participation of BCR and CR1/CR2 receptors for bacterial internalization [63]. B lymphocytes from mice infected with the live vaccine strain of *F. tularensis* (LVS), especially the B1-a lymphocytes uptake the bacteria; produce numerous proinflammatory cytokines such as IFN-γ, IL-1β, IL-12, IL-17, and TNF-α; decrease amounts of IL-10; and express costimulatory molecules like CD80 and CD86; mice were able to clear bacterial burden 10 days postinfection [129]. Recent studies confirm that the involvement of B lymphocytes is critical for the control of *F. novicida* infections [130] and that *Francisella* internalization into B cells requires cell membrane integrity [63].

4.4. *Salmonella* B-cell infection

The role of B lymphocytes among the bacterial infections has been studied the most for the case of *Salmonella* infection, and the evidences demonstrate the importance of these cells in the pathogenesis of diseases caused by this bacterial genus. Infections caused by *Salmonella* genus can be differentiated into two types: typhoid and non-typhoid. Gastroenteritis are caused by non-typhoidal serovars such as *Salmonella enterica* serovar Typhimurium, *S. enterica* serovar Enteritidis, and *S. enterica* serovar Newport, while the enteric fever is caused by typhoidal *Salmonella* serovars like *Salmonella enteritidis* serovar Typhi and *S. enteritidis* serovar Paratyphi [131]. The infection caused by *S. Typhimurium* in mouse is very similar to that caused by *Salmonella* Typhi in the human, and much of the knowledge of this infection is due to studies in the murine model with *S. Typhimurium* [132]. *Salmonella* are facultative intracellular pathogens; both serovars share many virulence factors (flagella, lipopolysaccharide, and pathogenicity islands) but differ in clinical manifestations: typhoid fever occurs within 2 weeks and has systemic manifestations, and gastroenteritis occurs in a shorter period (12–72 h), with a rapid accumulation of neutrophils at the intestinal level [133]. After *S. enterica* enters the organism orally, it is rapidly captured by the epithelial cells of the intestine and M cells and after a few hours is found in the lamina propria of the intestine and in the Peyer's plaques [134]. Already in the intestinal tissue, Salmonella is internalized by various phagocytic cell types such as macrophages, dendritic cells, and neutrophils [135], and it has been suggested that Salmonella is internalized also by B lymphocytes, which are abundant in Peyer's plaques adjacent to intestinal M cells [43, 136]. *Salmonella* epithelial cell invasion is an active process triggered by the bacterium, in which cell cytoskeleton rearrangements OCCUR, resulting in the formation of membranal protrusions that allow bacterial internalization, a phenomenon known as macropinocytosis [137]; *Salmonella* has developed very specialized systems to promote this event, within these is the type III secretion system (TTSS), through which the bacteria injects to the host cell products derived from the pathogenicity islands I and 2 (SPI1, SPI2) [138], which promote the activation of Rho, Rac, and Cdc42 small GTPases, thus favoring cytoskeletal remodeling and stimulating the production of caspase-1 which catalytically activates proinflammatory cytokines such as IL-1β and IL -18 [133]. Once internalized, *Salmonella* resides intracellularly in membranes called *Salmonella*-containing vacuole (SCV), which protects the bacteria by avoiding fusion with lysosomes and avoiding the reactivity of reactive oxygen metabolites [139, 140]. *Salmonella* can infect several cell types, from macrophage and dendritic cells to non-phagocytic like epithelial cells and hepatocytes [141]. *Salmonella* can be internalized in and infect B lymphocytes [43]. Evidence has shown that *Salmonella* is internalized into B lymphocytes through a macropinocytosis process [72, 73]. Bacterial recognition by B cells is also required for internalization; *Salmonella* may be recognized by BCR [88], by TLR [142], or by products derived from SPI-1 [143]. Depending on the internalization mechanism, *Salmonella* survival will occur, for instance, bacteria opsonized with complement or internalized by a mechanism triggered by products of the SPI-1 survive a replicate few hours after internalization, whereas bacteria opsonized with IgG or not opsonized will be eliminated soon after internalization [139]. Once internalized, the bacterium resides in SCV vacuoles, which in the case of B lymphocytes allow the cross-presentation of the Salmonella antigens to major histocompatibility complex molecules class one (MHC-I), by the vacuolar or cytosolic pathways [144]. This cross-presentation would promote infected-B-cell recognition and elimination by CD8 + T lymphocytes; however, this elimination does not occur, and it has been described that in both B1 and B2 lymphocytes infected with *Salmonella*, the PD1-PD1L pathway (programmed death-1; programmed death-1 ligand) is expressed, resulting in a reduction in the signaling required for activation of the T-cell receptor (TCR) and consequently avoiding B-cell death [145–147]. One of the characteristics of *Salmonella* is its ability to persist, and the use of the PD1 system in B lymphocytes makes them an ideal niche for prolonged stay in the body.

Thus, B lymphocytes play a key role in *Salmonella* infections, functioning as bacteria reservoir, acting as immunoregulatory cell through IL-10 production [148], facilitating bacterial systemic dissemination [43], and promoting a proinflammatory intestinal state characteristic of non-typhoidal infections through the production of proinflammatory cytokines such as IL-1β [135].

4.5. *Mycobacterium* B-cell infection

The genus *Mycobacterium* comprises a large number of species, some of which are highly pathogenic as *Mycobacterium tuberculosis* (MTB), being also the most studied species of all mycobacteria. MTB is a facultative intracellular pathogen; macrophages are the main cells where the mycobacteria reside and multiply [149], being able to infect other cells such as pulmonary epithelial cells [93, 150], fibroblasts [151], adipocytes [152], or endothelial cells [153]; bacterial replication into the non-phagocytic cells is discrete, so they have been suggested as niches where the bacteria may persist. In mycobacterial infections, the protective response is cellular, mediated by T helper (Th) lymphocytes and activated macrophages [154]. The involvement of antibodies and B lymphocytes has recently begun to be recognized. For example, B lymphocytes are required to control pulmonary inflammation and bacterial load [155] and antibodies and cytokine production by B lymphocytes mainly IL-10 and contribute to these activities [156]. Lymphocytes have been considered as non-phagocytic cells or with less interiorization capacity than macrophages [70, 71]. *Mycobacteria* promote their internalization in non-phagocytic cells, including B lymphocytes [72]. One way to establish the low phagocytic activity of B lymphocytes is to incubate them in the presence of inert particles like zymosan (**Figure 4**).

Macropinocytosis is an internalization process triggered by several inductors [157]; experimentally, phorbol esters trigger macropinocytosis even in phagocytic cells [158]. Pathogens use this internalization mechanism to achieve their entry into cells, by producing factors that trigger cytoskeleton reorganization [93]; for the case of mycobacteria, our group has suggested that pathogenic mycobacteria such as *M. tuberculosis* or nonpathogenic *Mycobacterium smegmatis* produce soluble factors present in the culture medium that trigger this phenomenon in B lymphocytes (**Figure 5**). Some of the reported mycobacterial products that facilitate adhesion and internalization into non-phagocytic cells are fibronectin-binding protein (FBP) and heparin-binding hemagglutinin adhesin (HBHA) [159, 160], among others [161, 162]. The internalization of mycobacteria in immortalized B lymphocytes (cell lines) has been described by some authors [72, 74, 163]; these studies show that *M. tuberculosis* survives and multiplies intracellularly in B lymphocytes, and as a consequence of infection, there is lymphocyte activation, resulting in antibody production of IgM class mainly and expression of co-stimulatory molecules like CD80 and CD86 [74]. There are scarce studies on human in vivo B-lymphocyte infection [164], so establishing the precise involvement of B lymphocytes in mycobacterial infections is an area of great interest.

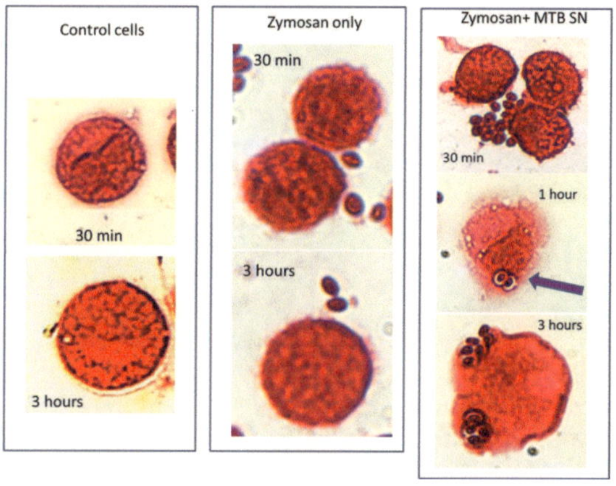

Figure 4. Is the B cell a "phagocytic cell"? B cells from the Raji cell line were incubated with zymosan without any further treatment, during 3 h; then cells were fixed with paraformaldehyde and stained with Giemsa dye. Control cells: cells did not receive any treatment. Zymosan only: cells were incubated with zymosan without any treatment. Zymosan and MTB SN: cells were incubated with zymosan and *Mycobacterium tuberculosis* filtrated growth bacterial culture medium (0.22 mm) for complete removal of the bacteria. Zymosan only: zymosan particles were observed bound to B-cell membrane; 3 h after, zymosan was not observed into the B cells. Zymosan + MTB SN: culture medium collected after 2 weeks of incubation at 37°C was placed with B lymphocyte; more zymosan particles were observed bound to B cell; after one h it was possible to observe intracellular zymosan.

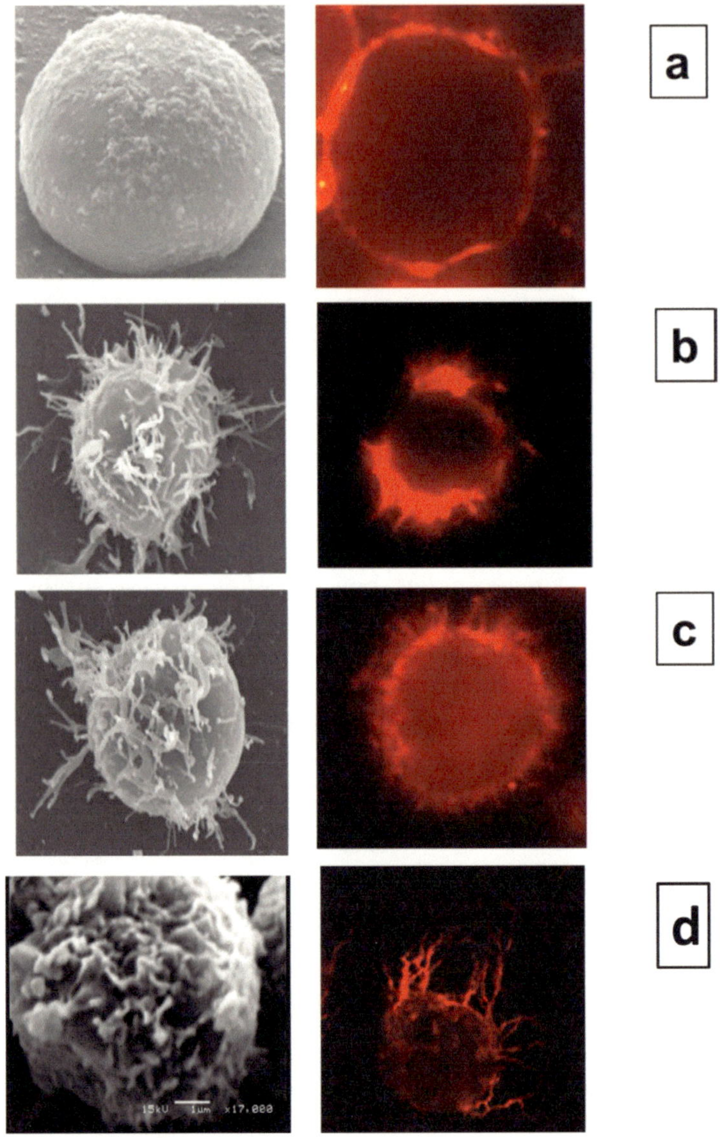

Figure 5. B-cell membrane changes after 1 h of incubation with PMA or mycobacteria derivatives. Scanning electron microscopy (SEM) and fluorescence microscopy images of Raji B cells. (Panel a) Control cells. (Panel b) Cells treated with phorbol-myristate-acetate (PMA), a classical macropinocytosis inductor. (Panel c) Cells treated with filtrated supernatant from growth culture medium of *Mycobacterium smegmatis*. (Panel d) Cells infected with *Mycobacterium tuberculosis*. Fluorescence images correspond to actin cytoskeleton labeled with phalloidin rhodamine. SEM images were 17,000× (panels a and d) or 15,000× (panels b and c); all fluorescence images were observed at 1200×.

5. Implications of B-cell response in bacterial infections

B lymphocytes are involved in various stages of the immune response against pathogens; the traditional role of these cells has been associated with adaptive immune response, characterized by the production of antibodies and the generation of immune memory. In bacterial infection, the role of these cells in the innate response has recently been recognized; in this sense, it has been demonstrated that B cells express receptors capable to recognize bacterial structures (TLRs, CR, dectin-1, etc.) [55, 165–167] and produce the effectors of the immune response—cytokines and antimicrobial peptides [168–171]—also activating mechanisms that prompt pathogen control like nitric oxide (NO) and antimicrobial peptides, among other [168]. The immune response induced in B lymphocytes often depends on the type of pathogen and the way in which B cell is activated, so B-cell response may be regulated by the bacteria to favor its intracellular survival. The B lymphocytes possess an endocytic capability that allows them to internalize pathogens; the mechanisms that these cells use to internalize bacteria can be endocytosis dependent or independent of clathrin, macropinocytosis, phagocytosis, etc. [72, 73, 88, 88, 168, 172]. As a result of this internalization, B lymphocytes produce a series of mediators of the innate response that will be described.

5.1. Cytokines

B cells recognize pathogens in an infectious process through the BCR or PRR receptors; this recognition may induce the cell activation and the production of inflammatory cytokines such as IL-1, IL-6, IL-8, TNFα, and IFNγ and suppressor cytokines as IL-10 and transforming growth factor beta (TGF-β), in addition to participating in Th2 profile events characterized by the production of IL-4, IL-5, IL-13, granulocyte-colony stimulating factor (GCSF), and granulocyte-macrophage colony-stimulating factor (GMCSF). B-cell plasticity is so extensive that any of these profiles can be induced by B cells depending on how they are activated [173–176].

Although B cells can show an inflammatory profile in response to bacterial infections, they cannot control infection at all times; some pathogens, especially intracellular ones, are able to occupy B cells as reservoirs of infection and can modulate the immune response of these cells to survive or even multiply within B lymphocytes. In the case of B-lymphocyte interaction with some Gram-negative bacteria such as *Brucella abortus* [69], *M. catarrhalis* [112, 166], and *Salmonella spp* [148, 177, 178], induce a high production of IL-10 which activates an immunosuppressive response characterized in addition by the simultaneous production of TGF-β, under this stage the bacteria rapidly spread. *Listeria monocytogenes* infection shows an IL-10-producing B-cell profile at very early stages of infection, which promotes bacteria persistence and dissemination [179–181]. Another example of B lymphocyte-bacteria interaction is the infection caused by *F. tularensis* which in B cell (particularly B1-a subtype) induces a clearly inflammatory profile characterized by the production of IL1-b, IFNγ, IL-6, IL-12, IL-17, and TNF-α [128, 129]. Regarding the activation of the inflammasome complex in B cells infected with *Salmonella*, it has been described that although this system is functional in B cells, the IL1-β is not secreted because this bacterium inhibits its production by a mechanism of negative regulation of the NLRC4 protein, which favors bacterial intracellular persistence [182].

5.2. Nitric oxide (NO)

Nitric oxide is one of the important mediators of the immune response that plays a fundamental role in the elimination of pathogens. This molecule is produced by classical phagocytic cells; however, its production has also been described by cells classified as non-phagocytic including B lymphocytes. During respiratory burst, NO in conjunction with the reactive oxygen species (ROS) participates in the formation of peroxynitrites, which are highly oxidizing agents of many components of the bacteria. NO increases its expression and activity in B lymphocytes infected with intracellular pathogens such as *M. tuberculosis*, *S. Typhimurium*, and *Citrobacter rodentium* [183–185]. The subclass of B1 lymphocytes constitutively produces nitric oxide inducible synthase (iNOS); however, in infectious events this enzyme increases its expression levels and therefore its activity, such as the LBs infected with *Cryptococcus neoformans*; in this infection, NO has a fundamental role in the elimination of the pathogen [186]. NO production in B1 lymphocytes appears to be linked to the stimulation of various TLRs, since some studies have shown that the stimulation of these receptors and their ligands resulted in production of higher NO levels by B lymphocytes. Of the Toll receptor ligands that have been studied, the major enhancer of NO expression was bacterial LPS; other agonists such as Poly I: C (TLR3), Imiquimod (TLR4), and CpG DNA (TLR9) also induce their expression [168, 187].

5.3. Antimicrobial peptides

Antimicrobial peptides are innate response effectors present in most human cells; these molecules are classified into alpha-defensins (HNP1-6) beta-defensins (hBD 1-4), and cathelicidins such as LL37. Its mechanisms of action include the direct lysis of the microorganisms, the generation of a proinflammatory environment, or the modulation of the immune response. There are very few studies on B-lymphocyte expression of antimicrobial peptides; however, there are some evidences demonstrating that B cells express antimicrobial peptides in constitutive and inducible fashion; under stimulation with some PAMPS, B lymphocytes express alpha defensins (HNPs 1–3), hBD2, and the cathelicidin LL-37 [170, 188].

5.4. Reactive oxygen species

B cells participate actively in the control of microorganisms, and although many authors have considered them as non-phagocytic cells, it seems that these cells possess microbicidal capacities, since they are able to produce antibacterial mediators like ROS. The Nox family of enzymes is responsible for regulating the production of ROS in several cell types like neutrophils and macrophages; the Nox2 isoform is particularly essential in the elimination of bacteria in these cells. Recently Nox2 production was described by splenic and peritoneal B lymphocytes; the absence in Nox2 production decreases the production of ROS resulting in a deficient elimination of *Staphylococcus aureus* by B lymphocytes; contrarily normal B cell controlled intracellular bacteria growth [171].

5.5. Regulation of B-cell survival during bacterial infection

The ability of several pathogens to regulate the death pathways of the host cell has been described for most of the pathogens that infect different cells, and actually this situation is recognized for B lymphocytes. For example, *L. monocytogenes* is known to induce apoptosis in B cells through various mechanisms such as activation of caspases 3, 8, and 9 [179, 189]. Apoptosis induction during bacterial infection of B cells has been reported for *F. tularensis, S. flexneri,* and *Helicobacter pylori* [55, 128, 190]; in all three cases, apoptosis of B cells is a mechanism that can facilitate the survival and dissemination of pathogens in their host due to the death of B lymphocytes that could have a protective effect. In comparison, during B-cell infection with *Salmonella,* the bacteria promote B-cell survival by engaging different mediators like PD-1 [145] or through the negative regulation of the protein NLRC4 [182], avoiding in both cases cell death. In this way, B cell becomes an intracellular niche for bacterial survival, persistence, and dissemination; the bacteria have a major role in promoting this situation [43, 182].

6. Concluding remarks

B lymphocytes are fascinating cells, far beyond being precursors of plasma cells; they represent a heterogenic cell population with an ample range of activities; beside antibody synthesis, they act as antigen-presenting cells; they produce pro- and anti-inflammatory cytokines acting as modulators of the immune response; and also they can uptake bacterial pathogens for latter processing and presenting them to T cells. Recent findings have left behind the old idea that B lymphocytes were not able to internalize bacterial or particulate antigens, but not all the B lymphocyte subsets have this ability. The B1-a subset is the major B-cell subset that is able to internalize bacterial pathogens; in the beginning, the antigen is recognized by PRRs like BCRs, TLRs, CRs, etc. After recognition, B cell will be activated, internalizing the bacteria, and depending on antigen′s nature (pathogenic or no pathogenic), the B lymphocyte will be activated to contribute in the establishment of a protective immune response. In some cases (specially for pathogenic bacteria), the B cell will not be able to control the pathogen; then the B cell becomes a pathogen niche or reservoir, acting as a "Trojan horse" that allows bacteria dissemination in the organism; in other cases, the pathogen modulates B-cell death, allowing cell and pathogen survival and making the B cell as an excellent host for bacterial persistence. The endocytic pathways performed by B lymphocytes to uptake bacteria, so far reported, are macropinocytosis and phagocytosis; still, there exists controversy regarding the ability of B lymphocyte to perform one, the other, or both mechanisms. It has been proposed that the B1-a cell subset has the double lineage lymphocyte/macrophage, making the B1-a cell prompt to respond to bacterial challenges and to respond to them in conjunction with the T cells; then these cells represent a bridge between the innate and the adaptive responses. Still, the B cells have many "secrets" that have to be revealed.

Acknowledgements

This work was supported by CONACYT-SEP-180401 and SIP/IPN project 20170126. JICS, MLDL, and JLH are SNI fellows. MLDL and JLH received fellowships from COFAA and EDI. The authors would also like to acknowledge the Electron Microscopy Central of ENCB/IPN for technical assistance and the Departamento de Sistemas Biológicos- Universidad Autónoma Metropolitana Xochimilco, for financial support for chapter publication.

Author details

Jorge Ismael Castañeda-Sánchez[1], Ana Rosa Muñoz Duarte[2], María Lilia Domínguez-López[2], Juan José de la Cruz-López[3] and Julieta Luna-Herrera[2*]

*Address all correspondence to: julietalunah@hotmail.com

1 Department of Biological Systems, Universidad Autonoma Metropolitana – Xochimilco Unit, Mexico City, Mexico

2 Department of Immunology, Escuela Nacional de Ciencias Biologicas, Instituto Politecnico Nacional, Mexico City, Mexico

3 Mesoamerican Center for Public Health and Disaster Studies, Universidad Autonoma de Chiapas, Tuxtla Gutiérrez, Chiapas, Mexico

References

[1] Tan SY, Dee MK. Elie Metchnikoff (1845-1916): Discoverer of phagocytosis. Singapore Medical Journal. 2009;**50**:456-458

[2] Bracha A, Tan SY. Emil von Behring (1854-1917): Medicine's first Nobel laureate. Singapore Medical Journal. 2011;**52**;1

[3] Bochner R. Paths to the discovery of antivenom serotherapy in France. Journal of Venomous Animals and Toxins including Tropical Diseases. 2016;**22**:20. DOI: 10.1186/s40409-016-0074-7

[4] Coons AH, Leduc EH, Connolly JM. Studies on antibody production: I. A method for the histochemical demonstration of specific antibody and its application to a study of the hyperimmune rabbit. Journal of Experimental Medicine. 1955;**102**:49-60

[5] Tiselius A, Kabat EA. An electrophoretic study of immune sera and purified antibody preparations. Journal of Experimental Medicine. 1939;**69**:119-131

[6] Fagraeus A. The plasma cellular reaction and its relation to the formation of antibodies in vitro. Journal of Immunology. 1948;**58**:1-13

[7] Nossal GJ, Lederberg J. Antibody production by single cells. Nature. 1958;**181**:1419-1420

[8] Bruton OC. Agammaglobulinemia. Pediatrics. 1952;**9**:722-728

[9] Varco RL, MacLean LD, Aust JB, Good RA. Agammaglobulinemia: An approach to homovital transplantation. Annals of Surgery. 1955;**142**:334-344

[10] Black CA. Delayed type hypersensitivity: Current theories with a historic perspective. Dermatology Online Journal. 1999;**5**:1-7

[11] Miller JFAP, Mitchell GF. Cell to cell interaction in the immune response : I. hemolysin-forming cells in neonatally thymectomized mice reconstituted with thymus or thoracic duct lymphocytes. Journal of Experimental Medicine. 1968;**128**:801-820

[12] Cross AM, Leuchars E, Miller JFAP. Studies on the recovery of the immune response in irradiated mice thymectomized in adult life. Journal of Experimental Medicine. 1964;**119**:837-850

[13] Glick B, Chang TS, Jaap RG. The bursa of fabricius and antibody production. Poultry Science. 1956;**35**:224

[14] Cooper MD, Peterson RDA, Good RA. Delineation of the thymic and bursal lymphoid systems in the chicken. Nature. 1965;**205**:143-146 DOI: 10.1038/205143a0

[15] Gowans, J, Knight, E. The route of re-circulation of lymphocytes in the rat. Proceedings of the Royal Society of London. Series B, Biological Sciences. 1964;**159**:257-282

[16] Cohen EP, Talmage DW. Onset and duration of dna synthesis in antibody-forming cells after antigen. Journal of Experimental Medicine. 1965;**121**:125-132

[17] Roitt IM, Greaves MF, Torrigiani G, Brostoff J, Playfair JH. The cellular basis of immunological responses. A synthesis of some current views. Lancet. 1969;**16**:367-371

[18] Mitchell GF, Miller JFAP. Cell to cell interaction in the immune response : II. The source of hemolysin-forming cells in irradiated mice given bone marrow and thymus or thoracic duct lymphocytes. Journal of Experimental Medicine. 1968;**128**:821-837

[19] Crotty S. A brief history of T cell help to B cells. Nature Reviews Immunology. 2015;**15**:185-189. DOI: 10.1038/nri3803

[20] LeBien TW, Tedder TF. B lymphocytes: How they develop and function. Blood. 2008;**112**:1570-1580. DOI: 10.1182/blood-2008-02-078071

[21] Baumgarth N, Herman OC, Jager GC, Brown L, Herzenberg LA, Herzenberg LA. Innate and acquired humoral immunities to influenza virus are mediated by distinct arms of the immune system. Proceedings of the National Academy of Sciences of the United States of America. 1999;**96**:2250-2255

[22] Baumgarth N, Tung JW, Herzenberg LA. Inherent specificities in natural antibodies: A key to immune defense against pathogen invasion. Springer Seminars in Immunopathology. 2005;**26**:347. DOI: 10.1007/s00281-004-0182-2

[23] Tung JW, Herzenberg LA. Unraveling B-1 progenitors. Current Opinion in Immunology. 2007;**19**:150-155. DOI: 10.1016/j.coi.2007.02.012

[24] Lopes JD, Mariano M. B-1 cell: The precursor of a novel mononuclear phagocyte with immuno-regulatory properties. Anais da Academia Brasileira de Ciências. 2009;**81**:489-496. DOI: https://dx.DOI.org/10.1590/S0001-37652009000300013

[25] Gao J, Ma X, Gu W, Fu M, An J, Xing Y, et al. Novel functions of murine B1 cells: Active phagocytic and microbicidal abilities. European Journal of Immunology. 2012;**42**:982-992. DOI: 10.1002/eji.201141519

[26] Sunyer JO. Evolutionary and functional relationships of B cells from fish and mammals: insights into their novel roles in phagocytosis and presentation of particulate antigen. Infectious Disorders Drug Targets. 2012;**12**:200-212

[27] Panda S, Ding JL. Natural antibodies bridge innate and adaptive immunity. Journal of Immunology. 2015;**194**:13-20. DOI: 10.4049/jimmunol.1400844

[28] Martin F, Kearney JF. B-cell subsets and the mature preinmmune repertoire. Marginal zone and B1 B cells as part of a "natural immune memory". Immunological Reviews. 2000;**175**:70-79. DOI: 10.1111/j.1600-065X.2000.imr017515.x

[29] Haas KM, Poe JC, Steeber DA, Tedder TF. B-1a and B-1b cells exhibit distinct developmental requirements and have unique functional roles in innate and adaptive immunity to *S. pneumoniae*. Immunity. 2005;**23**:7-18. DOI: 10.1016/j.immuni.2005.04.011

[30] Berland R, Wortis HH. Origins and functions of B-1 cells with notes on the role of CD5. Annual Review of Immunology. 2002;**20**:253-300. DOI: 10.1146/annurev.immunol.20.100301.064833

[31] Duan B, Morel L. Role of B-1a cells in autoimmunity. Autoimmunity Reviews. 2006;**5**:403-408. DOI: 10.1016/j.autrev.2005.10.007

[32] Baumgarth N. The double life of a B-1 cell: Self-reactivity selects for protective effector functions. Nature Reviews Immunology. 2011;**11**:34-46. DOI: 10.1038/nri2901

[33] Merino MC, Gruppi A. Origin and development of B1 lymphocytes. A cell population involved in defence and autoimmunity. Medicina (B Aires). 2006;**66**:165-172

[34] Baumgarth N. B-1 cell heterogeneity and the regulation of natural and antigen-induced IgM production. Frontiers in Immunology. 2016;**9**:324. DOI: 10.3389/fimmu.2016.00324

[35] Grupp SA, Mitchell RN, Schreiber KL, McKean DJ, Abbas AK. Molecular mechanisms that control expression of the B lymphocyte antigen receptor complex. Journal of Experimental Medicine. 1995 Jan 1;**181**:161-168

[36] Treanor B. B-cell receptor: From resting state to activate. Immunology. 2012;**136**:21-27. DOI: 10.1111/j.1365-2567.2012.03564.x

[37] Rogers J, Early P, Carter C, Calame K, Bond M, Hood L, Wall R. Two mRNAs with different 3' ends encode membrane-bound and secreted forms of immunoglobulin mu chain. Cell. 1980 Jun;**20**:303-311

[38] Fleire SJ, Goldman JP, Carrasco YR, Weber M, Bray D, Batista FD, et al. B cell ligand discrimination through a spreading and contraction response. Science. 2006;**312**:738-741. DOI: 10.1126/science.1123940

[39] Tolar P, Hanna J, Krueger PD, Pierce SK. The constant region of the membrane immunoglobulin mediates B cell-receptor clustering and signaling in response to membrane antigens. Immunity. 2009;**30**:44-55. DOI: 10.1016/j.immuni.2008.11.007

[40] Depoil D, Fleire S, Treanor BL, Weber M, Harwood NE, Marchbank KL, et al. CD19 is essential for B cell activation by promoting B cell receptor-antigen microcluster formation in response to membrane-bound ligand. Nature Immunology 2008;**9**:63-72. DOI: 10.1038/ni1547

[41] Batista FD, Neuberger MS. B cells extract and present immobilized antigen: Implications for affinity discrimination. EMBO Journal. 2000;**19**:513-520

[42] Wingren GA, Hadzic R, Forsgren A, Riesbeck K. The novel IgD binding protein from *Moraxella catarrhalis* induces human B lymphocyte activation and Ig secretion in the presence of Th2 cytokines. Journal of Immunology. 2002;**168**:5582-5588

[43] Souwer Y, Griekspoor A, de Wit J, Martinoli C, Zagato E, Janssen H, Jorritsma T, Bar-Ephraïm YE, Rescigno M, Neefjes J, van Ham SM. Selective infection of antigen-specific B lymphocytes by Salmonella mediates bacterial survival and systemic spreading of infection. PLoS One. 2012;**7**:e50667. DOI: 10.1371/journal.pone.0050667.

[44] Ghosh D, Stumhofer JS. Do you see what I see: Recognition of protozoan parasites by Toll-like receptors. Current Immunology Reviews. 2013;**9**:129-140

[45] Peng SL. Signaling in B cells via Toll-like receptors. Current Opinion in Immunology. 2005;**17**:230-236. DOI: 10.1016/j.coi.2005.03.003

[46] Dasari P, Nicholson IC, Hodge G, Dandie GW, Zola H. Expression of Toll-like receptors on B lymphocytes. Cellular Immunology. 2005;**236**:140-145. DOI: 10.1016/j.cellimm.2005.08.020

[47] Underhill DM, Toll-like receptors and microbes take aim at each other. Current Opinion in Immunology. 2004;**16**:483-487. DOI: 10.1016/j.coi.2004.05.012

[48] Gururajan M, Jacob J, Pulendran B. Toll-like receptor expression and responsiveness of distinct murine splenic and mucosal B-cell subsets. PLoS One. 2007;**2**:e863. DOI: 10.1371/journal.pone.0000863.

[49] Bernasconi NL, Onai N, Lanzavecchia A. A role for Toll-like receptors in acquired immunity: Up-regulation of TLR9 by BCR triggering in naive B cell sand constitutive expression in memory B cells. Blood. 2003;**101**:4500-4504. DOI: 10.1182/blood-2002-11-3569

[50] Leadbetter EA, Rifkin IR, Hohlbaum AM, Beaudette BC, Shlomchik MJ, Marshak-Rothstein A. Chromatin-IgG complexes activate B cells by dual engagement of IgM and Toll-like receptors. Nature. 2002;**416**:603-607. DOI: 10.1038/416603a

[51] Lin L, Gerth AJ, Peng SL. CpG DNA redirects class-switching towards "Th1-like" Ig isotype production via TLR9 and MyD88. European Journal of Immunology. 2004;**34**:1483-1487. DOI: 10.1002/eji.200324736

[52] Viglianti GA, Lau CM, Hanley TM, Miko BA, Shlomchik MJ, Marshak-Rothstein A: Activation of autoreactive B cells by CpG dsDNA. Immunity. 2003;**19**:837-847. DOI: 10.1016/S1074-7613(03)00323-6

[53] Genestier L, Taillardet M, Mondiere P, Gheit H, Bella C, Defrance T. TLR agonists selectively promote terminal plasma cell differentiation of B cell subsets specialized in thymus-independent responses. Journal of Immunology. 2007;**178**:7779-7786. DOI: https://DOI.org/10.4049/jimmunol.178.12.7779

[54] Picard C, von Bernuth H, Ghandil P, Chrabieh M, Levy O, Arkwright PD, et al. Clinical features and outcome of patients with IRAK-4 and MyD88 deficiency. Medicine. 2010;**89**:403-425. DOI: 10.1097/MD.0b013e3181fd8ec3

[55] Nothelfer K, Sansonetti PJ, Phalipon A. Pathogen manipulation of B cells: The best defence is a good offence. Nature Reviews Microbiology. 2015;**13**:173-184. DOI: 10.1038/nrmicro3415

[56] Plato A, Willment JA, Brown GD. C-type lectin-like receptors of the dectin-1 cluster: Ligands and signaling pathways. International Reviews of Immunology. 2013;**32**:134-156. DOI: 10.3109/08830185.2013.777065.

[57] Ali MF, Driscoll CB, Walters PR, Limper AH, Carmona EM. Beta-glucan activated human B-lymphocytes participate in innate immune responses by releasing pro-inflammatory cytokines and stimulating neutrophil chemotaxis. Journal of Immunology. 2015;**195**:5318-5326. DOI: 10.4049/jimmunol.1500559

[58] Sancho D, Reis e Sousa C. Signaling by myeloid C-type lectin receptors in immunity and homeostasis. Annual Review of Immunology. 2012;**30**:491-529. DOI: 10.1146/annurev-immunol-031210-101352

[59] Geijtenbeek TB, Gringhuis SI. Signalling through C-type lectin receptors: Shaping immune responses. Nature Reviews Immunology. 2009;**9**:465-479. DOI: 10.1038/nri2569

[60] Carroll MC. The complement system in B cell regulation, Molecular Immunology. 2004;**41**:141-146. DOI: 10.1016/j.molimm.2004.03.017

[61] Kremlitzka M, Polgár A, Fülöp L, Kiss E, Poór G, Erdei A. Complementreceptor type 1 (CR1, CD35) is a potent inhibitor of B-cell functions in rheumatoid arthritis patients. International Immunology. 2013;**25**:25-33. DOI: 10.1093/intimm/dxs090

[62] Józsi M, Prechl J, Bajtay Z, Erdei A. Complement receptor type 1 (CD35) mediates inhibitory signals in human B lymphocytes. Journal of Immunology. 2002;**168**:2782-2788. DOI: https://DOI.org/10.4049/jimmunol.168.6.2782

[63] Plzakova L, Krocova Z, Kubelkova K, Macela A. Entry of *Francisella tularensis* into murine B cells: The role of B cell receptors and complement receptors. PLoS One. 2015;**10**:e0132571. DOI: 10.1371/journal.pone.0132571

[64] Nimmerjahn F, Ravetch JV. Fcg receptors: Old friends and new family members. Immunity. 2006;**24**:19-28. DOI: 10.1016/j.immuni.2005.11.010

[65] Ravetch JV, Bolland S. IgG Fc receptors. Annual Review of Immunology. 2001;**19**:275-290. DOI: 10.1146/annurev.immunol.19.1.275

[66] Ravetch JV, Lanier LL. Immune inhibitory receptors. Science. 2000;**90**:84-89. DOI: 10.1126/science.290.5489.84

[67] Hayes JM, Wormald MR, Rudd PM, Davey GP. Fc gamma receptors: glycobiology and therapeutic prospects. Journal of Inflammation Research. 2016;**9**:209-219. DOI: 10.2147/JIR.S121233

[68] Jarasch-Althof N, Wiesener N, Schmidtke M, Wutzler P, Henke A. Antibody-dependent enhancement of coxsackievirus B3 infection of primary CD19+ B lymphocytes. Viral Immunology. 2010 Aug;**23**:369-376. DOI: 10.1089/vim.2010.0018

[69] Goenka R, Guirnalda PD, Black SJ, Baldwin CL. B lymphocytes provide an infection niche for intracellular bacterium *Brucella abortus*. Journal of Infectious Diseases. 2012;**206**:91-98. DOI: 10.1093/infdis/jis310

[70] Galelli A, Charlot B, Dériaud E, Leclerc C. B cells do not present antigen covalently linked to microsphere. Immunology. 1993;**79**:69-76.

[71] Vidard L, Kovacsovics-Bankowski M, Kraeft SK, Chen LB, Benacerraf B, Rock KL. Analysis of MHC class II presentation of particulate antigens of B lymphocytes. Journal of Immunology. 1996;**15**(156):2809-2818

[72] García-Pérez BE, De la Cruz-López JJ, Castañeda-Sánchez JI, Muñóz-Duarte AR, Hernández-Pérez AD, Villegas-Castrejón H, García-Latorre E, Caamal-Ley A, Luna-Herrera J. Macropinocytosis is responsible for the uptake of pathogenic and non-pathogenic mycobacteria by B lymphocytes (Raji cells). BMC Microbiology. 2012;**12**:246. DOI: 10.1186/1471-2180-12-246

[73] Rosales-Reyes R, Pérez-López A, Sánchez-Gómez C, Hernández-Mote RR, Castro-Eguiluz D, Ortiz-Navarrete V, et al. Salmonella infects B cells by macropinocytosis and formation of spacious phagosomes but does not induce pyroptosis in favor of its survival. Microbial Pathogenesis. 2012;**52**:367-374. DOI: 10.1016/j.micpath.2012.03.007

[74] Zhu Q, Zhang M, Shi M, Liu Y, Zhao Q, Wang W, et al. Human B cells have an active phagocytic capability and undergo immune activation upon phagocytosis of *Mycobacterium tuberculosis*. Immunobiology. 2016;**221**:558-567. DOI: 10.1016/j.imbio.2015.12.003

[75] Rohatgi S, Pirofski LA. Molecular characterization of the early B cell response to pulmonary *Cryptococcus neoformans* infection. Journal of Immunology. 2012;**189**:5820-5830. DOI: 10.4049/jimmunol.1201514. Epub 2012

[76] Parra D, Rieger AM, Li J, Zhang YA, Randall LM, Hunter CA, Barreda DR, Sunyer JO. Pivotal advance: Peritoneal cavity B-1 B cells have phagocytic and microbicidal capacities and present phagocytosed antigen to CD4+ T cells. Journal of Leukocyte Biology. 2012;**91**:525-536. DOI: 10.1189/jlb.0711372. Epub Nov 4, 2011.

[77] Mills SD, Finlay BB. Comparison of *Salmonella typhi* and *Salmonella typhimurium* invasion, intracellular growth and localization in cultured human epithelial cells. Microbial Pathogenesis. 1994;**17**:409-423

[78] Mao Y, Finnemann SC. Regulation of phagocytosis by Rho GTPases. Small GTPases. 2015;**6**:89-99. DOI: 10.4161/21541248.2014.989785. Epub May 5, 2015.

[79] May RC, Machesky LM. Phagocytosis and the actin cytoskeleton. Journal of Cell Science. 2001;**114**:1061-1077

[80] Qualmann B, Mellor H. Regulation of endocytic traffic by Rho GTPases. Biochemical Journal. 2003;**371**:233-241. DOI: 10.1042/BJ20030139

[81] Doherty GJ, McMahon HT. 2009. Mechanisms of endocytosis. Annual Review of Biochemistry. 2009;**78**:857-902. DOI: 10.1146/annurev.biochem.78.081307.110540

[82] Saffarian S, Cocucci E, Kirchhausen T. Distinct dynamics of endocytic clathrin-coated pits and coated plaques. PLoS Biology. 2009;**7**:1337-1341. DOI: 10.1371/journal.pbio.1000191

[83] Natkanski E, Lee WY, Mistry B, Casal A, Molloy JE, Tolar P. B cells use mechanical energy to discriminate antigen affinities. Science 2013;**340**:1587-1590. DOI: 10.1126/science.1237572

[84] Stoddart A, Dykstra ML, Brown BK, Song W, Pierce SK, Brodsky FM. Lipid rafts unite signaling cascades with clathrin to regulate BCR internalization. Immunity. 2002;**17**:51-462. DOI: http://dx.DOI.org/10.1016/S1074-7613(02)00416-8

[85] Putnam MA, Moquin AE, Merrihew M, Outcalt C, Sorge E, Caballero A, Gondré-Lewis TA, Drake JR. Lipid raft-independent B cell receptor-mediated antigen internalization and intracellular trafficking. Journal of Immunology. 2003 Jan 15;**170**:905-912

[86] Caballero A, Katkere B, Wen XY, Drake L, Nashar TO, Drake JR. Functional and structural requirements for the internalization of distinct BCR-ligand complexes. European Journal of Immunology. 2006;**36**:3131-3145. DOI: 10.1002/eji.200636447

[87] Salisbury JL, Condeelis JS, Satir P. Role of coated vesicles, microfilaments, and calmodulin in receptor-mediated endocytosis by cultured B lymphoblastoid cells. Journal of Cell Biology. 1980;**87**:132-141

[88] Souwer Y, Griekspoor A, Jorritsma T, de Wit J, Janssen H, Neefjes J, et al. B cell receptor-mediated internalization of Salmonella: A novel pathway for autonomous B cell activation and antibody production. Journal of Immunology. 2009;**182**:7473-7481. DOI: 10.4049/jimmunol.0802831

[89] Lewis WH. Pinocytosis. Johns Hopkins Hospital Bulletin. 1931;**49**:17-23

[90] Cardelli J. Phagocytosis and macropinocytosis in dictyostelium: Phosphoinositide-based processes, biochemically distinct. Traffic. 2001;**2**:311-320

[91] Lim PJ, Gleeson PA. Macropinocytosis: An endocytic pathway for internalising large gulps. Immunology and Cell Biology. 2011;**89**:836-843

[92] Jones AT. Macropinocytosis: Searching for an endocytic identity and a role in the uptake of cell penetrating peptides. Journal of Cellular and Molecular Medicine. 2007;**1**:670-684. DOI: 10.1111/j.1582-4934.2007.00062.x

[93] Kerr MC, Teasdale RD. Defining macropinocytosis. Traffic. 2009;**10**:364-371. DOI: 10.1111/j.1600-0854.2009.00878.x.

[94] Cain RJ, Hayward RD, Koronakis V. Deciphering interplay between Salmonella invasion effectors. PLOS Pathogens. 2008;**4**(4):e1000037. DOI: 10.1371/journal.ppat.1000037

[95] Carayol N, Tran Van Nhieu G. The inside story of *Shigella* invasion of intestinal epithelial cells. Cold Spring Harbor Perspectives in Medicine. 2013;**1**(3):a016717. DOI: 10.1101/cshperspect.a016717

[96] Tran Van Nhieu G, Kai Liu B, Zhang J, Pierre F, Prigent S, Sansonetti P, Erneux C, Kuk Kim J, Suh PG, Dupont G, Combettes L. Actin-based confinement of calcium responses during *Shigella* invasion. Nature Communications. 2013;**4**:1567. DOI: 10.1038/ncomms2561.

[97] García-Pérez BE, Mondragón-Flores R, Luna-Herrera J. Internalization of *Mycobacterium tuberculosis* by macropinocytosis in non-phagocytic cells. Microbial Pathogenesis. 2003;**35**:49-55

[98] Cossart P, Helenius A. Endocytosis of viruses and bacteria. Cold Spring Harbor Perspectives in Medicine. 2014;**6**(8). pii: a016972. DOI: 10.1101/cshperspect.a016972

[99] Bloomfield G, Kay RR. Uses and abuses of macropinocytosis. Journal of Cell Science. 2016 Jul 15;**129**:2697-2705. DOI: 10.1242/jcs.176149

[100] Shen P, Roch T, Lampropoulou V, O'Connor RA, Stervbo U, Hilgenberg E, et al. IL-35-producing B cells are critical regulators of immunity during autoimmune and infectious diseases. Nature. 2014;**507**:366-370. DOI: 10.1038/nature12979.

[101] Selvaraj UM, Poinsatte K, Torres V, Ortega SB, Stowe AM. Heterogeneity of B Cell functions in stroke-related risk, prevention, injury, and repair. Neurotherapeutics. 2016;**13**:729-747

[102] Young KA, Chen XS, Holers VM, Hannan JP. Isolating the Epstein-Barr virus gp350/220 binding site on complement receptor type 2 (CR2/CD21). Journal of Biological Chemistry. 2007;**14**(282):36614-36625. DOI: 10.1074/jbc.M706324200

[103] Hatton OL, Arnold-Harris A, Schaffert S, Krams SM, Martinez OM. The interplay between Epstein-Barr virus and B lymphocytes: Implications for infection, immunity, and disease. Immunologic Research. 2014;**58**:268-276. DOI: 10.1007/s12026-014-8496-1

[104] Meier U-C, Giovannoni G, Tzartos JS, Khan G. Translational mini-review series on B cell subsets in disease. B cells in multiple sclerosis: Drivers of disease pathogenesis and Trojan horse for Epstein-Barr virus entry to the central nervous system? Clinical & Experimental Immunology. 2012;**167**:1-6. DOI: 10.1111/j.1365-2249.2011.04446.x

[105] Olding LB, Jensen FC, Oldstone MBA. Pathogenesis of cytomegalovirus infection. I. Activation of virus from bone marrow-derived lymphocytes by in vitro allogenic reaction. Journal of Experimental Medicine. 1975;**141**:561-572.

[106] Rice GP, Schrier RD, Oldstone MB. Cytomegalovirus infects human lymphocytes and monocytes: virus expression is restricted to immediate-early gene products. Proceedings of the National Academy of Sciences of the United States of America. 1984;**81**:6134-6138

[107] McChesney MB, Bankhurst AD. Cytotoxic mechanisms in vitro against Epstein-Barr virus infected lymphoblastoid cell lines in rheumatoid arthritis. Annals of the Rheumatic Diseases. 1986;**45**:546-552

[108] McChesney MB, Oldstone MB. Viruses perturb lymphocyte functions: selected principles characterizing virus-induced immunosuppression. Annual Review of Immunology. 1987;**5**:279-304. DOI: 10.1146/annurev.iy.05.040187.001431

[109] Kubelkova K, Krocova Z, Plzakova L, Macela A. The role of B cells in intracellular bacterial pathogen infection. In: Montes RL, Reyes L, editors. B cells: Molecular Biology, Developmental Origin and Impact on the Immune System. Nova Science Publishers; 2013. pp. 1-43. DOI: 10.13140/2.1.1078

[110] Murphy TF, Parameswaran GI. *Moraxella catarrhalis*, a human respiratory tract pathogen. Clinical Infectious Diseases. 2009;**49**:124-131. DOI: 10.1086/599375

[111] Karalus R, Campagnari A. *Moraxella catarrhalis*: A review of an important human mucosal pathogen. Microbes and Infection. 2000;**2**:547-559. DOI: 10.1016/S1286-4579(00)00314-2

[112] Jendholm J, Mörgelin M, Perez Vidakovics ML, Carlsson M, Leffler H, Cardell LO, et al. Superantigen- and TLR-dependent activation of tonsillar B cells after receptor-mediated endocytosis. Journal of Immunology. 2009;**182**:4713-4720. DOI: 10.4049/jimmunol.080303

[113] Hua Z, Hou B. TLR signaling in B-cell development and activation. Cellular & Molecular Immunology. 2013;**10**:103-106. DOI: 10.1038/cmi.2012.61

[114] Heiniger N, Spaniol V, Troller R, Vischer M, Aebi C. A reservoir of *Moraxella catarrhalis* in human pharyngeal lymphoid tissue. Journal of Infectious Diseases. 2007;**196**:1080-1087. DOI: 10.1086/521194

[115] Ahmed W, Zheng K, Liu Z-F. Establishment of chronic infection: Brucella's stealth strategy. Frontiers in Cellular and Infection Microbiology. 2016;**6**:30. DOI: 10.3389/fcimb.2016.00030

[116] De Figueiredo P, Ficht TA, Rice-Ficht A, Rossetti CA, Adams LG. Pathogenesis and immunobiology of Brucellosis: Review of Brucella – host interactions. The American Journal of Pathology. 2015;**185**:1505-1517. DOI: 10.1016/j.ajpath.2015.03.003

[117] Guzmán-Verri C, Chaves-Olarte E, von Eichel-Streiber C, López-Goñi I, Thelestam M, Arvidson S, et al. GTPases of the Rho subfamily are required for *Brucella abortus* internalization in nonprofessional phagocytes: Direct activation of Cdc42. Journal of Biological Chemistry. 2001;**276**:44435-44443. DOI: 10.1074/jbc.M105606200

[118] McCaffrey RL, Allen L-AH. Pivotal advance: *Francisella tularensis* LVS evades killing by human neutrophils via inhibition of the respiratory burst and phagosome escape. Journal of Leukocyte Biology. 2006;**80**:1224-1230. DOI: 10.1189/jlb.0406287

[119] Rabadi SM, Sanchez BC, Varanat M, Ma Z, Catlett SV, Melendez JA, et al. Antioxidant defenses of *Francisella tularensis* modulate macrophage function and production of proinflammatory cytokines. Journal of Biological Chemistry. 2016;**291**:5009-5021. DOI: 10.1074/jbc.M115.681478.

[120] Hall JD, Woolard MD, Gunn BM, Craven RR, Taft-Benz S, Frelinger JA, et al. Infected-host-cell repertoire and cellular response in the lung following inhalation of *Francisella tularensis* Schu S4, LVS, or U112. Infection and Immunity. 2008;**76**:5843-5852. DOI: 10.1128/IAI.01176-08

[121] Rennert K, Otto P, Funke H, Huber O, Tomaso H, Mosig AS. A human macrophage – hepatocyte co-culture model for comparative studies of infection and replication of *Francisella tularensis* LVS strain and subspecies holarctica and mediasiatica. BMC Microbiology. 2016;**16**:2. DOI: 10.1186/s12866-015-0621-3

[122] Golovliov I, Baranov V, Krocova Z, Kovarova H, Sjöstedt A. An attenuated strain of the facultative intracellular bacterium *Francisella tularensis* can escape the phagosome of monocytic cells. Infection and Immunity. 2003;**71**:5940-5950. DOI: 10.1128/IAI.71.10.5940-5950.2003

[123] Checroun C, Wehrly TD, Fischer ER, Hayes SF, Celli J. Autophagy-mediated reentry of *Francisella tularensis* into the endocytic compartment after cytoplasmic replication. Proceedings of the National Academy of Sciences of the United States of America. 2006 Sep 26;**103**:14578-14583. Epub Sep 18, 2006

[124] Clemens DL, Lee BY, Horwitz MA. *Francisella tularensis* phagosomal escape does not require acidification of the phagosome. Infection and Immunity. 2009 May;**77**:1757-1773. DOI: 10.1128/IAI.01485-08. Epub Feb 2009

[125] Bosio, CM, Bielefeldt-Ohmann H, and Belisle JT. Active suppression of the pulmonary immune response by *Francisella tularensis* Schu4. Journal of Immunology. 2007;**178**:4538-4547. DOI: https://DOI.org/10.4049/jimmunol.178.7.4538

[126] Gillard JJ, Laws TR, Lythe G, Molina-París C. Modeling early events in *Francisella tularensis* pathogenesis. Frontiers in Cellular and Infection Microbiology. 2014;**4**:169. DOI: 10.3389/fcimb.2014.00169

[127] Elkins KL, Bosio CM, Rhinehart-Jones TR. Importance of B cells, but not specific antibodies, in primary and secondary protective immunity to the intracellular bacterium *Francisella tularensis* live vaccine strain. Infection and Immunity. 1999;**67**:6002e7

[128] Krocova Z, Härtlova A, Souckova D, Zivna L, Kroca M, Rudolf E, et al. Interaction of B cells with intracellular pathogen *Francisella tularensis*. Microbial Pathogenesis. 2008;**45**:79-85. DOI: 10.1016/j.micpath.2008.01.010

[129] Plzakova L, Kubelkova K, Krocova Z, Zarybnicka L, Sinkorova Z, Macela A. B cell subsets are activated and produce cytokines during early phases of *Francisella tularensis* LVS infection. Microbial Pathogenesis. 2014;**75**:9-58. DOI: 10.1016/j.micpath.2014.08.009.

[130] Chou AY, Kennett NJ, Melillo AA, Elkins KL.Murine survival of infection with Francisella novicida and protection against secondary challenge is critically dependent on B lymphocytes. Microbes and Infection. 2017;**19**:91-100. DOI: 10.1016/j.micinf.2016.12.001

[131] Dekker J, Frank K. Salmonella, Shigella, and Yersinia. Clinics in Laboratory Medicine. 2015;**35**:225-246. DOI: 10.1016/j.cll.2015.02.002

[132] Coburn B, Grassl GA, Finlay BB. Salmonella, the host and disease: A brief review. Immunology & Cell Biology. 2007;**85**:112-118. DOI: 10.1038/sj.icb.7100007

[133] Andrews-Polymenis HL, Bäumler AJ, McCormick BA, Fang FC. Taming the elephant: Salmonella biology, pathogenesis, and prevention. Infection and Immunity. 2010;**78**:2356-2369. DOI: 10.1128/IAI.00096-10.

[134] Eckmann L, Kagnoff MF. Cytokines in host defense against Salmonella. Microbes and Infection. 2001;**3**:1191-1200. DOI: http://dx.DOI.org/10.1016/S1286-4579(01)01479-4

[135] Santos RL, Zhang S, Tsolis RM, Bäumler AJ, Adams LG. Morphologic and molecular characterization of *Salmonella typhimurium* infection in neonatal calves. Veterinary Pathology. 2002;**39**:200-215. DOI: 10.1354/vp.39-2-200

[136] Verjans GM, Ringrose JH, van Alphen L, Feltkamp TE, Kusters JG. Entrance and survival of *Salmonella typhimurium* and *Yersinia enterocolitica* within human B- and T-cell lines. Infection and Immunity. 1994;**62**:2229-2235

[137] Patel JC, Galan JE. Manipulation of the host actin cytoskeleton by Salmonella – All in the name of entry. Current Opinion in Microbiology. 2005;**8**:10-15. DOI: 10.1016/j.mib.2004.09.001

[138] Hannemann S, Gao B, Galán JE. Salmonella modulation of host cell gene expression promotes its intracellular growth. PLOS Pathogens. 2013;**9**:e1003668. DOI: 10.1371/journal.ppat.1003668.

[139] Drecktrah D, Knodler LA, Ireland R, Steele-Mortimer O. The Mechanism of Salmonella entry determines the vacuolar environment and intracellular gene expression. Traffic. 2006;**7**:39-51. DOI: 10.1111/j.1600-0854.2005.00360.x

[140] van der Heijden J, Bosman ES, Reynolds LA, Finlay BB. Direct measurement of oxidative and nitrosative stress dynamics in Salmonella inside macrophages. Proceedings of the National Academy of Sciences of the United States of America 2015;**112**(2):560-565. DOI: 10.1073/pnas.1414569112. Epub Dec 29, 2014

[141] Lajarin F, Rubio G, Galvez J, Garcia-Peñarrubia P. Adhesion, invasion and intracellular replication of *Salmonella typhimurium* in a murine hepatocyte cell line. Effect of cytokines and LPS on antibacterial activity of hepatocytes. Microbial Pathogenesis. 1996;**21**:19-329. DOI: 10.1006/mpat.1996.0065

[142] Barr TA, Brown S, Mastroeni P, Gray D. TLR and B cell receptor signals to B cells differentially program primary and memory Th1 responses to *Salmonella enterica*. Journal of Immunology. 2010 Sep 1;**185**(5):2783-2789. DOI: 10.4049/jimmunol.1001431

[143] Kubori T, Galán JE. Salmonella type III secretion-associated protein InvE controls translocation of effector proteins into host cells. Journal of Bacteriology. 2002;**184**:4699-4708. DOI: 10.1128/JB.184.17.4699-4708.2002

[144] Lopez-Medina M, Perez-Lopez A, Alpuche-Aranda C, Ortiz-Navarrete V. Salmonella modulates B cell biology to evade CD8+ T cell-mediated immune responses. Frontiers in Immunology. 2014;**5**:586. DOI: 10.3389/fimmu.2014.00586

[145] Lopez-Medina M, Perez-Lopez A, Alpuche-Aranda C, Ortiz-Navarrete V. Salmonella induces PD-L1 expression in B cells. Immunology Letters. 2015;**167**:131-140. DOI: 10.1016/j.imlet.2015.08.004

[146] Freeman GJ, Long AJ, Iwai Y, Bourque K, Chernova T, Nishimura H, et al. Engagement of the Pd-1 immunoinhibitory receptor by a novel B7 family member leads to negative regulation of lymphocyte activation. Journal of Experimental Medicine. 2000;**192**:1027-1034. DOI: 10.1084/jem.192.7.1027

[147] Loke P, Allison JP. PD-L1 and PD-L2 are differentially regulated by Th1 and Th2 cells. Proceedings of the National Academy of Sciences of the United States of America. 2003;**100**:5336-5341. DOI: 10.1073/pnas.0931259100

[148] Neves P, Lampropoulou V, Calderon-Gomez E, Roch T, Stervbo U, Shen P, et al. Signaling via the MyD88 adaptor protein in B cells suppresses protective immunity during *Salmonella typhimurium* infection. Immunity. 2010;**33**:777-790. DOI: 10.1016/j.immuni.2010.10.016

[149] Amaral EP, Lasunskaia EB, D'Império-Lima MR. Innate immunity in tuberculosis: How the sensing of mycobacteria and tissue damage modulates macrophage death. Microbes and Infection. 2016;**18**(1):11-20. DOI: 10.1016/j.micinf.2015.09.005

[150] Chuquimia OD, Petursdottir DH, Rahman MJ, Hartl K, Singh M, Fernández C. The role of alveolar epithelial cells in initiating and shaping pulmonary immune responses: Communication between innate and adaptive immune systems. PLoS One. 2012;**7**(2):e32125. DOI: 10.1371/journal.pone.0032125

[151] Mariotti S, Sargentini V, Pardini M, Giannoni F, De Spirito M, Gagliardi MC, et al. *Mycobacterium tuberculosis* may escape helper T cell recognition by infecting human fibroblasts. Human Immunology. 2013 Jun;**74**(6):722-729. DOI: 10.1016/j.humimm.2013.02.005.

[152] Neyrolles O, Hernández-Pando R, Pietri-Rouxel F, et al. Is adipose tissue a place for *Mycobacterium tuberculosis* persistence? PLoS One. 2006;**1**(1):e43. DOI: 10.1371/journal.pone.0000043

[153] Mehta PK, Karls RK, White EH, Ades EW, Quinn FD. Entry and intracellular replication of *Mycobacterium tuberculosis* in cultured human microvascular endothelial cells. Microbial Pathogenesis. 2006;**41**:119-124. DOI: 10.1016/j.micpath.2006.05.002

[154] Andersen P, Urdahl KB. TB vaccines: promoting rapid and durable protection in the lung. Current Opinion in Immunology. 2015;**35**:55-62. DOI: 10.1016/j.coi.2015.06.001. Epub Jun 22, 2015

[155] Maglione PJ, Xu J, Chan J. B Cells moderate inflammatory progression and enhance bacterial containment upon pulmonary challenge with *Mycobacterium tuberculosis*. The Journal of Immunology. 2007;**178**:7222-7234. DOI: 10.4049/jimmunol.178.11.7222

[156] Maglione PJ, Chan J. How B cells shape the immune response against *Mycobacterium tuberculosis*. European Journal of Immunology. 2009;**39**:676-686

[157] Yoshida S, Gaeta I, Pacitto R, Krienke L, Alge O, Gregorka B, et al. Differential signaling during macropinocytosis in response to M-CSF and PMA in macrophages. Frontiers in Physiology. 2015;**6**:8. DOI: 10.3389/fphys.2015.00008

[158] Swanson JA. Phorbol esters stimulate macropinocytosis and solute flow through macrophages. Journal of Cell Science. 1989;**94**:135-142

[159] Schorey JS, Li Q, McCourt DW, Bong-Mastek M, Clark-Curtiss JE, Ratliff TL, et al. A Mycobacterium leprae gene encoding a fibronectin binding protein is used for efficient invasion of epithelial cells and Schwann cells. Infection and Immunity. 1995;**63**:2652-2657.

[160] Reddy VM, Hayworth DA. Interaction of *Mycobacterium tuberculosis* with human respiratory epithelial cells (HEp-2). Tuberculosis (Edinb). 2002;**82**:31-36. DOI: 10.1054/tube.2001.0320

[161] Garcia-Perez BE, Castrejon-Jimenez NS, Luna-Herrera J: The role of non-phagocytic cells in mycobacterial infections. In: Cardona PJ (ed): Understanding Tuberculosis – Analyzing the Origin of *Mycobacterium tuberculosis* Pathogenicity. Rijeka: InTech; 2012. pp. 149-178

[162] Scordo JM, Knoell DL, Torrelles JB. Alveolar epithelial cells in *Mycobacterium tuberculosis* infection: Active players or innocent bystanders?. Journal of innate immunity. 2016;**8**:3-14. DOI: 10.1159/000439275

[163] Lombardi G, del Gallo F, Vismara D, Piccolella E, de Martino C, Garzelli C, et al. Epstein-Barr virus-transformed B cells process and present *Mycobacterium tuberculosis* particulate antigens to T-cell clones. Cellular Immunology. 1987 Jul;**107**:281-292

[164] Chen P, Shi M, Feng GD, Liu JY, Wang BJ, Shi XD, et al. A highly efficient Ziehl-Neelsen stain: Identifying De Novo intracellular *Mycobacterium tuberculosis* and improving detection of extracellular *M. tuberculosis* in cerebrospinal fluid. Journal of Clinical Microbiology. 2012;**50**:1166-1170. DOI: 10.1128/JCM.05756-11.

[165] Hornung V, Rothenfusser S, Britsch S, Krug A, Jahrsdörfer B, Giese T, Endres S, Hartmann G. Quantitative expression of Toll-like receptor 1-10 mRNA in cellular subsets of human peripheral blood mononuclear cells and sensitivity to CpG oligodeoxynucleotides. Journal of Immunology. 2002;**168**:4531-4537. DOI: 10.4049/jimmunol.168.9.4531.

[166] Singh K, Bayrak B, Riesbeck K. A role for TLRs in Moraxella superantigen induced polyclonal B cell activation. Frontiers in Bioscience (Schol Ed). 2012;**4**:1031-1043. DOI: 10.2741/316

[167] Rawlings DJ, Schwartz MA, Jackson SW, Meyer-Bahlburg A. Integration of B cell responses through Toll-like receptors and antigen receptors. Nature Reviews Immunology. 2012;**12**:282-294. DOI: 10.1038/nri3190

[168] Fillatreau, S. Novel regulatory functions for Toll-like receptor-activated B cells during intracellular bacterial infection. Immunological Reviews. 2011;**240**:52-71. DOI: 10.1111/j.1600-065X.2010.00991.x

[169] Bao Y, Cao X. The immune potential and immunopathology of cytokine-producing B cell subsets: A comprehensive review. Journal of Autoimmunity. 2014;**55**:10-23. DOI: 10.1016/j.jaut.2014.04.001

[170] Agerberth B, Charo J, Werr J, Olsson B, Idali F, Lindbom L, Kiessling R, Jörnvall H, Wigzell H, Gudmundsson GH. The human antimicrobial and chemotactic peptides LL-37 and a-defensins are expressed by specific lymphocyte and monocyte populations. Blood. 2000;**96**:3086-3093

[171] Kovács I, Horváth M, Lányi Á, Petheő GL, Geiszt M. Reactive oxygen species-mediated bacterial killing by B lymphocytes. Journal of Leukocyte Biology. 2015;**97**:1133-1137. DOI: 10.1189/jlb.4AB1113-607RR

[172] Li J, Barreda DR, Zhang YA, Boshra H, Gelman AE, Lapatra S, Tort L, Sunyer JO. B lymphocytes from early vertebrates have potent phagocytic and microbicidal abilities. Nature Immunology. 2006;**7**:1116-1124. DOI: 10.1038/ni1389

[173] Mariño E, Grey ST. B cells as effectors and regulators of autoimmunity. Autoimmunity. 2012;**45**:377-387. DOI: 10.3109/08916934.2012.665527

[174] Bao Y, Liu X, Han C, et al. Identification of IFN-γ-producing innate B cells. Cell Research. 2014;**24**:161-176. DOI:10.1038/cr.2013.155

[175] Bao Y, Liu X, Han C, Xu S, Xie B, Zhang Q, Gu Y, Hou J, Qian L, Qian C, Han H, Cao X. Identification of IFN-γ-producing innate B cells. Cell Res. 2014;**24**:161-176. DOI: 10.1038/cr.2013.155.

[176] Saraiva M, O'Garra A. The regulation of IL-10 production by immune cells. Nature Reviews Immunology. 2010;**10**:170-181 DOI: 10.1038/nri2711

[177] Castro-Eguiluz D, Pelayo R, Rosales-Garcia V, Rosales-Reyes R, Alpuche-Aranda C, Ortiz-Navarrete V. B cell precursors are targets for Salmonella infection. Microbial Pathogenesis. 2009;**47**:52-56. DOI: 10.1016/j.micpath.2009.04.005

[178] Shen P, Fillatreau S. Suppressive functions of B cells in infectious diseases. International Immunology. 2015;**27**:513-559. DOI: 10.4049/jimmunol.1201247

[179] Menon A, Shroyer ML, Wampler JL, Chawan CB, Bhunia AK. In vitro study of *Listeria monocytogenes* infection to murine primary and human transformed B cells. Comparative Immunology Microbiology and Infectious Diseases. 2003;**26**:157-174. DOI: 10.1016/S0147-9571(02)00039-5

[180] Lee CC, Kung JT. Marginal zone B cell is a major source of Il-10 in *Listeria monocytogenes* susceptibility. Journal of Immunology. 2012;**189**:3319-3327. DOI: 10.4049/jimmunol.1201247

[181] Stavru F, Archambaud C, Cossart P. Cell biology and immunology of *Listeria monocytogenes* infections: novel insights. Immunological Reviews. 2011;**240**:160-184. DOI: 10.1111/j.1600-065X.2010.00993.x

[182] Perez-Lopez A, Rosales-Reyes R, Alpuche-Aranda CM, Ortiz-Navarrete V. Salmonella downregulates Nod-like receptor family CARD domain containing protein 4 expression to promote its survival in B cells by preventing inflammasome activation and cell death. Journal of Immunology. 2013;**190**:1201-1209. DOI: 10.4049/jimmunol.1200415.

[183] Maaser C, Housley MP, Iimura M, Smith JR, Vallance BA, Finlay BB, Schreiber JR, Varki NM, Kagnoff MF, Eckmann L. Clearance of *Citrobacter rodentium* requires B cells but not secretory immunoglobulin A (IgA) or IgM antibodies. Infection and Immunity. 2004;**72**:3315e24. DOI: 10.1128/IAI.72.6.3315-3324.2004

[184] Setta AM, Barrow PA, Kaiser P, Jones MA. Early immune dynamics following infection with *Salmonella enterica* serovars Enteritidis, Infantis, Pullorum and Gallinarum: Cytokine and chemokine gene expression profile and cellular changes of chicken cecal tonsils. Comparative Immunology Microbiology and Infectious Diseases. 2012;**35**:397-410. DOI: 10.1016/j.cimid.2012.03.004

[185] du Plessis WJ, Walzl G, Loxton AG. B cells as multi-functional players during *Mycobacterium tuberculosis* infection and disease. Tuberculosis (Edinb). 2016;**97**:118-125. DOI: 10.1016/j.tube.2015.10.007

[186] Ghosn EE, Russo M, Almeida SR. Nitric oxide-dependent killing of *Cryptococcus neoformans* by B-1-derived mononuclear phagocyte. Journal of Leukocyte Biology. 2006;**80**:36-44. DOI: 10.1189/jlb.1005603

[187] Tumurkhuu G, Koide N, Dagvadorj J, Noman AS, Khuda II, Naiki Y, Komatsu T, Yoshida T, Yokochi T. B1 cells produce nitric oxide in response to a series of Toll-like receptor ligands. Cellular Immunology. 2010;**261**:122-127. DOI: 10.1016/j.cellimm.2009.11.009

[188] Han SH, Kim YE, Park JA, Park JB, Kim YS, Lee Y, Choi IG, Kwon HJ. Expression of human b-defensin-2 gene induced by CpG-DNA in human B cells. Biochemical and Biophysical Research Communications. 2009;**389**:443-448. DOI: 10.1016/j.bbrc.2009.08.162

[189] Bhunia AK, Feng X. Examination of Cytopathic effect and apoptosis in *Listeria monocytogenes*-infected hybridoma B-lymphocyte (Ped-2E9) line in vitro. Journal of Microbiology and Biotechnology. 1999;**9**:398-403

[190] Singh M, Prasad KN, Saxena A, Yachha SK. *Helicobacter pylori* induces apoptosis of T- and B cell lines and translocates mitochondrial apoptosis-inducing factor to nucleus. Current Microbiology. 2006;**52**:254-260. DOI: 10.1007/s00284-005-0103-1